International Review of
RESEARCH IN
MENTAL RETARDATION

Personality and Motivational Systems in
Mental Retardation

VOLUME 28

International Review of
RESEARCH IN MENTAL RETARDATION

EDITED BY

LARAINE MASTERS GLIDDEN

DEPARTMENT OF PSYCHOLOGY
ST. MARY'S COLLEGE OF MARYLAND
ST. MARY'S CITY, MARYLAND

Board of Associate Directors

Phillip Davidson
UNIVERSITY OF ROCHESTER MEDICAL CENTER

Elisabeth Dykens
VANDERBILT UNIVERSITY

Michael Guralnick
UNIVERSITY OF WASHINGTON

Linda Hickson
COLUMBIA UNIVERSITY

Rathe Karrer
UNIVERSITY OF KANSAS MEDICAL CENTER

Connie Kasari
UNIVERSITY OF CALIFORNIA, LOS ANGELES

William McIlvane
E.K. SHRIVER CENTER

Glynis Murphy
UNIVERSITY OF KENT AT CANTERBURY

Ted Nettelbeck
UNIVERSITY OF ADELAIDE

Marsha M. Seltzer
UNIVERSITY OF WISCONSIN-MADISON

Jan Wallander
UNIVERSITY OF ALABAMA-BIRMINGHAM

Personality and Motivational Systems in Mental Retardation

A Volume in

International Review of
RESEARCH IN MENTAL RETARDATION

VOLUME 28

EDITED BY

Harvey N. Switzky

DEPARTMENT OF EDUCATIONAL ADMINISTRATION,
EDUCATIONAL PSYCHOLOGY & FOUNDATIONS
NORTHERN ILLINOIS UNIVERSITY
DEKALB, ILLINOIS

CONSULTING EDITORS

Linda Hickson

COLUMBIA UNIVERSITY

Robert L. Schalock

HASTINGS COLLEGE

Michael L. Wehmeyer

UNIVERSITY OF KANSAS

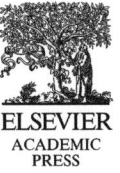

ELSEVIER
ACADEMIC
PRESS

AMSTERDAM • BOSTON • HEIDELBERG • LONDON
NEW YORK • OXFORD • PARIS • SAN DIEGO
SAN FRANCISCO • SINGAPORE • SYDNEY • TOKYO

Academic Press is an imprint of Elsevier

Image Copyright © 2003 Photo Researchers, Inc. All Rights Reserved.

Elsevier Academic Press
525 B Street, Suite 1900, San Diego, California 92101-4495, USA
84 Theobald's Road, London WC1X 8RR, UK

This book is printed on acid-free paper. ∞

Copyright © 2004, Elsevier Inc. All Rights Reserved.

No part of this publication may be reproduced or transmitted in any form or by any means, electronic or mechanical, including photocopy, recording, or any information storage and retrieval system, without permission in writing from the Publisher.

The appearance of the code at the bottom of the first page of a chapter in this book indicates the Publisher's consent that copies of the chapter may be made for personal or internal use of specific clients. This consent is given on the condition, however, that the copier pay the stated per copy fee through the Copyright Clearance Center, Inc. (www.copyright.com), for copying beyond that permitted by Sections 107 or 108 of the U.S. Copyright Law. This consent does not extend to other kinds of copying, such as copying for general distribution, for advertising or promotional purposes, for creating new collective works, or for resale. Copy fees for pre-2004 chapters are as shown on the title pages. If no fee code appears on the title page, the copy fee is the same as for current chapters.
0074-7750/2004 $35.00

Permissions may be sought directly from Elsevier's Science & Technology Rights Department in Oxford, UK: phone: (+44) 1865 843830, fax: (+44) 1865 853333, E-mail: permissions@elsevier.com.uk. You may also complete your request on-line via the Elsevier homepage (http://elsevier.com), by selecting "Customer Support" and then "Obtaining Permissions."

For all information on all Academic Press publications
visit our Web site at www.academicpress.com

ISBN: 0-12-366228-1

PRINTED IN THE UNITED STATES OF AMERICA
04 05 06 07 08   9 8 7 6 5 4 3 2 1

Contents

Contributors ix
Foreword xi
Preface xiii

Promoting Intrinsic Motivation and Self-Determination in People with Mental Retardation

Edward L. Deci

I. Introduction 1
II. Self-Determination Theory 2
III. Human Needs, Social Contexts, and Motivation 9
IV. Self-Determination, Learning, and Adjustment 14
V. Possible Implications of SDT for the Field of MR 19
VI. Conclusions 24
    References 25

Applications of a Model of Goal Orientation and Self-Regulated Learning to Individuals with Learning Problems

Paul R. Pintrich[†] and Juliane L. Blazevski

I. A General Framework for Self-Regulated Learning 32
II. Goal Orientation and Self-Regulated Learning 57
III. Conclusions and Future Directions for Theory and Research 71
     References 73

[†]Deceased

Learner-Centered Principles and Practices: Enhancing Motivation and Achievement for Children with Learning Challenges and Disabilities

Barbara L. McCombs

I. The LCPS as a Foundational Knowledge Base	87
II. What are Practice and Policy Implications of the Learner-Centered Framework for Serving the Needs of Students with Disabilities and Learning Challenges?	92
III. Implications for Research	112
IV. Conclusions	115
References	117

Why Pinocchio Was Victimized: Factors Contributing to Social Failure in People with Mental Retardation

Stephen Greenspan

I. A Case Study Drawn from Children's Literature	122
II. Use of an Action Model to Explain Pinocchio's Incompetence	125
III. Can Social Incompetence Be Remediated?	139
References	142

Understanding the Development of Subnormal Performance in Children from a Motivational-Interactionist Perspective

Janne Lepola, Pekka Salonen, Marja Vauras, and Elisa Poskiparta

I. Scaffolding and the Socially Mediated Development of Cognition and Motivation	148
II. Cognitive and Motivational Factors in the Development of Subnormal Reading Achievement	162
III. Summary and Conclusions	177
References	182

Toward Inclusion Across Disciplines: Understanding Motivation of Exceptional Students

Helen Patrick, Allison M. Ryan, Eric M. Anderman, and John Kovach

I. Barriers to Integrating Research within Fields of Motivation and Special Education	193
II. Importance of Integrating Motivation and Special Education Research	196
III. Examining Motivation of Exceptional and Non-Exceptional Students	197
IV. Motivation of Early Adolescents in Special Education Classes	208

V. The Classroom Environment and Student Motivation	213
VI. Directions for Future Research	216
References	218

Loneliness and Developmental Disabilities: Cognitive and Affective Processing Perspectives

Malka Margalit

I. Definitions	226
II. The Contribution of Genetic and Family Factors	227
III. The Loneliness Construct	230
IV. Loneliness and Social Difficulties in Developmental Disabilities	230
V. Self-Reports of Social Competence and Loneliness	231
VI. Developmental Trends	232
VII. Sources of Social Difficulties	234
VIII. The Affective-Cognitive Model of Loneliness	235
IX. Social Status and Companionship	240
X. Coping and Intervention	241
XI. Loneliness and Technology	247
References	249

The Motivation to Maintain Subjective Well-Being: A Homeostatic Model

Robert A. Cummins and Anna L. D. Lau

I. Issues of Nomenclature and Measurement	256
II. Generic Versus Specific Instrumentation	258
III. Normative Values	259
IV. SWB Homeostasis	261
V. A Model for Homeostasis	265
VI. Personality	266
VII. The Cognitive Buffering System	273
VIII. Met and Unmet Needs	281
IX. Adaptation	285
X. Homeostatic Maintenance and Failure	288
XI. Conclusions	291
References	292

Quality of Life from a Motivational Perspective

Robert L. Schalock

I. Our Current Understanding of the Concept of Quality of Life	304
II. The Focus on Effectance and Intrinsic Motivation	305
III. The Motivational Aspects of the Core Quality-Of-Life Domains	306

IV. Quality of Life and Motivational Strategies 308
V. Implications of Viewing Quality of Life from a Motivational Perspective 309
VI. Conclusions 316
   References 317

Index 321
Contents of Previous Volumes 333

Contributors

Numbers in parentheses indicate the pages on which the authors' contributions begin.

Eric M. Anderman (191), *Department of Educational and Counseling Psychology, University of Kentucky, Lexington, Kentucky 40506*

Juliane L. Blazevski (31), *Combined Program in Education and Psychology, University of Michigan, Ann Arbor, Michigan 48109*

Robert A. Cummins (255), *School of Psychology, Deakin University, Melbourne 3125, Victoria, Australia*

Edward L. Deci (1), *Department of Clinical and Social Psychology, University of Rochester, Rochester, New York 14627*

Stephen Greenspan (121), *University of Colorado Health Sciences Center, Littleton, Colorado 80127*

John Kovach (191), *Department of Leadership, Educational Psychology, and Foundations, Northern Illinois University, DeKalb, Illinois 60115*

Anna L. D. Lau (255), *Department of Rehabilitation Sciences, Hong Kong Polytechnic University, Hong Kong, China*

Janne Lepola (145), *Department of Education, University of Turku, Turku Fin-20014, Finland*

Malka Margalit (225), *Constantiner School of Education, Tel-Aviv University, Tel-Aviv, Israel*

Barbara L. McCombs (85), *University of Denver Research Institute, Denver, Colorado 80208*

Helen Patrick (191), *Department of Educational Studies, Purdue University, West Lafayette, Indiana 47907*

Paul R. Pintrich (31), *Combined Program in Education and Psychology, University of Michigan, Ann Arbor, Michigan 48109*

Elisa Poskiparta (145), *Department of Psychology and Centre for Learning Research, University of Turku, Turku Fin-20014, Finland*

Allison M. Ryan (191), *Department of Educational Psychology, University of Illinois, Champaign, Illinois 61820*

Pekka Salonen (145), *Department of Teacher Education and Centre for Learning Research, University of Turku, Turku Fin-20014, Finland*

Robert L. Schalock (303), *Robert Schalock & Associates; Hastings College, Chewelah, Washington 99109*

Marja Vauras (145), *Department of Teacher Education, University of Turku, Turku Fin-20014, Finland*

Foreword

This volume on *Motivation and Mental Retardation*, the first of two, returns to a subject that was at the heart of mental retardation research 40 years ago, but which has only recently begun to reassume its former prominence, as guest editor Harvey N. Switzky writes in his preface. The centrality of motivation becomes quite obvious as one scans the chapter titles of this volume and realizes that motivation is discussed within the usual context of learning and instruction, but also in the less typical contexts of subjective well-being, loneliness, and social competence. Taken together, these contributors guide us through the tangle of theories, models, and data that a complex construct of motivation spawns.

The field owes its gratitude to guest editor Harvey Switzky for conceptualizing this volume, assembling a remarkable array of contributors whose theorizing and research about motivation and mental retardation is at the forefront, and for bringing the volume to fruition. It is not surprising that he was able to accomplish this task so expeditiously since his own work in motivation is extensive and well-known. Among his recent accomplishments are the publication of a chapter on individual differences in personality and motivational systems in persons with mental retardation in the 3rd edition of *Ellis' Handbook of Mental Deficiency, Psychological Theory and Research* edited by Bill MacLean, Jr. (1997, Hillsdale, NJ: Lawrence Erlbaum); his own 2001 edited book, *Personality and Motivational Differences in Persons with Mental Retardation* (Mahwah, NJ: Lawrence Erlbaum); and a chapter on cognitive-motivational perspectives on mental retardation in the 2003 *What is MR?* that he co-edited with Stephen Greenspan (Washington, DC: American Association on Mental Retardation. July 2003, http: *www.disabilitybooksonline.com*). His expertise in the field made him an excellent choice for guest editor and his own intrinsic motivation assured that the product would be both timely and valuable. I look forward to working with him on the next special volume on motivation, currently in preparation.

LARAINE MASTERS GLIDDEN

SERIES EDITOR

Preface

Motivational processes are the energizing vectors that drive all other psychological, cognitive, memorial, learning, and self-regulatory operators that underpin all outcome performance, all individualized effort, and all attentional focus. Without motivational operators no learning can occur. Motivational processes influence what information gets stored in the long-term memory system, and how that information is organized and retrieved to enable individuals to solve problems. Motivational processes drive the intrinsic curiosity to learn new things. Motivation is the fulcrum of behavior. Motivation permeates everything one does in all areas of life activities, in all life endeavors. When motivation falls to low levels for whatever reason, the individual becomes inert, lonely and nonfunctional and can't solve problems related to survival. The individual's quality of life is low or the individual may have a mental illness. Many obstacles can cause the motivational system to become inoperable, especially failure in meeting the expected roles that the individual has to satisfy through out life which may be typical in persons with mental retardation and other allied learning problems. The constitutive and operational definition of mental retardation is currently in great flux and there is the increasing realization that there is much overlap among disability conditions such as learning disabilities, behavior disorders, and children at-risk for school failure especially in the milder forms (Jacobson, 2001; MacMillan, Siperstein, Gresham, & Bocian, 1997; MacMillan, Siperstein, & Leffert, 2003; Switzky, 2003a; Switzky and Greenspan, 2003) and that is represented in the chapters presented here.

Considering all the papers written in the last 40 years in the area of mental retardation and persons with allied learning difficulties, the area of individual differences in personality and motivational systems has been a neglected one because of the historical reliance of the field on both Skinnerian behavioral models with their emphases on external stimuli as modulators of outcome performance and on the rise of cognitive models that stressed that internal "thinking processes" mediated behavior but left out the influence of mediational personality and self-regulatory motivational processes on outcome performances as well as the physical and social contexts in which learning and performance occurs. Happily in the current period this has ended and a vast array of scholarship has exploded both within the general field of disability research and within mainstream psychology reflecting the accelerating integration between a psychology of mental retardation and a developmental and contextual psychology of human growth for all human beings (Switzky, 2001).

When this series was being planned, many authors were contacted in the forefront of research in motivation. Time, circumstance, and luck determined which papers were received and developed and the volumes were organized thematically within certain page limitations. This accounts very much for the organization of the volumes since enough papers were submitted for two volumes, volume 28 and its sister volume 30. These volumes concern various facets of the emerging international literature regarding individual differences in personality and motivational systems and allied learning problems, and expand on the earlier work reviewed by MacLean (1997), Burack, Hodapp, and Zigler (1998), Switzky and Greenspan (2003), and more specifically by Zigler and Bennett-Gates (1999), and Switzky (2001). Volume 28 represents chapters from the reaching out of motivational theorists from educational psychology to the problems of persons with mental retardation and related learning problems, which is a significant achievement. From the area of mental retardation and disability research, chapters regarding personality characteristics and quality of life are represented.

Edward Deci's chapter extends self-determination theory (SDT) which was developed by Deci and Ryan and their colleague (Deci & Ryan, 2000; Ryan & Deci, 2000) over the last 30 years on primarily nonhandicapped groups to people with mental retardation, and represents a giant step in providing a useful process model regarding the degree to which behaviors are *autonomous* (i.e., self-determined and representative of one's sense of self) versus being *controlled* (i.e., determined by an external agent or a strong internal demand alien to the self) for guiding future research and improving the life circumstances of persons with mental retardation and allied learning problems. This line of thinking substantially extends and augments the earlier work of the Yale group (Zigler & Bennett-Gates, 1999) and the Peabody-Vanderbilt Group (Haywood & Switzky, 1986; Switzky, 1997; Switzky, 2001) on intrinsic-extrinsic motivation.

Paul R. Pintrich and Juliane Blazevski's chapter extends their model of goal orientations and self-regulated academic learning developed for nonhandicapped learners to individuals with mental retardation and allied learning problems. A hallmark of this model is the importance of integrating both cognitive and motivational components in learning and performance, a theme that permeates all current theories of modern educational, psychological, and cognitive motivational theories (Bandura, 1997; Boekaerts, Pintrich, & Zeidner, 2000, Gollwitzer & Bargh, 1996; Sansone & Harackiewicz, 2000), but is largely ignored in current constitutive process models of mental retardation (Borkowski, 2003; Switzky, 2003b). Another assumption of Pintrich's model is that all learners actively construct their own meanings, goals, and strategies from the information available in the "external" environment as well as information in the "internal" environment of their minds. Another assumption is that learners can self-regulate, i.e., monitor, control, and regulate aspects of their cognition, motivation, and behavior, and their environments in accordance with an internal self-standard, a goal, or reference value against which comparisons are made in order to assess whether processes should continue or if change is necessary. Individuals with mental retardation and allied learning problems may have impairments in setting "realistic" standards or goals to strive for in their learning. They may similarly have impairments in monitoring their progress toward these goals, or adapting and regulating their cognitions, motivations, and behavior in order to reach their goals. These self-regulatory activities mediate between personal and contextual characteristics and actual achievement or performance discussed by modern theories of self-regulated learning (Winne & Perry, 2000; Zimmerman, 2000). Pintrich and Blazevski's chapter provide all the details useful to enhance the learning and performance of persons with mental retardation and allied learning problems.

Barbara McCombs' chapter focuses on instructional practices and contexts that can enhance motivation, learning, and achievement for nonhandicapped learners. These instructional practices are represented by the research-validated Learner-Centered Psychological Principles (APA, 1997) as a foundational knowledge base, which she extends to individuals with mental retardation and allied learning problems. Learner-Centered education is focused on how learning occurs and what teaching practices are most effective in promoting the highest levels of motivation, learning, and achievement for *all* learners. Students' performance and motivation depends on their perceptions of their teachers' instructional practices, so that fostering an interpersonal climate supportive of learning is vital if learning is to occur (McCombs, 2001). McCombs' chapter is a brilliant exposition of her model based on many years of work by herself and her colleagues (Alexander & Murphy, 1998; Lambert & McCombs, 1998; McCombs & Whisler, 1997) and the special Task Force on Psychology in Education of the American Psychological Association (APA, 1993, 1997).

Stephen Greenspan in his chapter uses the story of Pinocchio as an illustration of his model of social competence (Greenspan, 2003; Greenspan, Loughlin, & Black, 2001; Greenspan, Switzky, & Granfield, 1996) and the motivational operators that determine performances illustrative of socially competent outcome behaviors. It is Greenspan's contention that "incompetence", particularly gullibility, is the defining characteristic in the taxon of mental retardation and his chapter expands and presents a multidimensional motivational action model of social competence building from the ideas of Martin Ford (1992) and Greenspan and colleagues' earlier models (Greenspan, 1999; Greenspan & Driscoll, 1997; Greenspan, Loughlin, & Black, 2001).

The chapter from Janne Lepola, Pekka Salonen, Marja Vauras, and Elisa Poskiparta, all from the University of Turku, Finland provide an interesting new integrative perspective regarding "subnormal performance" in children from an ethological motivational-contextualist-interactionist-functionalist perspective (Olkinuora & Salonen, 1992; Salonen, Lehtinen, & Olkinuora, 1998; Tinbergen & Tinbergen, 1983), and dysfunctionalities in the operation of the Zone of Proximal Development (Palinscar, 1986; Rogoff & Gardner, 1984). In the normal operation of the Zone of Proximal Development (Vygotsky, 1978), adults and more skilled peers, through social mediation, initially take responsibility for organizing and developing the child's cognitive processes and then gradually the child is required to take charge of her own thinking processes. At least three types of aberrations can occur: (a) over-controlling teaching strategies with heavy reliance on external reinforcers, and externally coercive forms of control, (b) premature withdrawal of support combined with ineffective teaching leading to chronic failure, and (c) inconsistent, indeterminate, or asynchronous strategies of instruction consisting of over-compliance (extreme compliance to the child's momentary demands and refusals), asynchronous feedback (responses lacking reciprocity and coordination to the child's activity), randomly given aversive and positive responses (punishing and rewarding as a function of the adult's current mood) and unresponsiveness to the child's learning activities.

The authors have developed from this analysis of the situational and developmental transactions between a child's adaptive efforts and the "teacher's" controlling and rewarding styles, a three-part model of motivational orientation dimensions (Task orientation, Ego-defensive orientation, and Social dependence orientation), corresponding sets of coping strategies and emotional behaviors, and a related constellation of self-efficacy beliefs or perceived competences (Lehtinen et al., 1995; Olkinuora & Salonen, 1992; Salonen, 2000; Salonen, Lehtinen, & Olkinuora, 1998). The operation of this model and the research, which supports it, is illustrated by the author's longitudinal studies of motivation and reading in preschool to eighth grade children.

The chapter from Helen Patrick, Allison Ryan, Eric Anderman, and Eric Kovach, all from the field of educational psychology, investigates why there has been little rapprochement between motivational researchers from mainstream psychology and those in disability studies, followed by a review of theoretical models of motivation including theories of: intrinsic motivation, goal-theory, expectancy-value theory, and theories of social motivation (Murphy & Alexander, 2000; Pintrich & Schunk, 2002). The chapter ends with the author's own research on the motivation of early adolescents in both regular and special education classes.

Malka Margalit's chapter investigates the subjective experience of loneliness often experienced by children and youth with developmental disabilities and tries to identify factors that predict the subjective experience of social connectedness within a developmental and cognitive-affective model, the Sense of Coherence model (Margalit, 1994; Margalit & Efrati, 2003). The chapter concludes with strategies for empowering students with developmental disabilities. Margalit's chapter is a wonderful addition to the literature.

Robert Cummins and Anna Lau's chapter is devoted to the measurement and assessment of subjective well-being and presents their model of homeostasis and the motivational linkages to personality of the individual and her needs to engage in personally enhancing activities (Carver, 2000; Cummins, 1997, 2000, 2001; Edgerton, 1990; Mallard, Lance, & Michalos, 1997; Roberts & Del Vecchio, 2000). They propose a general model suitable for all people to maintain an adequate quality of life. The issue of well-being is of great importance to disability researchers because individuals with developmental disabilities are at very high risk of experiencing a poor quality of life (Switzky, 2003a). This chapter provides a very thorough integrative review of the literature.

Robert Schalock's chapter provides a related but overlapping model regarding the Quality of Life construct (Schalock, 2001; Schalock & Verdugo, 2002) and its motivational determinants viewed as a Personalized Quality of Life Hierarchy (Elorriaga et al., 2000; Maslow, 1954) and operationalized in a path model of the Quality of Life Hierarchy (Schalock et al., 2002; Schalock & Bonham, in press). The Cummins & Lau chapter and the Schalock chapter together, provide the reader with cutting edge thinking regarding the Quality of Life construct and the research that supports their thinking.

HARVEY N. SWITZKY
GUEST EDITOR

I would like to dedicate Volume 28 to Paul R. Pintrich, who reached out to all learners.

REFERENCES

Alexander, P. A., & Murphy, P. K. (1998). The research base for APA's Learner-Centered Psychological Principles. In N. Lambert & B.L. McCombs (Eds.), *How students learn: Reforming schools through learner-centered education.* Washington, DC: American Psychological Association.

APA Task Force on Psychology in Education (1993, January). *Learner-centered psychological principles: Guidelines for school design and reform.* Washington, DC: American Psychological Association and Mid-Continent Regional Educational Laboratory.

APA Work Group of the Board of Educational Affairs (1997, November). *Learner-centered psychological principles: A framework for school reform and design.* Washington, DC: American Psychological Association.

Bandura, A. (1997). *Self-efficacy: The exercise of control.* New York: W.H. Freeman & Company.

Boekaerts, M., Pintrich, P. R., & Zeidner (Eds.) (2000). *Handbook of self-regulation.* San Diego, CA.: Academic Press.

Borkowski, J. G. (2003, August). *Redefining mental retardation: The role of executive functioning.* Paper presented at the meeting of the American Psychological Association, Toronto, Canada.

Burack, J. A., Hodapp, R. M., & Zigler, E. (Eds.) (1998). *Handbook of mental retardation and development.* New York, NY: Cambridge University Press.

Carver, C. S. (2000). On the continuous calibration of happiness. *American Journal of Mental Retardation,* 105, 336–341.

Cummins, R. A. (1997). Self-rated quality of life scales for people with an intellectual disability: A review. *Journal of Applied Research in Intellectual Disability,* 10, 199–216.

Cummins, R. A. (2000). A homeostatic model for subjective quality of life. *Proceedings, Second Conference of Quality of Life in Cities* (pp. 51–59). Singapore: National University of Singapore.

Cummins, R. A. (2001). Self-rated quality of life-scales for people with an intellectual disability: A reply to Ager and Hatton. *Journal of Applied Research in Intellectual Disabilities,* 14, 1–11.

Deci, E. L., & Ryan, R. M. (2000). The "what" and "why" of goal pursuits: Human needs and the self-determination of behavior. *Psychological Inquiry,* 11, 227–268.

Edgerton, R. B. (1990). Quality of life from a longitudinal research perspective. In R. L. Schalock (Ed.), *Quality of life: Perspectives and issues* (pp. 149–160). Washington: American Association on Mental Retardation.

Elorriaga, J., Garcia, L., Martinez, J., & Unamunzaga, E (2000). Quality of life of people with mental retardation in Spain: One organization's experience. In K. D. Keith & R. L. Schalock (Eds.), *Cross-cultural perspectives on quality of life* (pp. 113–124). Washington, DC: American Association on Mental Retardation.

Ford, M. E. (1992). *Motivating humans: Goals, emotions, and personal agency beliefs.* Newbury Park, CA: Sage.

Gollwitzer, P. M. & Bargh, J. A. (Eds.) (1996). *The psychology of action: Linking cognition and motivation to behavior.* New York: The Guilford Press.

Greenspan, S. (1999). A contextualist perspective on adaptive behavior. In R. Schalock (Ed.), *Adaptive behavior: Conceptual basis, measurement and use* (pp. 61–80). Washington, DC: American Association on Mental Retardation.

Greenspan, S. (2003). Perceived risk status as a key to defining mental retardation: Social and everyday vulnerability in the natural prototype. In Switzky, N. Harvey, Greenspan, & Stephen (Eds.), *What is Mental Retardation? Ideas for an Evolving Disability* [On-line]. Washington, DC: American Association on Mental Retardation. Retrieved July 2003 from http://www.disabilitybooksonline.com.

Greenspan, S., & Driscoll, J. (1997). The role of intelligence in a broad model of personal competence. In D. P. Flanagan, J. L. Genshaft, & P. L. Harrison (Eds.), *Contemporary intellectual assessment: Theories, tests and issues* (pp. 131–150). New York: Guilford.

Greenspan, S., Loughlin, G., & Black, R. S. (2001). Credulity and gullibility in persons with mental retardation: A proposed framework for future research. In L. Masters-Glidden (Ed.), *International review of research in mental retardation* (Vol. 24, pp. 101–135). New York: Academic Press.

Greenspan, S., Switzky, H. N., & Granfield, J. (1996). Everyday intelligence and adaptive behavior: A theoretical framework. In J. Jacobson & J. Mulick (Eds.), *Manual on diagnosis and professional practice in mental retardation* (pp. 127–135). Washington, DC: American Psychological Association.

Haywood, H. C., & Switzky, H. N. (1986). Intrinsic motivation and behavioral effectiveness in retarded persons. In N. Ellis & N. Bray (Eds.), *International review of research in mental retardation* (Vol. 14, pp. 1–46). New York: Academic Press.

Jacobson, J. W. (2001). Environmental postmodernism and rehabilitation of the borderline of mental retardation. *Behavioral Interventions, 16*, 209–234.

Lambert, N. & McCombs, B. L. (Eds.) (1998). *How students learn: Reforming schools through learner-centered education.* Washington, DC: APA Books.

Lehtinen, E., Vauras, M., Salonen, P., Olkinuora, E., & Kinnunen, R. (1995). Long-term development of learning activity: motivational, cognitive, and social interaction. *Educational Psychologist, 30*, 21–35.

MacLean, W. M. (Ed.) (1997). *Ellis' handbook of mental deficiency, psychological theory and research* (3rd ed.). Mahwah, NJ: Lawrence Erlbaum Associates.

MacMillan, D. L., Siperstein, G., Gresham, F. M., & Bocian, K. M. (1997). Mild mental retardation: A concept that may have lived out its usefulness. *Psychology in Mental Retardation and Developmental Disabilities, 23*(1), 5–12.

MacMillan, D. L., Siperstein, G. N., & Leffert, J. S. (2003). Children with mild mental retardation: A challenge for classification practices. In H. N. Switzky & S. Greenspan (Eds.), *What is Mental Retardation?: Ideas for an Evolving Disability* [On-line]. Washington, DC: American Association on mental Retardation. Retrieved: July 2003 from *http://www.disabilitybooksonline.com.*

Mallard, A. G. C., Lance, C. E., & Michalos, A. C. (1997). Culture as a moderator of overall life satisfaction-Life facet of satisfaction relationships. *Social Indicators Research, 40*, 259–284.

Margalit, M. (1994). *Loneliness among children with special needs: Theory, research, coping and intervention.* New York: Springer-Verlag.

Margalit, M., & Efrati, M. (2003, April). Self-perception and mood of students with Learning Disabilities (LD). Paper presented at the SRCD Biennial Meeting at the symposium "Self-perceptions of children and adolescents with LD," Tampa, Florida, USA.

Maslow, A. H. (1954). *Motivation and personality.* New York: Harper & Row.

McCombs (2001). What do we know about learners and learning? The learner-centered framework: Bringing the educational system into balance. *Educational Horizons, 79*(4), 182–193.

McCombs, B. L., & Whisler, J. S. (1997). *The learner-centered classroom and school: Strategies for increasing student motivation and achievement*. San Francisco: Jossey-Bass.

Murphy, P. K., & Alexander, P. A. (2000). A motivated exploration of motivation terminology. *Contemporary Educational Psychology, 25*, 3–53.

Olkinuora, E., & Salonen, P. (1992). Adaptation, motivational orientation, and cognition in a subnormally-performing child: A systemic perspective for training. In B. Wong (Ed.), *Intervention research in learning disabilities: An international perspective* (pp. 190–213). New York: Springer-Verlag.

Palinscar, S. A. (1986). The role of dialogue in providing scaffolded instruction. *Educational Psychologist, 21*, 73–98.

Pintrich, P. R., & Schunk, D. H. (2002). *Motivation in education: Theory, research, and applications* (2nd ed.). Englewood Cliffs, NJ: Merrill Prentice-Hall.

Roberts, B. W., & DelVecchio, W. F. (2000). The rank-order consistency of personality traits from childhood to old age: A quantitative review of longitudinal studies. *Psychological Bulletin, 126*, 3–25.

Rogoff, B., & Gardner, W. (1984). Adult guidance and cognitive development. In B. Rogoff & L. Lave (Eds.), *Everyday cognition: Its development in social contexts* (pp. 95–116). Cambridge, MA: Harvard University Press.

Ryan, R. M., & Deci, E. L. (2000). Self-determination theory and the facilitation of intrinsic motivation, social development, and well-being. *American Psychologist, 55*, 68–78.

Salonen, P. (2000). *Subnormally performing children's coping strategies in situational; context: Field-theoretical foundations, taxonomy, and case analysis*. Centre for Learning Research, University of Turku (unpublished manuscript).

Salonen, P., Lehtinen, E., & Olkinuora, E. (1998). Expectations and beyond: The development of motivation and learning in a classroom context. In J. Brophy (Ed.), *Advances in research on teaching* (Vol. 7, pp. 111–150). Greenwich, CT: JAI Press.

Sansone, C. & Harackiewicz, J. M. (Eds.) (2000). *Intrinsic motivation and extrinsic motivation*. San Diego, CA: Academic Press.

Schalock, R. L. (2001). *Outcome-based evaluation: Second edition*. New York: Kluwer Academic/Plenum Publishers.

Schalock, R. L. & Bonham, G. S. (in press). Measuring outcomes and managing for results. *Evaluation and Program Planning*

Schalock, R. L., Brown, I., Brown, R., Cummins, R. A., Felce, D., Matikka, L., Keith, K. D., & Parmenter, T. (2002). Conceptualization, measurement, and application of quality of life for persons with intellectual disabilities: Results of an international panel of experts. *Mental Retardation, 40*(6), 457–470.

Schalock, R. L., & Verdugo, M. A. (2002). *Handbook on quality of life for human service practitioners*. Washington, DC: American Association on Mental Retardation.

Switzky, H. N. (1997). Individual differences in personality and motivational systems in persons with mental retardation. In W. E. MacLean Jr. (Ed.), *Ellis' handbook of mental deficiency, psychological theory and research* (3rd ed., pp. 343–377). Hillsdale, NJ: Lawrence Erlbaum Associates.

Switzky, H. N. (Ed.) (2001). *Personality and motivational differences in persons with mental retardation*. Mahwah, NJ: Lawrence Erlbaum Associates.

Switzky, H. N. (2003a). The plight of adults with mild cognitive limitation: Still forgotten? *Contemporary Psychology, APA Review of Books, 48*(30), 363–365.

Switzky, H. N. (2003b). A cognitive-motivational perspective on mental retardation. In H. N. Switzky, & Greenspan Stephen (Eds.), *What is Mental Retardation?: Ideas for a Evolving Disability* [On-Line]. Washington, DC: American Association on Mental Retardation. Retrieved: July 2003 from http: *www.disabilitybooksonline.com.*

Switzky, H. N., & Greenspan, Stephen (Eds.) (2003). *What is Mental Retardation?: Ideas for an Evolving Disability* [On-Line]. Washington, DC: American Association on Mental Retardation. Retrieved: July 2003 from http: *www.disabilitybooksonline.com.*

Tinbergen, N., & Tinbergen, E. (1983). *'Autistic' children: New hope for cure.* London: Allen & Unwin.

Vygotsky, L. S. (1978). *Mind in society.* Cambridge, MA: Harvard University Press.

Winne, P., & Perry (2000). Measuring self-regulated learning. In M. Boekaerts, P. R. Pintrich, & M. Zeidner (Eds.), *Handbook of self-regulation* (pp. 531–566). San Diego, CA: Academic Press.

Zigler, E., & Bennett-Gates, D. (Eds.) (1999). *Personality development in individuals with mental retardation.* New York, NY: Cambridge University Press.

Zimmerman, B. J. (2000). Attaining self-regulation: A social cognitive perspective. In M. Boekaerts, P. R. Pintrich, & M. Zeidner (Eds.), *Handbook of self-regulation* (pp. 13–39). San Diego, CA: Academic Press.

Promoting Intrinsic Motivation and Self-Determination in People with Mental Retardation

EDWARD L. DECI

UNIVERSITY OF ROCHESTER

Self-determination theory (SDT) is outlined and used as a basis for discussing the facilitation of education and adjustment of individuals with mental retardation (MR). The theory differentiates intrinsic and extrinsic motivation with respect to the concept of self-determination. The innate psychological needs for competence, autonomy, and relatedness are used as a basis for specifying how ongoing social contexts as well as intervention programs will affect self-determined motivation and, in turn, learning, adjustment, and life circumstances. Laboratory experiments and field studies are reviewed indicating that: (1) social contexts that facilitate satisfaction of the three basic needs—by providing optimal challenge, informational feedback, interpersonal involvement, and autonomy support—promote both intrinsic motivation and self-determined forms of extrinsic motivation; and (2) intrinsic motivation and self-determined extrinsic motivation are positively associated with high-quality learning and personal adjustment. Although most of the SDT research has been done with normal samples, the relevance of this work for the field of MR is readily apparent. Further, some specific work in the field of MR is discussed as it relates to SDT.

I. INTRODUCTION

The emerging view of mental retardation (MR) considers it to be a condition involving a complex interaction of cognitive deficits and self-relevant motivational processes, which places developmentally disabled individuals at a relative disadvantage for learning and adjustment (e.g., Haywood & Switzky, 1986; Switzky, 2001). Stated differently, people with MR tend to have diminished cognitive abilities as well as less intrinsic motivation and self-determination than matched individuals without MR, and these motivational deficiencies exacerbate the cognitive deficits resulting in negative consequences for life circumstances, academic performance, psychological well-being, and subsequent development of motivation and self-determination (Harter & Zigler, 1972, 1974; Haywood, 1968; Schultz & Switzky, 1993; Silon & Harter, 1985).

Recent federal legislation, such as the Americans with Disabilities Act of 1990, has emphasized that individuals with MR have greater rights to determine their own life circumstances than had previously been granted. A view of MR which recognizes the importance of motivational and self-relevant processes for outcomes in the lives of individuals with MR provides a meaningful basis for designing and interpreting research on interventions aimed at the promotion of self-determination among the mentally retarded.

This chapter uses self-determination theory (SDT) (Deci & Ryan, 2000; Ryan & Deci, 2000) to focus on motivational processes as they relate to learning and adjustment in individuals with MR. Much of the discussion extrapolates from the SDT research with normal samples and samples of individuals with learning disabilities and emotional handicaps (e.g., Grolnick & Ryan, 1990), but some studies of people with MR which employed other perspectives are also considered. In reviewing theory and research, I argue that SDT provides a useful process model for guiding future research and program development concerned with improvement of the life circumstances of the developmentally disabled.

The plan for this chapter is: to differentiate motivational processes in terms of the concept of self-determination or relative autonomy; to review evidence about the enhancement versus impairment of self-determined motivation; to relate the types of motivation to learning and adjustment outcomes; and to draw inferences about the education of individuals with MR.

II. SELF-DETERMINATION THEORY

In SDT, as in many current theories of motivation that have evolved in the cognitive tradition, the concept of *intention* is the central defining feature of motivated behavior (e.g., Lewin, 1951); people are said to be *motivated* for a specific behavior to the extent that they intend to perform it. Intentions, in turn, are theorized to be a function of: (1) desiring some outcome, (2) believing the behavior is instrumental to obtaining the outcome, and (3) possessing the necessary competencies to do the behavior. The concept of *amotivation,* in contrast, refers to a lack of intention and motivation. People are amotivated for a behavior to the extent that they lack an intention to do it.

The distinction between motivation and amotivation, although referred to by different terms, is pivotal in the theories of Heider (1958), Locke and Latham (1990), Bandura (1997), Seligman (1975), and numerous others. Heider, for example, used the term "impersonal causation" to describe amotivation and "personal causation" to refer to motivated behavior. In each of these theories, motivation is viewed as a unitary concept that differs in amount but not in type. Thus, people are said to have greater or lesser motivation for some behavior, but there is no distinction about the type or orientation of motivation they might have for the behavior.

Although the distinction between motivation and amotivation is extremely important, SDT has focused more attention on differentiating the concept of motivation—that is, on exploring different types of motivation that underlie intentional actions and differ in the degree to which they are the basis for self-determination.

A. Autonomous Versus Controlled Motivation

Central to SDT is the idea that behaviors differ in the extent to which they are *autonomous* (i.e., self-determined) versus *controlled*—that is, in the degree to which they are freely chosen and representative of one's sense of self versus pressured or controlled by some interpersonal or intrapsychic force. To the extent that behaviors are experienced as freely chosen, they are autonomous, whereas, to the extent that they are experienced as seduced or coerced, whether by an external agent or by a strong internal demand, they are controlled. The concepts of autonomy and control, therefore, describe types of motivated actions that differ in terms of the degree to which they emanate from one's self and are self-determined. Within the tradition of Heider (1958), deCharms (1968) used the concept of an internal versus an external perceived locus of causality to label this continuum, suggesting that when people are acting with an internal perceived locus of causality they are "origins" of their behavior, but when they are acting with an external perceived locus of causality they are "pawns" to some force that is operating on them. According to SDT, this distinction between autonomous and controlled behavior is important because the theory proposes that the quality of performance and affect varies as a function of whether the behavior tends to be more autonomous versus more controlled.

An example of controlled behavior would be the girl who does her schoolwork because she fears her teacher's disapproval if she did not. In contrast, self-determined behavior would be evident in a classmate who does the assignment because she finds it interesting or personally valuable. The former student would be complying with demands and pressures, whereas the latter student would be behaving with a much fuller sense of choice and self-initiation. In both cases, the behavior would be intentional—that is, it would be motivated, as opposed to amotivated—but the different degrees of self-determination experienced in the two cases would likely be associated with different antecedents, correlates, and consequences.

Conceptualization and empirical exploration of the distinction between autonomous and controlled behavior began with the differentiation of intrinsic and extrinsic motivation (e.g., deCharms, 1968; Deci, 1975).

B. Intrinsic and Extrinsic Motivation

Intrinsically motivated behaviors are those that are performed out of interest and require no "reward" other than the spontaneous experience of interest and enjoyment (Deci, 1975). When intrinsically motivated, people behave freely and willingly with no external or intrapsychic prods, promises, or threats. Csikszentmihalyi (1975) described these behaviors as "autotelic," meaning, as the word implies, that they are self-directed. Intrinsic motivation entails curiosity, spontaneity, and interest. It is readily evident, for example, in the play, exploration, and mastery strivings of children and in the delight that accompanies those behaviors (White, 1959).

In contrast to intrinsic motivation, extrinsic motivation is defined in terms of behaviors that are performed instrumentally to attain some specific outcome or reinforcement. Generally, extrinsically motivated behaviors are ones that would not occur spontaneously and, therefore, must be initially prompted by a reward contingency or other instrumentality.

Intrinsically motivated behaviors represent the prototype of self-determination. They are experienced as wholly volitional, as representative of and emanating from one's sense of self, and they are the activities people pursue out of interest when they are free from demands, constraints, and instrumentalities.

Early research on intrinsic motivation examined the effects of extrinsic rewards on people's intrinsic motivation for some interesting activity. This research question arose because some motivational theories had begun to advocate creating conditions (e.g., in the workplace) that would stimulate both intrinsic and extrinsic motivation (e.g., Porter & Lawler, 1968). The assumption was that they would be additive, yielding total motivation. Examination of the effects of extrinsic rewards on intrinsic motivation represented a way to test this assumption. Results of the first few studies, done with college students and with nursery school children, indicated that giving extrinsic rewards, such as money or prizes, for doing an intrinsically interesting activity tended to decrease people's intrinsic motivation for the activity (e.g., Deci, 1971, 1972; Lepper, et al., 1973). After people had been rewarded for performing an interesting activity they were less likely to do it again in a free-choice period and they expressed less interest in the activity than did people who had performed the activity without being rewarded.

In interpreting these findings, Deci (1975) suggested that the introduction of extrinsic motivators for performing an intrinsically motivated (and thus self-determined) behavior tends to leave people feeling controlled. Their behavior becomes dependent on the reward contingency, which diminishes their experience of autonomy or self-determination. Thus, people experience the rewards, rather than their own interest, as the reason for performing the activity; in the words of deCharms (1968), the rewards induce a shift in people's perceived locus of causality from internal to external, leaving them feeling like pawns to the extrinsic controls. They will subsequently be less willing to do the activity simply for its intrinsic satisfaction.

Since publication of the initial experiment (Deci, 1971), nearly 100 others have examined the effects of tangible rewards on intrinsic motivation, and a recent meta-analysis of these studies (Deci et al., 1999) concluded definitively that, overall, extrinsic rewards do undermine intrinsic motivation, thus indicating that extrinsically motivated behavior tends to be less self-determined than intrinsically motivated behavior.

The finding that extrinsic rewards tend to undermine intrinsic motivation has been controversial (e.g., Eisenberger et al., 1999) from the time the first studies were published. Presumably, because rewards are relatively easy to use and are reasonably effective in controlling behavior, the critics prefer not to acknowledge any negative consequences to the use of rewards. The problem, however, is that when rewards control behavior there are indeed costs to the people being controlled. For one, the rewards co-opt people's sense of autonomy. They make the instrumental behaviors dependent on the continued presence of the rewards, so the behaviors do not persist when the rewards are no longer present. The reason this is a problem is that, in life, most parents, teachers, and other socializing agents would like to facilitate their children and students being self-initiating and self-regulating—that is, being self-motivated even when rewards are not present.

It is true, of course, that some tangible-reward experiments have shown that, under certain limited circumstances, tangible extrinsic rewards sustain rather than undermine intrinsic motivation (e.g., Harackiewicz, 1979; Ryan, 1982; Ryan et al., 1983), which suggests that extrinsically motivated behaviors *can* be self-determined. In other words, being extrinsically motivated does not necessarily imply that one is controlled. Accordingly, SDT (Deci & Ryan, 1985) includes a developmental analysis of extrinsic motivation which differentiates the concept of extrinsic motivation and explains when and how extrinsically motivated activities can be self-determined. Specifically, this analyses focuses on activities that a person does not find interesting and, thus, is not intrinsically motivated to do—that is, it addresses how people can become autonomous for activities that they begin doing because of extrinsic contingencies.

C. Internalization of Extrinsic Motivation

Extrinsically motivated behaviors—those done to attain a specific outcome, such as parental approval—can become autonomous or self-determined through the developmental processes of *internalization* and *integration*. Internalization involves people receiving the external regulatory processes so the behavior no longer requires the presence of an external demand or contingency (Schafer, 1968), and integration is the process through which these now internalized values and regulations are assimilated and made part of one's integrated sense of self (Ryan, 1993).

Integration is a central developmental process within organismic theories of behavior (e.g., Piaget, 1971; Ryan & Deci, 2000). It is based on the assumption that people are inherently active and naturally inclined toward growth and development. Thus, from this perspective, development is not something that happens to people by the environment but rather is something that people *do* when they have the nutrients necessary to support the active, inherent developmental process of organismic integration (Deci & Ryan, 1985).

According to SDT, internalizing regulations represents an instance of the natural trajectory toward integration in personality. People internalize socially sanctioned activities in order to feel related to others and effective in the social world, and they integrate those regulatory processes into their sense of self in order to maximize their experience of self-determination. Stated differently, individuals seek to feel related to others, socially competent, and autonomous in their actions by taking in and integrating the regulation of those behaviors that were initially externally prompted within a social milieu (Deci & Ryan, 2000). The experience of relatedness, competence, and autonomy, therefore, are the nutrients that are important for facilitating internalization and integration. Accordingly, the integrative process may be more or less effective with respect to any particular behavioral regulation as a function of the degree to which people experience relatedness, competence, and autonomy while performing the behavior. To the extent that more integration occurs, the subsequent behavior will be more self-determined, whereas to the extent that less occurs, the subsequent behavior will be more controlled.

More specifically, SDT posits four types of extrinsic regulation that result from different degrees of internalization and integration of extrinsic motivation. These regulatory processes underlie intentional, extrinsically motivated behaviors, but they differ in the extent to which they are autonomous versus controlled. As such, the theory places the four regulatory processes along a continuum of relative autonomy or self-determination. The four types of regulation are as follows.

External regulation involves behaviors being regulated by contingencies overtly external to the individual. When people engage in behaviors to attain rewards or avoid punishments, their behavior is being externally regulated. This is the classic type of extrinsic motivation that is central to operant behaviorism (e.g., Skinner, 1953), and the initial discussions of and experiments on extrinsic reward were concerned with this type of extrinsic motivation. Externally regulated behaviors are intentional—that is, they are motivated—but they are dependent on external contingencies and are thus said to be controlled by the contingencies. In fact, external regulation represents the most controlled form of extrinsic motivation.

Introjected regulation refers to behaviors that are motivated by internal prods and pressures such as self-esteem–relevant contingencies. When people behave because they think they *should* or because they would feel guilty if they did not, they are displaying introjected regulation. This type of regulation results when an external contingency has been taken in by the person but not really accepted as his or her own. The regulation has to some extent been internalized, but it has not become part of the person's sense of self. When a regulation has been introjected, it is thus internal to the person in the sense that it no longer requires external contingencies. However, the behavior is dependent on the internalized contingencies that are still separate from or external to the person's sense of self. Metaphorically, it is as if one part of the person—namely, the introjected contingencies—were controlling the rest of the person. Introjected regulation thus describes a form of internal motivation in which actions are considered *controlled* or coerced by internal contingencies that are external to the self. As such, the behaviors still have an external perceived locus of causality even though the regulation is within the person (Ryan & Connell, 1989). This is a very interesting form of extrinsic motivation, because most theories of internalization would consider this type of regulation to constitute self-motivation and to reflect fully successful internalization, but SDT views it as a relatively ineffective type of internalization whose qualities have considerable similarity to those of regulation by external contingencies.

Identified regulation results when a behavior or regulation is accepted by individuals as being personally important or valuable for themselves. They identify with the value of the activity and thus do the behavior with a sense of personal endorsement, even though they do not find the activity interesting. With identified regulation, people do not behave because they feel they should; rather, they do the behavior because it has personal relevance and meaning to their lives. In other words, they have accepted the regulation as their own. Thus, through identification, people begin to incorporate an extrinsic motivation into their sense of self. An example of an identified regulatory style might be a boy who identifies with the importance of studying subjects he finds uninteresting so he will be able to attend an excellent university that offers the program he truly wants to pursue. This example stands in contrast to the student who studies hard because he believes he "should" go to college like everyone else and will feel unworthy if he does not (introjected regulation), or to another student who studies because his parents pressure him to do so (external regulation).

Integrated regulation is the most self-determined form of extrinsic motivation. It results from the integration of identified values and regulations into one's coherent sense of self. When people have integrated a regulation, they not only value that behavior but they have brought it into harmony with other aspects of themselves. For example, a high-school girl might identify with becoming a doctor and also with being a serious soccer player, two identifications that she might value equally but feel conflict about, at least with respect to time commitment and peer pressure. However, she could integrate these identifications, although doing so might necessitate making adjustments, such as changing how she spends her time or who her friends are. In such a case, the two values could co-exist harmoniously along with other aspects of her self. A creative synthesis would have occurred and she would no longer feel psychological stress about holding these two identifications. Regulation resulting from integration is the most autonomous and mature form of extrinsic motivation.

In the example of the boy who had identified with the value of studying subjects he finds uninteresting because he understands their importance for getting into a university, it was not made clear the degree to which he had integrated that identification. Insofar as he experiences some resistance and conflict, at times wanting to *not* do his assignments so he can be with his friends who are not invested in learning, the identification is likely to be relatively unintegrated. But if he is easily able to do his studying and not experience ambivalence and discomfort with respect to his friends who are not invested in learning, the identification would be relatively integrated.

Integrated extrinsic motivation and intrinsic motivation represent the two bases for self-determined functioning. They share the qualities that constitute self-determination, namely, a total involvement of the self and an experience of personal endorsement and choice. Nonetheless, these two types of motivation are different in that intrinsically motivated behaviors are based on a person's *interest* in the activity for its own sake, whereas integrated behaviors are based on the *importance* or instrumental value of the activity for the person's self-selected goals. Behaviors for which a person is intrinsically motivated typically did not require initial extrinsic prompts—the person found them interesting and pursued them willingly from the start—but behaviors whose regulation is integrated did require initial external prompts that were gradually internalized and integrated. Thus, integrated regulation involves a person coming to the point of personally endorsing values and behaviors that socializing agents believe to be important for that person.

Summary. SDT differentiates motivation into intrinsic motivation, which involves doing an activity out of interest, and extrinsic motivation, which involves doing it because of some instrumental relation to a desired outcome. Intrinsic motivation is the prototype of self-determined activity, and extrinsic motivation, in its classic form of dependence on external reward contingencies, represents the prototype of controlled behavior. However, SDT has specified four types of extrinsic motivation that differ in the degree to which the relevant behavioral regulation has been internalized and integrated. Ordered from the least to the most self-determined form of extrinsic motivation, the four types are: (1) external regulation, (2) introjected regulation, (3) identified regulation, and (4) integrated regulation. As we will see later, these various types of motivation are associated with very different learning and well-being outcomes, so understanding what social-contextual conditions facilitate or inhibit the various types of motivation is a matter of considerable importance.

III. HUMAN NEEDS, SOCIAL CONTEXTS, AND MOTIVATION

SDT has proposed that there are a set of three innate psychological needs, which are defined as essential nutriments for healthy psychological development. The specification of these fundamental needs was important in part because it provided a means of integrating the results of a large body of research concerning the effects of social contexts on intrinsic and extrinsic motivation (Deci & Ryan, 1985). The three needs are: *competence* or effectance (White, 1959); *autonomy* or self-determination (deCharms, 1968); and *relatedness* or affiliation (Harlow, 1958). SDT suggests that people are inherently motivated to feel connected to others within a social milieu, to function effectively in that milieu, and to feel a sense of personal initiative while doing so. Without these experiences, SDT proposes, people will suffer some negative psychological consequences.

The integration of extrinsic motivation has been analyzed in terms of all three needs (e.g., Deci & Ryan, 1991), whereas intrinsic motivation has been linked most directly to the needs for competence and autonomy (e.g., Deci,

1975). As pointed out by Deci and Ryan (2000), the experience of relatedness can facilitate intrinsic motivation, but there are many intrinsically motivated activities where proximal experiences of relatedness are not necessary for maintaining a high level of the motivation.

According to SDT, a consideration of these innate human needs allows prediction of how variables in the social context will affect people's intrinsic motivation and the development of their extrinsic motivation. Simply stated, social-contextual factors that afford people the opportunity to satisfy their needs for autonomy, competence, and relatedness are theorized to facilitate intrinsic motivation and the integration of extrinsic motivation, whereas those that thwart satisfaction of these needs are expected to diminish intrinsic motivation and impair the integration of extrinsic motivation.

Numerous studies that have examined the effects of social contextual factors on motivational processes are reviewed in the remainder of this section. First, the effects of contexts on intrinsic motivation are considered, followed by contextual effects on internalization and integration of extrinsic motivation.

A. The Social Context and Intrinsic Motivation

The initial studies of social-contextual influences were the laboratory experiments already discussed that examined the effects of extrinsic rewards on intrinsic motivation and found the general tendency for tangible extrinsic rewards to undermine intrinsic motivation. Additional studies also investigated the effects of other specific external events such as deadlines, threats of punishment, and performance feedback on intrinsic motivation. In each case, participants in an experimental group who worked on an interesting task when the event was manipulated were compared to those in a control group who also worked on the same task but without the manipulated event being present (e.g., without a reward or a deadline). Of interest were the participants' levels of intrinsic motivation subsequent to the period when the experimental manipulation was done.

The studies confirmed that events which are experienced as controlling (i.e., as pressure to perform in specific ways) undermined intrinsic motivation, whereas those that are experienced as autonomy supportive (i.e., as encouragement for self-initiation and choice) maintained or enhanced intrinsic motivation. With some limiting conditions, these experiments indicated that not only tangible rewards (Deci, 1971) but also threats of punishment (Deci & Cascio, 1972), evaluations (Smith, 1975), deadlines (Amabile et al., 1976), imposed goals (Mossholder, 1980), and good player awards (Lepper et al., 1973) all tended to undermine intrinsic motivation because they were experienced as controlling. In contrast, providing people with a choice (Zuckerman et al., 1978) and acknowledging their feelings (Koestner et al., 1984) tended to be experienced as autonomy supportive and thus enhanced intrinsic motivation.

Subsequent work indicated that, although certain events tend to be experienced as controlling (e.g., tangible rewards) while others tend to be experienced as autonomy supportive (e.g., choice), the style and language with which the events are administered significantly influence their effects. For example, Ryan et al. (1983) found that performance-contingent rewards, when administered in a controlling style using language such as "you should" or "you have to," undermined intrinsic motivation, but when administered with a more autonomy supportive style (i.e., with supportive non-pressuring language) tended not to be undermining. Similar results were found with respect to setting limits on children's behavior (Koestner et al., 1984). When limits were set without using pressuring language and in a way that provided a choice and acknowledged feelings, they were not detrimental to intrinsic motivation, although they were undermining when administered in a more controlling way.

Other studies have focused on contextual factors that tend to enhance versus undermine intrinsic motivation by increasing versus decreasing people's experience of competence. To be intrinsically motivating an activity must provide an optimal challenge (Csikszentmihalyi, 1975; Deci, 1975). Thus, when a target activity is optimally discrepant from one's skill level, it tends to be intrinsically motivating relative to easier or harder tasks. A study by Danner and Lonky (1981) confirmed this hypothesis. The researchers found that when children were left on their own to choose what activities to work on, they chose ones that were slightly beyond their current levels of mastery.

Other studies showed that positive feedback tended to strengthen perceived competence and enhance intrinsic motivation (e.g., Deci, 1971). These effects, however, were found to depend on the feedback being administered in a relatively autonomy-supportive way. Positive feedback has been found to enhance intrinsic motivation by strengthening perceived competence only when the positive feedback resulted from a relatively self-determined activity and was presented in a non-controlling style (Fisher, 1978; Ryan, 1982; Usui, 1991). We refer to positive feedback that is administered in an autonomy-supportive fashion as being *informational*.

In contrast to positive feedback, negative feedback, particularly if it is critical and evaluative or administered in a controlling context, tends to diminish perceived competence and decrease intrinsic motivation (e.g., Deci & Cascio, 1972; Vallerand & Reid, 1984). If administered in a non-evaluative, autonomy supportive way, however, negative feedback can represent a challenge and help people figure out how to do better. When provided in this way, negative feedback will not necessarily undermine intrinsic motivation, but in general negative feedback does tend to have detrimental effects.

Several theorists have proposed that the ability to control outcomes and the feeling that one can effectively interact with the environment are important motivational factors (Skinner, 1995), and some consider these to be the critical factors for promoting interest, behavior change, and learning (e.g., Bandura, 1997). The previously mentioned research by Ryan (1982) and others has shown, however, that although personal control over outcomes (i.e., self-efficacy) is important, it is not sufficient for intrinsic motivation; the feelings of competence must be accompanied by perceived autonomy in order for people to be intrinsically motivated.

Other studies of social contexts, which were performed in school classrooms, contrasted autonomy-supportive versus controlling interpersonal climates. Deci et al. (1981) developed a measure of autonomy support within the classroom which assesses the degree to which teachers attempt to motivate learning and behavior in an autonomy-supportive manner versus a controlling manner. Autonomy support involves taking the students' perspective, supporting exploration and self-initiation, and encouraging the students to develop and implement solutions for their own problems, whereas control involves telling the students what they should do and using sanctions to ensure that they do as told. The researchers found that children in more autonomy-supportive classrooms displayed greater curiosity, more independent mastery attempts, and higher self-esteem than students in the more controlling classrooms where teachers tended to pressure them to behave in particular ways. Ryan and Grolnick (1986) also found autonomy-supportive teaching environments to be associated with the students' reports of greater intrinsic interest in learning; however, whereas the Deci et al. (1981) study was done with the teachers' reports about their orientations, the Ryan and Grolnick (1986) study was done with students' perceptions of how autonomy-supportive versus controlling their teachers were. Thus, whether focusing on the teachers' self-reports or the students' reports about the teachers, the results converge on a negative relation between teachers being controlling and their students being less intrinsically motivated and engaged.

The finding that autonomy support plays an important role in increasing motivation and satisfaction of students is not limited to the influence of teachers. Grolnick and Ryan (1989) interviewed parents to assess whether they tended to be autonomy supportive versus controlling with respect to their children's learning. An autonomy-supportive parenting style was evidenced by a willingness to offer choice and to consider the child's perspective when making decisions about his or her homework and other school-related activities. In contrast, a controlling parental style was characterized by the use of extrinsic contingencies such as rewards, punishments, and pressure to motivate the child. Results revealed that parental autonomy support was positively correlated with children's self-reported intrinsic motivation for schoolwork.

In general, then, the results of a range of laboratory experiments and field studies support the view that contextual supports for competence and autonomy are the key ingredients for maintaining intrinsic motivation.

B. The Social Context and Internalization

A central proposition of SDT is that individuals have an innate tendency to internalize the regulation of extrinsically motivated behaviors that are useful for effective functioning in the social world. Internalization allows people to feel related to others and to feel competent within the social matrix. As already noted, however, internalization can take the form of introjection or it can lead to greater integration of the internalized regulation with other aspects of the self. Although people may feel both relatedness and competence when their behavior is regulated by introjects, they will feel autonomous only when the regulations have been more fully integrated.

Consider these examples: people might introject the regulation of behaviors endorsed by an attractive group and thus feel accepted by that group's members; or they might introject parental demands to do homework and thus feel competent at school. With these introjects, the people would feel satisfaction of their needs for relatedness and competence, but they would not experience a sense of volition, of doing the activities in a truly autonomous or self-initiated way.

As predicted by SDT, several studies have shown that the processes of internalization and integration are facilitated in conditions that support satisfaction of the basic psychological needs. Thus, autonomy support and interpersonal involvement of significant adults in children's lives have been associated with the more autonomous forms of internalization. For example, Ryan and Connell (1989) found that the levels of teacher autonomy support and relatedness were associated with the degree to which the students were self-regulating in doing their schoolwork, and Grolnick and Ryan (1989) found that parental autonomy support and involvement also influenced children to be autonomously self-regulating. When teachers and parents were more autonomy-supportive and involved, students displayed greater internalized motivation and were rated by teachers as being more competent and better adjusted.

Deci et al. (1994) hypothesized that three factors in the social environment, which tend to support self-determination, therefore, should facilitate internalization and integration of the regulation of an uninteresting activity: (1) a meaningful rationale for requested behaviors so individuals will understand the personal importance of the behavior for themselves; (2) an acknowledgement of their perspective so they will feel understood; and (3) an interpersonal style that conveys choice rather than control. The researchers performed a laboratory experiment showing that these three facilitating factors led to greater internalization as reflected in greater subsequent performance of the target activity than did the conditions which were not supportive of self-determination. This, then, was an experimental complement to the findings in the Grolnick and Ryan (1989) field study.

Further, the Deci et al. (1994) experiment also showed that internalization which occurred in the self-determination–supporting conditions was integrated, as evidenced by positive correlations between behavioral self-regulation and self-reports of perceived choice and enjoyment of the activity, whereas the internalization which occurred in the more controlling conditions was introjected, as reflected by negative correlations between behavioral self-regulation and the same affective self-report variables. In other words, when people perform an activity and feel endorsement and enjoyment from the activity it is likely that they have integrated the activity's regulation; however, when they perform the activity in spite of not feeling free and not enjoying it, they display a lack of integration suggesting that they have merely introjected the regulation. In short, it seems that controlling contexts not only decrease the likelihood of internalization, but they also ensure that whatever internalization does occur will be only introjected rather than integrated.

IV. SELF-DETERMINATION, LEARNING, AND ADJUSTMENT

Numerous studies have related the motivational processes outlined in SDT to people's learning and performance—that is, to their acquisition and integration of information as well as the flexible, creative use of that information. We began with the hypothesis that high-quality learning would be maximized by intrinsic motivation and integrated self-regulation. Some studies predicted learning outcomes from intrinsic motivation and autonomous self-regulation, while others predicted the outcomes from social contexts that facilitate intrinsic motivation and autonomous self-regulation.

A. Motivation and Learning

Ryan et al. (1990) asked students to read a passage and rate their interest and enjoyment (i.e., their intrinsic motivation) for the material. Subsequently, the students were tested on the material although they had not been informed about the test until after they had read the material and completed their ratings. Results revealed a strong positive correlation between students' interest/enjoyment and both their self-reported comprehension and their actual recall of the material. These findings suggest that intrinsic motivation for learning, as reflected in interest and enjoyment, are important contributors to the learning process. Research by Schiefele (1991) similarly found interest to be positively correlated with depth of text processing and thus quality of learning.

Grolnick and Ryan (1987) found that greater self-determination, as evidenced by higher intrinsic motivation and more identified regulation, was positively associated with conceptual learning in late elementary-school children. Further, Grolnick et al. (1991) reported a positive relation between children's self-determined motivation and both objective measures of achievement and teacher reports of the children's competence.

Several studies have reported results which buttress and expand the findings that self-determined forms of motivation are related to high-quality learning. For example, Vallerand and Bissonnette (1992) reported that more autonomous forms of motivation (that is, integrated regulation and intrinsic motivation) were negatively associated with dropping out of school, whereas more controlling forms (viz., external regulation and introjected regulation) were positively correlated with dropping out of school. A very interesting finding by Ryan and Connell (1989) was that although both introjected regulation (i.e., controlled motivation) and identified regulation (i.e., autonomous motivation) were correlated with children's self-reports of trying hard and parents' reports of their children being motivated, introjection was positively correlated with anxiety in school and maladaptive coping with failures, whereas identification was positively correlated with interest and enjoyment of school and positive coping with failures. Thus, children who are either controlled or autonomous may try hard in school and will look motivated to others, but the quality of their motivation is very different and these different motivations are associated with very different affective and adjustment consequences.

To summarize, people can be motivated to learn in relatively controlled ways or relatively self-determined ways, and it is the self-determined forms of motivation that positively predict school persistence, high-quality learning, and personal adjustment.

B. Social Contexts, Learning, and Adjustment

Other studies focused on the extent to which the contextual factors of autonomy support and involvement promote high-quality learning and adjustment. For example, Grolnick and Ryan (1987) hypothesized that autonomy-supportive contexts would result in greater depth of processing and better comprehension of learned material for elementary school students than would controlling contexts. They examined a learning condition in which the experimenter was autonomy-supportive and stated that the students would be asked some questions about their reactions to the material, relative to a condition in which the experimenter was controlling and emphasized that the students' learning would be tested and graded. After reading the text, all students were given the same test, and results showed that the controlling condition led to poorer conceptual learning of the material than did the autonomy-supportive condition. In contrast, children in the controlling condition performed slightly better on rote memorization than the children whose autonomy was supported, but the controlled group evidenced greater deterioration in their recall over the subsequent week. Thus, at the end of the week the rote recall of the two groups was equal but the conceptual understanding of the students in the autonomy-supportive group was still significantly greater. In short, autonomy support led to better performance on conceptual understanding and comparable performance on rote memorization.

Research in Japanese schools by Kage (1991) provided additional support to the SDT formulation. Among other things, the study showed that junior high school students who were given a series of five quizzes to be counted as part of their grade for the subject of medieval history (thus, a controlling evaluative condition) expressed less interest in the material, rated themselves as less competent, and reported greater anxiety than similar students who had been given the quizzes as a means of monitoring their own learning without having the quizzes count in their final grades (thus, an autonomy-supportive condition). Furthermore, the students whose quiz scores comprised part of their course grade actually performed significantly worse on a summary exam at the end of the course segment. This work suggests that the use of graded quizzes, which is a prevalent, controlling means of motivating students' learning, may actually be counterproductive, not only causing negative affective reactions but also poorer learning.

The importance of autonomy-support and autonomous motivation for enhanced learning has also been demonstrated at the university level. A study by Black and Deci (2000) showed that college students who had instructors who were more autonomy-supportive displayed increases in their autonomous motivation for organic chemistry over the semester-long course and, furthermore, those who were more autonomously motivated in the course enjoyed it more and got higher grades than students who were more controlled in their motivation.

A laboratory experiment with college students also provided support. Specifically, Benware and Deci (1984) asked participants to learn material so they could put it to actual use by teaching it to others (the active-involvement condition) or were asked to learn the material because they would be tested on it (the passive-involvement condition). Students in the active-involvement condition expressed greater intrinsic motivation to learn the material and showed greater conceptual understanding of the material than did students in the passive-involvement condition. The two groups did not differ in terms of the amount of rote memorization.

The importance of self-determination for learning has also been demonstrated with respect to flexible thinking. McGraw and McCullers (1979) found that participants who were controlled with the offer of a financial reward for solving a series of problems had a harder time breaking mental set when presented with a novel problem than did participants who were not offered a reward. The researchers interpreted the result as an indication that the reward undermined intrinsic motivation for the problem-solving, resulting in less cognitive flexibility.

Amabile (1983) reported research linking intrinsic motivation to creativity. She found that when individuals created artistic products in response to controlling contingencies (e.g., evaluations, competition with others, or promised rewards), their work was judged to be less creative compared to those who created artwork in the absence of these controlling pressures. This research lends support to the notion that motivation for creativity, which is one component of high-quality learning and performance, can be enhanced by providing autonomy support, thus affording the individual a greater sense of self-determination.

Thus far, we have focused on the importance of autonomy support for high-quality learning, although the studies by Grolnick and Ryan (1989) and Grolnick et al. (1991) also found that parents' involvement (that is, being concerned about the related to their children about the children's school work) facilitated autonomous self-regulation and learning. The importance of involvement in the learning process was further demonstrated in a study of adolescents by Ryan et al. (1994). Results showed significant positive correlations between the quality of the parents' relatedness to their children and various indices of school functioning, including self-esteem, positive coping, autonomous self-regulation, and engagement in learning.

In sum, studies have indicated that when learning climates are characterized by autonomy support and involvement students are more autonomously motivated and in turn evidence higher quality learning and better psychological adjustment than when learning climates are more controlling.

C. Learning and Adjustment in Special Education Students

In 1986, the *Journal of Learning Disabilities* published a series of articles on the future of the field of learning disabilities (LD). The guest editors, Howard Adelman and Linda Taylor, asked me and Cristine Chandler to read and provide a commentary on the papers written by distinguished researchers in the field of LD. The papers were interesting and informative in many ways. However, one thing that struck us very strongly was that the treatment approaches discussed in these articles focused very heavily on applied behavior analysis. In other words, work in the LD field had been using behavioral approaches to treat individuals with LD, which assume that individuals (at least individuals with LD) are relatively passive and are controlled by contingencies in the environment. Thus, in terms of promoting learning and behavior changes in these individuals, the approaches employed reinforcement-based behavioral interventions to promote change.

As noted earlier in this chapter, SDT perspective acknowledges that rewards and reinforcements can work effectively to control behavior; however, the theory also maintains that the rewards and reinforcements often carry with them negative affective and motivational consequences, most notably the diminishment or thwarting of self-determination. Thus, a consideration of the work that had been done in the LD field prompted us to conduct studies of SDT-related processes in students with learning disabilities or emotional handicaps.

In the first of these, Grolnick and Ryan (1990) assessed four groups of late elementary-aged students: (1) children with LD; (2) children matched for IQ but without LD; (3) children without LD who were randomly selected; and (4) children who were low achievers who did not have LD. Results of this study showed that the children with LD perceived themselves to be less competent and were less autonomously motivated than the second and third groups who were nondisabled, but that the students with LD did not differ from the low-achieving students on these variables. This would seem to imply that it is the level of achievement, rather than the fact of being learning disabled, per se, that has the negative consequences for the levels of the children's motivational variables.

Another study was done with 457 students who had primary handicapping codes of either LD or emotional handicap (EH). The students came from elementary, middle, and high schools in a state-operated special education system. The study linked autonomy support and involvement from teachers and parents, as well as the students' perceived competence and autonomous motivation, to adjustment and learning outcomes for the disabled students (Deci et al., 1992). The mean IQ for students classified as LD was 88 at the elementary level and 83 at the middle and high school levels, whereas the students classified as EH had average IQs that were 10 points higher.

There were several interesting aspects to the results of this study. First, for students with both handicapping codes, the motivation of those who were in elementary school were more strongly related to variables in the home (i.e., parents' autonomy support and involvement) than to variables in the school (i.e., teachers' autonomy support and warmth), whereas the opposite was true for middle and high school students. In these latter groups, the classroom-context variables were more strongly related to the students' motivation than were the home-context variables.

In general, the results showed that the students' perceptions of their mothers and teachers providing autonomy support (rather than being controlling) were associated with the students' perceived academic competence and self-esteem, among other motivation and affective variables. Further, maternal autonomy support also predicted students' scores on the Stanford Achievement Test, as did the students' competence and autonomy. Thus, this study indicated that social-context variables concerning satisfaction of basic psychological needs predicted important educational outcomes for the students with LD and EH, just as the studies reviewed earlier indicated that autonomy support and involvement from parents and teachers were an important influence on educational outcomes for students without handicaps who were in standard classrooms.

There was a further interesting result. Specifically, there was a tendency for autonomy support from mothers and teachers to be stronger predictors of motivation and educational outcomes for the students with EH, whereas involvement/warmth from mothers and teachers were stronger predictors of motivation and educational outcomes for the students with LD. This suggests that autonomy disturbances may be more central to students with EH whereas competence disturbances may be more central for students with LD.

V. POSSIBLE IMPLICATIONS OF SDT FOR THE FIELD OF MR

Although SDT-based studies of special education students did not include students with MR, it is reasonable to infer that learning environments and interventions that are designed to provide autonomy support and involvement—in other words, that would allow satisfaction of the students' basic needs for autonomy, competence, and relatedness—would also lead to more positive outcomes for developmentally disabled students.

There is another intriguing possible implication of these studies which have linked motivation variables to outcomes for special education students, an implication that concerns the concept of MR itself. The traditional view of MR considers it to be a deficiency in innate cognitive abilities, as reflected in level of IQ. However, as noted throughout this volume, the emerging view considers MR to be a condition involving a complex interaction of cognitive deficits and self-relevant motivational processes which conduce toward poorer learning and adjustment outcomes for individuals with MR. This newer view would imply that the disadvantaged outcomes associated with MR are, to a significant degree, a function of the social environments provided for developmentally disabled individuals; in other words, the social environments could be understood as contributing to the condition itself. Simply stated, to the extent that individuals with below average intelligence are deprived by the social environment of opportunities to satisfy their needs for autonomy, competence, and relatedness, the environment would be contributing to their MR. This seems like an important issue that deserves greater consideration from MR researchers.

Although little work has attempted to apply SDT directly to the learning and well-being of MR individuals, I will now briefly consider research using other perspectives that has examined issues related to motivation and self-determination among the mentally retarded. This work has tended to fall into two general categories. The first is pioneering basic research on the intrinsic and extrinsic motivation of individuals with MR done by the Peabody-Vanderbilt group (Haywood & Switzky, 1986) and the Yale group (Zigler, 2001), both of which view students with MR as being relatively deficient in intrinsic motivation and overly reliant on environmental cues and reinforcements. The second is a set of intervention studies that are intended to teach individuals with MR to be more self-reliant.

A. Intrinsic Motivation in Students With MR

In the first category, Haywood & Switzky (1992) have differentiated motivation into intrinsic and extrinsic, treating this as a dichotomy. In doing so, the concept of extrinsic motivation was undifferentiated and was essentially equivalent to what is called external regulation within SDT. Further, Haywood and Switzky (1992) conceptualized intrinsic and extrinsic motivation for learning as individual differences or learned personality traits, much as was done by Harter (1981). Thus, from this perspective, students are considered either intrinsically motivated or extrinsically motivated, and research indicates that students with MR tend to be less intrinsically motivated than students without MR, and that the intrinsic motivation deficits lead to less effective learning (e.g., Schultz & Switzky, 1993).

Switzky (2001) suggested that motivational orientations of students with MR interact with incentive systems such that intrinsically motivated students will be optimally reinforced by rewards intrinsic to the activity itself, whereas extrinsically motivated students will be optimally reinforced by extrinsic rewards. This perspective, which is common to the work in other domains as well, represents what can be termed a match hypothesis. If people are intrinsically motivated or autonomous in their own orientation, the most effective way to motivate them is through autonomy support, whereas, if people are extrinsically motivated or controlled in their own orientation, this perspective advocates the use of extrinsic rewards or other types of control. This is a point about which there is disagreement between SDT perspective and that of the Peabody-Vanderbilt group. Specifically, SDT perspective suggests that regardless of the children's orientation, which SDT viewpoint agrees is learned, the use of rewards and controls will have negative psychological consequences. That is, it will diminish autonomy and be associated with poorer well-being. Of course, it is possible that the use of rewards with extrinsically oriented individuals will control their behavior and produce the intended behavior while the controls are in effect, but as so much research has documented, this will further undermine their own capacities and motivation to be self-motivating. In fact, SDT research has continually found that all students respond positively to autonomy support and involvement from teachers and parents regardless of their initial levels of intrinsic motivation or self-determination. In other words, we have repeatedly found positive main effects for autonomy support with no interactions between autonomy support and autonomous (or intrinsic) motivation when the outcomes are self-determination, maintained behavior change, or well-being. It is precisely because autonomy support and involvement allow satisfaction of the individuals' needs for autonomy, competence, and relatedness that this approach has a more positive effect.

Central to SDT is a developmental perspective, which maintains that it is possible to facilitate greater autonomous motivation in all students and that the enhanced autonomous motivation will result in higher quality learning and enhanced well-being for all students. Of course, if individuals' predominant experiences have been ones of being controlled by rewards and other external events, such as threats or deadlines, the process of facilitating these individuals' becoming more self-initiating and self-sustaining and of decreasing their reliance on rewards and controls will take concerted effort and time. Becoming more self-determined is, after all, a developmental process that needs to be stimulated and supported, but it is a process that is worthwhile to facilitate. Thus, although some students may be strongly desirous of extrinsic rewards, SDT maintains that it is important to support basic psychological need satisfaction in all students, regardless of their initial motivations, so they will gradually become more self-determined in their motivation and behavior.

B. Self-Determination Interventions for Individuals With MR

Prompted in part by the Americans with Disabilities Act of 1990 and by other legislative actions and federal funding opportunities in recent years, there has been increasing interest in promoting self-determination among individuals with MR and other disabilities. In large part, the federal actions have prompted more intervention programs than research, but there have been a number of studies relevant to these efforts. For example, several studies have evaluated programs referred to as self-determination interventions (e.g., Hoffman & Field, 1995), although the definitions of self-determination and other key concepts have varied among the studies and are not always consistent with SDT definition of self-determination. In other words, the term self-determination in much of this literature refers to specific behaviors related to people taking care of themselves rather than to psychological processes that might underlie such behaviors. Further, the quality of the studies has varied greatly, with some using control groups and others not, some using sample sizes large enough for reasonable statistical inferences and others not, and so on. Still, some studies have compared a so-called self-determination intervention with a suitable control group for participants with MR (e.g., Bregman, 1984; Tymchuk et al., 1988). The Bregman (1984) study, for example, targeted adults with MR and introduced a curriculum intended to promote self-advocacy. Results showed significant improvement in the communications of the intervention group relative to the control group.

With this enhanced interest in the self-determination of disabled individuals, it seems highly appropriate to be developing and evaluating interventions intended to facilitate self-determination, as is being done. Such interventions and evaluations would benefit greatly from the use of process models of change that specify: (1) the intervention in terms of both the external conditions that are to be affected and the psychological or experiential interpretation of those changes; (2) the mediating processes through which the intervention is expected to have positive effects on learning, well-being, or life circumstance of the participants; and (3) concrete indicators of the outcomes that are expected to be affected. SDT represents one such process model that has guided interventions to promote more self-determination in other domains ranging from the workplace to the medical clinic (e.g., Deci et al., 1989; Williams et al., 2002, 2004) and could provide a basis for fine-tuning interventions in the field of MR and for clarifying the psychological processes through which the interventions are affecting the lives of the individuals with MR. For example, SDT has isolated many factors that enhance versus diminish self-determined motivation, and it has proposed clearly that any intervention will have a more positive effect if administered in an autonomy-supportive way so that participants will experience greater satisfaction of the needs for competence, autonomy, and relatedness. Further, SDT specifies that one could focus either on the perceptions of competence, autonomy, and relatedness or on types of motivation (i.e., intrinsic motivation and autonomous extrinsic motivation) as the mediating processes through which interventions are expected to have their positive effects, and instruments have been developed to assess each of the constructs of SDT which could either be used as they are or be easily adapted for use in research with MR samples. There are, of course, other theories that could also guide such efforts, yet SDT seems particularly suited to the issues being addressed in the MR field at this time.

Recently, the clinical and research work being done on self-determination among individuals with MR by various teams have become increasingly sophisticated and grounded in research and theory, thus representing important steps in the right direction. A new volume by Wehmeyer et al. (2003) presents several of these programs. There are numerous points of agreement, as well as a number of points of disagreement, between SDT and the perspectives presented in the Wehmeyer et al. (2003) book. Space does not allow a detailed consideration of each of those perspectives, in terms of their points of agreement and disagreement with SDT, but I will mention just one point of disagreement in an attempt to clarify a theoretical point that highlights a fairly prevalent difference between SDT and the perspectives in the book.

In a chapter by Abery and Stancliffe (2003) a tripartite-ecological approach to self-determination is presented. These authors draw on many psychological theories to formulate their position, as well as present a compelling case for providing MR individuals with greater control over their own lives. Much of what these authors argue is consistent with SDT; however, I will now highlight one point of divergence that is worth noting for theoretical as well as practical reasons. Abery and Stancliffe (2003) emphasized that "personal control" is one of the most powerful factors facilitating self-determination, and they further suggested that reinforcing attempts to be self-determining is an additionally important contributor to self-determination.

SDT takes a somewhat different perspective concerning the concepts of "personal control" and "reinforcement." The concept of personal control (e.g., Skinner, 1995) which derived from the work of Rotter (1966) refers to having control over outcomes. Thus, developmentally disabled individuals would have personal control if a contingency in the environment allows them to attain an outcome—for example, to obtain a monetary reward or avoid a punishment—by performing an instrumental behavior. In contrast, self-determination is about the self-initiation and self-regulation of one's own behavior. Of course, one needs to have control over outcomes in order to be self-determining, but personal control does not ensure self-determination. Indeed, many of the factors that provide personal control have been found to undermine autonomous motivation and self-determination.

Consider the following example. A statement to a developmentally disabled individual such as, "You will get a candy bar if you wash your face, comb your hair, and brush your teeth now," would provide that individual with personal control. The individual could control the outcome by doing the requisite behavior. Further, the outcome would represent a reinforcement, which is to say that it would increase the likelihood of the behavior being emitted again the next time the contingency is encountered. In SDT, however, we would characterize that statement to be controlling, and we would expect it to be undermining, rather than supportive, of self-determination. The person could attain the outcome (i.e., the candy bar) but the behaviors would tend to become dependent on that outcome, so the behaviors are less likely to be self-motivated in the future and displayed in the absence of the contingency. The SDT perspective would instead emphasize providing people with choices and opportunities for self-initiation in order to encourage them to take greater responsibility for themselves, and it would support development of the skills or capacities necessary to enact the behaviors. Thus, the approach would focus on allowing the individuals to choose when and how to do their daily activities rather than creating contingencies aimed at controlling their performance of the activities. Contingencies, with the resulting reinforcements, do provide personal control, but they are unlikely to promote self-determination. Simply stated, the concept of reinforcement, which according to Skinner (1953) is essentially synonymous with control, has been found to diminish self-determination rather than enhance it. In contrast, the SDT idea of being responsive to the initiations of developmentally disabled individuals, of taking their perspective and encouraging their self-initiation, is consistent with providing autonomy support, which has been found repeatedly to enhance autonomous motivation.

Central to SDT, then, is the idea of encouraging and supporting volition and self-initiation. Such encouragement involves providing optimal challenges and structures (Deci, 1975) as well as allowing people the opportunity to make choices and initiate their own behavior. And, for this to be autonomy-supportive it must all be done in a way that is geared to the developmental level of the individuals involved. In other words, choices and responsibilities offered to individuals need to represent optimal challenges in order to encourage those individuals to be autonomously engaged in learning and self-care.

VI. CONCLUSIONS

SDT proposes that people have an intrinsic desire to explore, understand, and assimilate aspects of their environment. This proactive motivation is present from the very earliest stages of development, does not depend on external pressures, and is essential for the acquisition of cognitive skills and the development of self. Optimal learning, development, and maintained behavior change, according to SDT, requires this intrinsic motivation along with extrinsic motivation that has been internalized and integrated with one's sense of self.

However, both intrinsic motivation and internalized extrinsic motivation require nutriments from the social environment. Specifically, social contexts that support satisfaction of individuals' innate psychological needs for autonomy, competence, and relatedness—that is, contexts in which significant others are involved and autonomy supportive—allow the individuals to maintain intrinsic motivation and facilitate integration of extrinsic motivation. In turn, such social contexts promote higher quality learning and better personal adjustment.

SDT maintains that individuals with MR, like other individuals whether disabled or non-disabled, will become more motivated and self-determined to the extent that teachers or caregivers are autonomy-supportive and involved. Regardless of the initial levels of intrinsic and extrinsic motivation of the individuals, healthy development and greater self-determination can be facilitated when interventions or educational programs are administered by involved and autonomy-supportive educators and providers.

REFERENCES

Amabile, T. M. (1983). *The social psychology of creativity.* New York: Springer-Verlag.
Amabile, T. M., DeJong, W., & Lepper, M. R. (1976). Effects of externally imposed deadlines on subsequent intrinsic motivation. *Journal of Personality and Social Psychology, 34,* 92–98.
Abery, B. H., & Stancliffe, R. J. (2003). A tripartite-ecological theory of self-determination. In M. L. Wehmeyer, B. Abery, D. E. Mithaug, & R. Stancliffe (Eds.), *Theory in self-determination: Foundations for educational practice* (pp. 43–78). Springfield, IL: Charles C. Thomas, Ltd.
Bandura, A. (1997). *Self-efficacy: The exercise of control.* New York: Freeman.
Benware, C., & Deci, E. L. (1984). Quality of learning with an active versus passive motivational set. *American Educational Research Journal, 21,* 755–765.
Black, A. E., & Deci, E. L. (2000). The effects of instructors' autonomy support and students' autonomous motivation on learning organic chemistry: A self-determination theory perspective. *Science Education, 84,* 740–756.
Bregman, S. (1984). Assertiveness training for mentally retarded adults. *Mental Retardation, 22,* 12–16.
Csikszentmihalyi, M. (1975). *Beyond boredom and anxiety.* San Francisco: Jossey-Bass.
Danner, F. W., & Lonky, E. (1981). A cognitive-developmental approach to the effects of rewards on intrinsic motivation. *Child Development, 52,* 1043–1052.
deCharms, R. (1968). *Personal causation: The internal affective determinants of behavior.* New York: Academic Press.

Deci, E. L. (1971). Effects of externally mediated rewards on intrinsic motivation. *Journal of Personality and Social Psychology, 18,* 105–115.

Deci, E. L. (1972). Intrinsic motivation, extrinsic reinforcement, and inequity. *Journal of Personality and Social Psychology, 22,* 113–120.

Deci, E. L. (1975). *Intrinsic motivation.* New York: Plenum.

Deci, E. L., & Cascio, W. F. (1972, April). *Changes in intrinsic motivation as a function of negative feedback and threats,* Paper presented at the meeting of the Eastern Psychological Association, Boston.

Deci, E. L., Connell, J. P., & Ryan, R. M. (1989). Self-determination in a work organization. *Journal of Applied Psychology, 74,* 580–590.

Deci, E. L., Eghrari, H., Patrick, B. C., & Leone, D. R. (1994). Facilitating internalization: The self-determination theory perspective. *Journal of Personality, 62,* 119–142.

Deci, E. L., Hodges, R., Pierson, L., & Tomassone, J. (1992). Autonomy and competence as motivational factors in students with learning disabilities and emotional handicaps. *Journal of Learning Disabilities, 25,* 457–471.

Deci, E. L., Koestner, R., & Ryan, R. M. (1999). A meta-analytic review of experiments examining the effects of extrinsic rewards on intrinsic motivation. *Psychological Bulletin, 125,* 627–668.

Deci, E. L., & Ryan, R. M. (1985). *Intrinsic motivation and self-determination in human behavior.* New York: Plenum.

Deci, E. L., & Ryan, R. M. (1991). A motivational approach to self: Integration in personality. In R. Dienstbier (Ed.), *Nebraska symposium on motivation: Perspectives on motivation* (Vol. 14, pp. 237–288). Lincoln, NE: University of Nebraska Press.

Deci, E. L., & Ryan, R. M. (2000). The "what" and "why" of goal pursuits: Human needs and the self-determination of behavior. *Psychological Inquiry, 11,* 227–268.

Deci, E. L., Schwartz, A. J., Sheinman, L., & Ryan, R. M. (1981). An instrument to assess adults' orientations toward control versus autonomy with children: Reflections on intrinsic motivation and perceived competence. *Journal of Educational Psychology, 73,* 642–650.

Eisenberger, R., Pierce, W. D., & Cameron, J. (1999). Effects of reward on intrinsic motivation—negative, neutral, and positive: Comment on Deci, Koestner, and Ryan (1999). *Psychological Bulletin, 125,* 677–691.

Fisher, C. D. (1978). The effects of personal control, competence, and extrinsic reward systems on intrinsic motivation. *Organizational Behavior and Human Performance, 21,* 273–288.

Grolnick, W. S., & Ryan, R. M. (1987). Autonomy in children's learning: An experimental and individual difference investigation. *Journal of Personality and Social Psychology, 52,* 890–898.

Grolnick, W. S., & Ryan, R. M. (1989). Parent styles associated with children's self-regulation and competence in school. *Journal of Educational Psychology, 81,* 143–154.

Grolnick, W. S., & Ryan, R. M. (1990). Self-perception, motivation, and adjustment in children with learning disabilities: A multiple group comparison study. *Journal of Learning Disabilities, 23,* 177–184.

Grolnick, W. S., Ryan, R. M., & Deci, E. L. (1991). The inner resources for school achievement: Motivational mediators of children's perceptions of their parents. *Journal of Educational Psychology, 83,* 508–517.

Harackiewicz, J. (1979). The effects of reward contingency and performance feedback on intrinsic motivation. *Journal of Personality and Social Psychology, 37,* 1352–1363.

Harlow, H. F. (1958). The nature of love. *American Psychologist, 13,* 673–685.

Harter, S. (1981). A new self-report scale of intrinsic versus extrinsic orientation in the classroom: Motivational and informational components. *Developmental Psychology, 17,* 300–312.

Harter, S., & Zigler, E. (1972). Effects of rate of stimulus presentation and penalty conditions on the discrimination learning of normal and retarded children. *Developmental Psychology, 6*, 85–91.

Harter, S., & Zigler, E. (1974). The assessment of effectance motivation in normal and retarded children. *Developmental Psychology, 10*, 169–180.

Haywood, C. I. (1968). Motivational orientation of overachieving and underachieving elementary school children. *Developmental Psychology, 10*, 169–180.

Haywood, C. I., & Switzky, H. N. (1986). Intrinsic motivation and behavioral effectiveness in retarded persons. In N. Ellis & N. Bray (Eds.), *International review of research in mental retardation* (Vol. 14, pp. 1–46). New York: Academic Press.

Haywood, C. I., & Switzky, H. N. (1992). Ability and modifiability: What, how and how much? In J. S. Carlson (Ed.), *Advances in cognition and educational practice: Theoretical issues: Intelligence, cognition, and assessment* (Vol. 1, Part A, pp. 25–85). Greenwich, CT: JAI Press.

Heider, F. (1958). *The psychology of interpersonal relations.* New York: Wiley.

Hoffman, A., & Field, S. (1995). Promoting self-determination through effective curriculum development. *Intervention in School and Clinic, 30*(3), 134–141.

Kage, M. (1991, September). *The effects of evaluation on intrinsic motivation,* Paper presented at the meetings of the Japan Association of Educational Psychology, Joetsu, Japan.

Koestner, R., Ryan, R. M., Bernieri, F., & Holt, K. (1984). Setting limits on children's behavior: The differential effects of controlling versus informational styles on intrinsic motivation and creativity. *Journal of Personality, 52*, 233–248.

Lepper, M. R., Greene, D., & Nisbett, R. E. (1973). Undermining children's intrinsic interest with extrinsic rewards: A test of the "overjustification" hypothesis. *Journal of Personality and Social Psychology, 28*, 129–137.

Lewin, K. (1951). Intention, will, and need. In D. Rapaport (Ed.), *Organization and pathology of thought* (pp. 95–153). New York: Columbia University Press.

Locke, E. A., & Latham, G. P. (1990). *A theory of goal setting and task performance.* Englewood Cliffs, NJ: Prentice-Hall.

McGraw, K. O., & McCullers, J. C. (1979). Evidence of a detrimental effect of extrinsic incentives on breaking a mental set. *Journal of Experimental Social Psychology, 15*, 285–294.

Mossholder, K. W. (1980). Effects of externally mediated goal setting on intrinsic motivation: A laboratory experiment. *Journal of Applied Psychology, 65*, 202–210.

Piaget, J. (1971). *Biology and Knowledge.* Chicago: University of Chicago Press.

Porter, L. W., & Lawler, E. E. III. (1968). *Managerial attitudes and performance.* Homewood, IL: Irwin-Dorsey.

Rotter, J. B. (1966). Generalized expectancies for internal versus external control of reinforcement. *Psychological Monographs, 80*(1, Whole No. 609), 1–28.

Ryan, R. M. (1982). Control and information in the intrapersonal sphere: An extension of cognitive evaluation theory. *Journal of Personality and Social Psychology, 43*, 450–461.

Ryan, R. M. (1993). Agency and organization: Intrinsic motivation, autonomy and the self in psychological development. In J. Jacobs (Ed.), *Nebraska symposium on motivation: Developmental perspectives on motivation* (Vol. 40, pp. 1–56). Lincoln, NE: University of Nebraska Press.

Ryan, R. M., & Connell, J. P. (1989). Perceived locus of causality and internalization: Examining reasons for acting in two domains. *Journal of Personality and Social Psychology, 57*, 749–761.

Ryan, R. M., Connell, J. P., & Plant, R. W. (1990). Emotions in non-directed text learning. *Learning and Individual Differences, 2*, 1–17.

Ryan, R. M., & Deci, E. L. (2000). Self-determination theory and the facilitation of intrinsic motivation, social development, and well-being. *American Psychologist, 55,* 68–78.

Ryan, R. M., & Grolnick, W. S. (1986). Origins and pawns in the classroom: Self-report and projective assessments of individual differences in children's perceptions. *Journal of Personality and Social Psychology, 50,* 550–558.

Ryan, R. M., Mims, V., & Koestner, R. (1983). Relation of reward contingency and interpersonal context to intrinsic motivation: A review and test using cognitive evaluation theory. *Journal of Personality and Social Psychology, 45,* 736–750.

Ryan, R. M., Stiller, J., & Lynch, J. H. (1994). Representations of relationships to teachers, parents, and friends as predictors of academic motivation and self-esteem. *Journal of Early Adolescence, 14,* 226–249.

Schafer, R. (1968). *Aspects of internalization.* New York: International Universities Press.

Schiefele, U. (1991). Interest, learning, and motivation. *Educational Psychologist, 26,* 299–323.

Schultz, G. F., & Switzky, H. N. (1993). The academic achievement of elementary and junior high school students with behavior disorders and their nonhandicapped peers as a function of motivational orientations. *Learning & Individual Differences, 5,* 31–42.

Seligman, M. E. P. (1975). *Helplessness: On depression, development, and death.* San Francisco: Freeman.

Silon, E. L., & Harter, S. (1985). Assessment of perceived competence, motivational orientation, and anxiety in segregated and main-streamed educable mentally retarded children. *Journal of Educational Psychology, 77,* 217–230.

Skinner, B. F. (1953). *Science and human behavior.* New York: Macmillan.

Skinner, E. A. (1995). *Perceived control, motivation, and coping.* Thousand Oaks, CA: Sage.

Smith, W. E. (1975). *The effects of social and monetary rewards on intrinsic motivation.* Cornell University.

Switzky, H. N. (2001). Personality and motivational self-system processes in people with mental retardation: Old memories and new perspectives. In H. N. Switzky (Ed.), *Personality and motivational differences in persons with mental retardation* (pp. 57–143). Mahwah, NJ: Lawrence Erlbaum Associates.

Tymchuk, A. J., Andron, L., & Rahbar, B. (1988). Effective decision-making/problem-solving training with mothers who have mental retardation. *American Journal of Mental Retardation, 92,* 510–516.

Usui, M. (1991, September). *The effects of perceived competence and self-determination on intrinsic motivation,* Paper presented at the Japanese Association of Educational Psychology, Joetsu, Japan.

Vallerand, R. J., & Bissonnette, R. (1992). Intrinsic, extrinsic, and amotivational styles as predictors of behavior: A prospective study. *Journal of Personality, 60,* 599–620.

Vallerand, R. J., & Reid, G. (1984). On the causal effects of perceived competence on intrinsic motivation: A test of cognitive evaluation theory. *Journal of Sport Psychology, 6,* 94–102.

Wehmeyer, M. L., Abery, B., Mithaug, D. E., & Stancliffe, R. (2003). *Theory in self-determination: Foundations for educational practice.* Springfield, IL: Charles C. Thomas, Ltd.

White, R. W. (1959). Motivation reconsidered: The concept of competence. *Psychological Review, 66,* 297–333.

Williams, G. C., McGregor, H. A., Zeldman, A., Freedman, Z. R., & Deci, E. L. (2004). Testing a self-determination theory process model for promoting glycemic control through diabetes self-management. *Health Psychology, 23,* 58–66.

Williams, G. C., Minicucci, D. S., Kouides, R. W., Levesque, C. S., Chirkov, V. I., Ryan, R. M., & Deci, E. L. (2002). Self-determination, smoking, diet, and health. *Health Education Research, 17,* 512–521.

Zigler, E. (2001). Looking back 40 years and still seeing the person with mental retardation as a whole person. In H. N. Switzky (Ed.), *Personality and motivational differences in persons with mental retardation* (pp. 3–55). Mahwah, NJ: Lawrence Erlbaum Associates.

Zuckerman, M., Porac, J., Lathin, D., Smith, R., & Deci, E. L. (1978). On the importance of self-determination for intrinsically motivated behavior. *Personality and Social Psychology Bulletin, 4,* 443–446.

Applications of a Model of Goal Orientation and Self-Regulated Learning to Individuals with Learning Problems

PAUL R. PINTRICH[†] AND JULIANE L. BLAZEVSKI

UNIVERSITY OF MICHIGAN

Self-regulated learning concerns the application of general models of regulation and self-regulation to issues of learning, in particular academic learning that occurs in school or classroom contexts. An important aspect of models of self-regulation is that individuals regulate towards a goal, thereby implicating the motivational system. Pintrich (2000) has proposed a general model that links different goal orientations to various self-regulatory processes related to academic learning. A hallmark of this model is the importance of integrating both cognitive and motivational components in learning. In this chapter, we will apply that general model to understanding how goal orientations and self-regulated learning processes might operate for individuals with learning problems. We first provide an overview of the general model of self-regulation and goal orientation, followed by a discussion of how different goal orientations might promote or constrain self-regulated learning. In these two different sections we note how these general processes might apply to individuals with learning problems. Given space constraints, this chapter does not include a comprehensive review of research in special education on how these processes might be related to individuals with learning problems, rather we include a few citations from the special education literature to illustrate potential applications.

[†]Deceased

I. A GENERAL FRAMEWORK FOR SELF-REGULATED LEARNING

There are many different models of self-regulated learning that propose different constructs and mechanisms, but they share some basic assumptions about learning and regulation. One common assumption might be called the *active, constructive assumption* which follows from a general cognitive perspective. That is, all the models view learners as active, constructive participants in the learning process. Learners are assumed to actively construct their own meanings, goals, and strategies from the information available in the "external" environment as well as information in their own minds (the "internal" environment). Learners are not just passive recipients of information from teachers, parents, or other adults, but rather active, constructive meaning-makers as they approach learning. Given the general behavioral perspective in much of the special education literature, this assumption may be controversial, but it is a common assumption in the more general current research on learning and motivation. Moreover in line with a general developmental perspective on developmental disabilities (e.g., Hodapp et al., 1998; Zigler, 1999), there is utility in making similar assumptions about the development of *all* individuals, regardless of their specific learning problem.

A second, but related, assumption is the *potential for control assumption*. All the models assume that learners can potentially monitor, control, and regulate certain aspects of their own cognition, motivation, and behavior as well as some features of their environments. This assumption does not mean that individuals will or can monitor and control their cognition, motivation, or behavior at all times or in all contexts, rather just that some monitoring, control, and regulation is possible. All of the models recognize that there are biological, developmental, contextual, and individual difference constraints that can impede or interfere with individual efforts at regulation. Accordingly, even learners with no specific learning problems still have difficulty regulating their own learning. Of course, those individuals with learning problems may have even more difficulties in controlling and regulating their own learning.

A third general assumption that is made in these models of self-regulated learning, as in all general models of regulation stretching back to Miller et al. (1960), is the *goal, criterion, or standard assumption*. All models of regulation assume that there is some type of criterion or standard (also called goals or reference value) against which comparisons are made in order to assess whether the process should continue as is or if some type of change is necessary. The common sense example is the thermostat operation for the heating and cooling of a house. Once a desired temperature is set (the goal, criterion, standard), the thermostat monitors the temperature of the house (monitoring process) and then turns on or off the heating or air conditioning units (control and regulation processes) in order to reach and maintain the standard. In a parallel manner, the general example for learning assumes that individuals can set standards or goals to strive for in their learning, monitor their progress towards these goals, and then adapt and regulate their cognition, motivation, and behavior in order to reach their goals. Of course, all individuals may have difficulties in regulating towards goals, but individuals with learning problems may have even more difficulties in this aspect of self-regulated learning.

A fourth general assumption of most of the models of self-regulated learning is that self-regulatory activities are *mediators between personal and contextual characteristics and actual achievement or performance*. That is, it is not just individuals' cultural, demographic, or personality characteristics that directly influence achievement and learning, nor just the contextual characteristics of the classroom environment that shape achievement, but the individuals' self-regulation of their cognition, motivation, and behavior that mediate the relations between the person, context, and eventual achievement. Most models of self-regulation assume that self-regulatory activities are directly linked to outcomes such as achievement and performance, although much of the research examines self-regulatory activities as outcomes in their own right. Accordingly, for individuals with learning problems, these self-regulatory processes mediate between other personal characteristics and their actual achievement or learning.

Given these assumptions, a general working definition of self-regulated learning is that it is an active, constructive process whereby learners set goals for their learning and then attempt to monitor, regulate, and control their cognition, motivation, and behavior, guided and constrained by their goals and the contextual features in the environment. These self-regulatory activities can mediate the relations between individuals and the context and their overall achievement. This definition is similar to other models of self-regulated learning (e.g., Butler & Winne, 1995; Zimmerman, 1989, 1998a,b, 2000). Although this definition is relatively simple, the remainder of this section outlines in more detail the various processes and areas of regulation and their application to learning and achievement in the academic domain that reveals the complexity and diversity of the processes of self-regulated learning.

Table I displays a framework for classifying the different phases and areas for regulation. The four phases that create the rows of the table are processes that many models of regulation and self-regulation share (e.g., Zimmerman, 1998a,b, 2000) and reflect goal-setting, monitoring, control, and regulation processes. Of course, not all academic learning follows these phases as there

TABLE I
PHASES AND AREAS FOR SELF-REGULATED LEARNING

Phases	Areas for Regulation			
	Cognition	Motivation/Affect	Behavior	Context
1) Forethought, planning, and activation	1) Target goal setting 2) Prior content knowledge activation 3) Metacognitive knowledge activation	1) Goal orientation adoption 2) Efficacy judgments 3) Perceptions of task difficulty 4) Task value activation 5) Interest activation	1) Time and effort planning 2) Planning for self-observations of behavior	1) Perceptions of task 2) Perceptions of context
2) Monitoring	1) Metacognitive awareness and monitoring of cognition	1) Awareness and monitoring of motivation and affect	1) Awareness and monitoring of effort, time use, need for help 2) Self-observation of behavior	1) Monitoring changing task and context conditions
3) Control	1) Selection and adaptation of cognitive strategies for learning and thinking	1) Selection and adaptation of strategies for managing motivation and affect	1) Increase/decrease effort 2) Persist, give up 3) Help-seeking behavior	1) Change or re-negotiate task 2) Change or leave context
4) Reaction and reflection	1) Cognitive judgments 2) Attributions	1) Affective reactions 2) Attributions	1) Choice behavior	1) Evaluation of task 2) Evaluation of context

are many occasions for students to learn academic material in more tacit, implicit, or unintentional ways without self-regulating their learning in such an explicit manner as suggested in the model. These phases are suggested as a heuristic to organize our thinking and research on self-regulated learning. Phase 1 involves planning and goal-setting as well as activation of perceptions and knowledge of the task, the context, and the self in relation to the task. Phase 2 concerns various monitoring processes that represent metacognitive awareness of different aspects of the self and task or context. Phase 3 involves efforts to control and regulate different aspects of the self or task and context. Finally, phase 4 represents various kinds of reactions and reflections on the self and the task or context.

The four phases do represent a general time-ordered sequence that individuals would experience as they perform a task, but there is no strong assumption that the phases are hierarchically or linearly structured such that earlier phases must always occur before later phases. In most models of self-regulated learning, monitoring, control, and reaction can occur simultaneously and dynamically as the individual progresses through the task, with the goals and plans being changed or updated based on the feedback from the monitoring, control, and reaction processes.

The four columns in Table I represent different areas for regulation that an individual learner can attempt to monitor, control, and regulate. The first three columns of cognition, motivation/affect, and behavior reflect the traditional tripartite division of the different areas of psychological functioning (Snow et al., 1996). As Snow et al. (1996) note, the boundaries between these areas may be observed, but there is utility in discussing them separately, particularly since much of traditional psychological research has focused on the different areas in isolation from the others. The first three areas in the columns in Table I represent aspects of the individual's own cognition, motivation/affect, and behavior that he or she can attempt to control and regulate. These attempts to control or regulate are "self-regulated" in that the individual is focused on trying to control or regulate his or her own cognition, motivation, and behavior. Of course, other individuals in the environment such as teachers, peers, or parents can try to "other" regulate an individual's cognition, motivation, or behavior as well, by directing or scaffolding the individual in terms of what, how, and when to do a task. More generally, other task and contextual features (e.g., task characteristics, feedback systems, positive and negative reinforcers, evaluation structures) can facilitate or constrain an individual's attempts to self-regulate his or her learning.

The cognition column in Table I concerns the different cognitive strategies individuals may use to learn and perform a task as well as the metacognitive strategies individuals may use to control and regulate their cognition. In addition, both content and strategic knowledge are included in the cognition column. The motivation affect column concerns the various motivational beliefs that individuals may have about themselves in relation to the task, such as self-efficacy beliefs and values for the task. In addition, interest or liking of the task would be included in this column as well as positive and negative affective reactions to the self or task. Finally, any strategies that individuals may use to control and regulate their motivation and affect would be included in this column. The behavior column reflects the general effort the individual may exert on the task as well as persistence, help-seeking, and choice behaviors.

The fourth column in Table I, context, represents various aspects of the task environment, general classroom, or cultural context where the learning is taking place. Individuals do try to monitor and control their environment to some extent and, in fact, in some models of intelligence (e.g., Sternberg, 1985) attempts to selectively control and change the context are seen as very adaptable. In the same manner, in this model, it is assumed that individual attempts to monitor and control the environment or context are an important aspect of self-regulated learning.

This general description of the rows and columns of Table I provides an overview of how the different phases of regulation relate to different areas for regulation. The next section describes in more detail the cells in the table, organized by column.

A. Regulation of Cognition

Table I displays the four general phases of self-regulation that can occur; within the column for cognition, there are four cells that represent how these different phases may be applied to the various aspects of cognition. Each cell is discussed separately for rhetorical and logical reasons including ease of presentation; although as noted above, the phases may overlap or occur simultaneously with multiple interactions among the different processes and components. There is no strong assumption of a simple linear, static process with separable non-interacting components.

1. COGNITIVE PLANNING AND ACTIVATION

As shown in Table I, there are three general types of planning or activation: (1) target goal setting; (2) activation of relevant prior content knowledge; and (3) activation of metacognitive knowledge. Target goal setting involves the setting of task-specific goals which can be used to guide cognition in general and monitoring in particular (Harackiewicz et al., 1998; Pintrich et al., 2000; Pressley & Afflerbach, 1995; Schunk, 1994; Zimmerman, 1989; Zimmerman & Martinez-Pons, 1986, 1988). As noted above, the goal acts as a criterion against which to assess, monitor, and guide cognition, just as the temperature setting of a thermostat guides the operation of the thermostat and the heating/cooling system. Of course, goal-setting is most often assumed to occur before starting a task, but goal-setting can actually occur at any point during performance. Learners may begin a task by setting specific goals for learning, goals for time use, and goals or criteria for eventual performance, but all of these can be adjusted and changed at any time during task performance as a function of monitoring, control, and reflection processes.

The second aspect of forethought and planning involves the activation of relevant prior knowledge. At some level, this process of activation of prior knowledge can and does happen automatically and without conscious thought. That is, as students approach a task in a particular domain, for example, mathematics, some aspects of their knowledge about mathematics will be activated automatically and quickly without conscious control. This type of process would not be considered self-regulatory and involves general cognitive processing, as it is not under the explicit control of the learner. At the same time, students who are more self-regulating or metacognitive, can actively search their memory for relevant prior knowledge before they actually begin performing the task. This prior knowledge can include content knowledge as well as metacognitive knowledge about the task and strategies (Alexander et al., 1991; Flavell, 1979; Pintrich et al., 2000).

The activation of prior knowledge of the content area can happen automatically, but it also can be done in a more planful and regulatory manner through various prompts and self-questioning activities, such as asking oneself, "What do I know about this domain, subject area, topic, problem type, etc.?" as well as the construction of better problem representations. It appears that both domain experts and self-regulating learners do engage in these types of planning activities (refer to, Chi et al., 1981; Larkin et al., 1980; Zimmerman & Martinez-Pons, 1986).

The third entry in the cell in Table I, the activation of metacognitive knowledge, includes the activation of knowledge about cognitive tasks and strategies and seems to be useful for learning (Pintrich et al., 2000; Schneider & Pressley, 1997). Again, as with prior content knowledge, this activation can be rather automatic, stimulated by individual, task, or contextual features, or it can be more controlled and conscious. Metacognitive task knowledge includes knowledge about how task variations can influence cognition. For example, if there is more information provided in a question or a test, then it will generally be more easily solved than when there is little information provided. Most students come to understand this general idea and it becomes part of their metacognitive knowledge about task features. Other examples include knowing that some tasks, or the goals for the task, are more or less difficult, like trying to remember the gist of a story versus remembering the story verbatim (Flavell, 1979).

Knowledge of strategy variables includes all the knowledge individuals can acquire about various procedures and strategies for cognition including memorizing, thinking, reasoning, problem solving, planning, studying, reading, writing, and so on. This is the area that has seen the most research and is probably the most familiar category of metacognitive knowledge. Knowledge that rehearsal strategies can help in recalling a telephone number, or that organizational and elaboration strategies can help in the memory and comprehension of text information, are examples of strategy knowledge.

Metacognitive knowledge has been further divided into declarative, procedural, and conditional metacognitive knowledge (Alexander et al., 1991; Paris et al., 1983; Schraw & Moshman, 1995). Declarative knowledge of cognition can be considered knowledge of the *what* of cognition, as it includes knowledge of different cognitive strategies that can be used for learning. For example, knowing about strategies such as rehearsal or elaboration would constitute declarative knowledge. Procedural knowledge includes knowing *how* to perform and use the various cognitive strategies. It may not be enough to only know that there are elaboration strategies, like summarizing and paraphrasing, but that it is important to know how to effectively use these strategies. Finally, conditional knowledge includes knowing *when* and *why* to use the various cognitive strategies. For example, elaboration strategies may be appropriate in some contexts for some types of tasks (learning from text); other strategies such as rehearsal may be more appropriate for different tasks or different goals (trying to remember a telephone number). This type of conditional knowledge is important for the flexible and adaptive use of various cognitive strategies.

2. COGNITIVE MONITORING

Cognitive monitoring involves the awareness and monitoring of various aspects of cognition and is an important component of what is classically labeled metacognition (Brown et al., 1983; Flavell, 1979; Koriat & Goldsmith, 1996; Pintrich et al., 2000; Schneider & Pressley, 1997). In contrast to metacognitive knowledge, which is more static and "statable" (individuals can tell if they know it or not), metacognitive judgments and monitoring are more dynamic and process-oriented and reflect metacognitive awareness and ongoing metacognitive activities individuals may engage in as they perform a task.

One type of metacognitive judgment or monitoring activity involves judgments of learning (JOLs) and comprehension monitoring (Nelson & Narens, 1990; Pintrich et al., 2000). These judgments may manifest themselves in a number of activities such as individuals becoming aware that they do not understand something they just read or heard or becoming aware that they are reading too quickly or slowly given the text and their goals. The JOLs also would be made as students actively monitor their reading comprehension by asking themselves questions. They also could be made when students try to decide if they are ready to take a test on the material they have just read and studied or in a memory experiment as they try to judge whether they have learned the target words (Nelson & Narens, 1990). Pressley and Afflerbach (1995) provide a detailed listing of monitoring activities that individuals can engage in while reading. In the classroom context, besides reading comprehension or memory judgments, JOLs could involve students making judgments of their comprehension of a lecture as the instructor is delivering it or whether they could recall the lecture information for a test at a later point in time.

Another type of metacognitive awareness process is termed the feeling-of-knowing (FOK) (Koriat, 1993; Nelson & Narens, 1990). A typical instance of FOK occurs when a person cannot recall something when called upon to do so, but they know they know it, or at least they have a strong feeling that they know it. In colloquial terms, this experience is often called the tip-of-the tongue phenomenon and occurs as a person is attempting to recall something. In the Nelson and Narens (1990) framework, FOKs are made after failure to recall an item and involve a determination of whether the currently unrecallable item will be recognized or recalled by the individual at a later point in time. Koriat (1993) points out that there is evidence that FOK judgments are better than chance predictors of future recall performance, albeit not a perfect correlate. In a reading comprehension task, FOKs would involve the awareness of reading something in the past and having some understanding of it, but not being able to recall it on demand. The FOKs in the classroom context could involve having some recall of the teacher lecturing on the material or the class discussing it, but not being able to recall it on the exam.

3. COGNITIVE CONTROL AND REGULATION

Cognitive control and regulation includes the types of cognitive and metacognitive activities that individuals engage in to adapt and change their cognition. In most models of metacognition and self-regulated learning, control and regulation activities are assumed to be dependent on, or at least strongly related to, metacognitive monitoring activities, although metacognitive control and monitoring are conceived as separate processes (Butler & Winne, 1995; Nelson & Narens, 1990; Pintrich et al., 2000; Zimmerman, 1989, 1994). As in any model of regulation, it is assumed that attempts to control, regulate, and change cognition should be related to cognitive monitoring activities that provide information about the relative discrepancy between a goal and current progress towards that goal. For example, if a student is reading a textbook with the goal of understanding (not just finishing the reading assignment), then as the student monitors his or her comprehension, this monitoring process can provide the student with information about the need to change reading strategies.

One of the central aspects of the control and regulation of cognition is the actual selection and use of various cognitive strategies for memory, learning, reasoning, problem-solving, and thinking. Numerous studies have shown that the selection of appropriate cognitive strategies can have a positive influence on learning and performance. These cognitive strategies range from the simple memory strategies very young children through adults use to help them remember (Schneider & Pressley, 1997) to sophisticated strategies that individuals have for reading (Pressley & Afflerbach, 1995), mathematics (Schoenfeld, 1992), writing (Bereiter & Scardamalia, 1987), problem-solving, and reasoning (Baron, 1994; Nisbett, 1993). Although the use of various strategies is probably deemed more "cognitive" than metacognitive, the decision to use them is an aspect of metacognitive control and regulation as is the decision to stop using them or to switch from one strategy type to another.

In research on self-regulated learning, the various cognitive and learning strategies that individuals use to help them understand and learn the material would be placed in this cell. For example, many researchers have investigated the various rehearsal, elaboration, and organizational strategies that learners can use to control their cognition and learning (refer to Pintrich & De Groot, 1990; Pintrich et al., 1993; Pressley & Afflerbach, 1995; Schneider & Pressley, 1997; Weinstein & Mayer, 1986; Zimmerman & Martinez-Pons, 1986). These strategies include the use of imagery to help encode the information on a memory task as well as imagery to help one visualize correct implementation of a strategy (e.g., visualization in sports activities as well as academic ones; refer to, Zimmerman, 1998a). The use of mnemonics would also be included in this cell as well as various strategies like paraphrasing, summarizing, outlining, networking, constructing tree diagrams, and notetaking (see Weinstein & Mayer, 1986).

4. COGNITIVE REACTION AND REFLECTION

The processes of reaction and reflection involve learners' judgments and evaluations of their performance on the task as well as their attributions for performance. As Zimmerman (1998b) has pointed out, good self-regulators do evaluate their performance in comparison to learners who avoid self-evaluations or are not aware of the importance of self-evaluation in terms of the goals set for the task. In addition, it appears that good self-regulators are more likely to make adaptive attributions for their performance (Zimmerman, 1998b). Adaptive attributions are generally seen as making attributions to low effort or poor strategy use, not lack of general ability (e.g., "I did poorly because I'm stupid or dumb.") in the face of failure (Weiner, 1986; Zimmerman & Kitsantas, 1997). These adaptive attributions have been linked to deeper cognitive processing and better learning and achievement (Pintrich & Schrauben, 1992) as well as a host of adaptive motivational beliefs and behaviors such as positive affect, positive efficacy and expectancy judgments, persistence, and effort (Weiner, 1986).

5. APPLICATION TO INDIVIDUALS WITH LEARNING PROBLEMS

The discussion of the applicability of this model to students with learning problems such as the developmentally disabled or learning disabled (LD) population, should be prefaced with the acknowledgment that there is significant variability in the metacognitive processing strengths and weaknesses among these students (Bebko & Luhaorg, 1998; Borkowski, Johnston, & Reid, 1987; Butler, 1998; Torgesen, 1980) as well as variability in their cognitive and information processing capacities (Goldstein & Dundon, 1987). For example, Goldstein and Dundon (1987) identify four possible "factors" that may impair academic performance in LD children. These factors include strategic deficits (children do not know the strategies, they lack metacognitive knowledge), metacognitive deficits (children are unaware of the need to use strategies and have difficulty in planning, monitoring, and controlling their cognition), structurally reduced cognitive capacity (e.g., minimal brain dysfunction), and functionally reduced cognitive capacity (children experience a temporary reduction in available cognitive capacity due to mediating affective factors). Any number or combination of these factors may affect LD students. This variability decreases the likelihood that any one specific cognitive or metacognitive strategy or any one recommended instructional approach will be beneficial for all LD students.

Despite this variability, some generalizations about the metacognitive weaknesses of these students can be made. It is widely accepted that most LD children experience difficulty in the selection, monitoring, and revision of strategies, especially when completing novel tasks (Borkowski et al., 1987; Paris & Myers, 1981). The LD students are also often characterized as "inactive learners" who employ primarily weak, general, and largely inefficient task strategies, if any, rather than strategies that are fine-tuned to the task demands (Hallahan & Kauffman, 1982; Swanson, 1990; Torgesen, 1980; Wong, 1985). As compared to their normally achieving peers, LD students are more likely to set inappropriate criteria for monitoring progress (Butler, 1998), are more likely to have difficulty with executive control processing and coordinating strategies (Swanson, 1990), and tend to be less thorough and exhaustive in their search for and use of appropriate strategies (Wong, 1982). They are also less likely to be aware of the value of using an effortful, strategic approach to academic tasks (Borkowski et al., 1987) and are less likely to generalize or transfer strategy instruction to different content areas or novel tasks (Gelzheiser, 1984; Hagan et al., 1982).

Bebko and Luhaorg (1998) make many of the same points about mentally retarded or developmentally disabled children in terms of their strategic and metacognitive difficulties. They note that mentally retarded children may have difficulties in acquiring different strategies. In particular, these individuals tend to encode strategies in a relatively unanalyzed form that is not personalized to his or her needs. These problems in controlled acquisition processes leads to less generalization of strategies and a limited repertoire of strategies to use for different tasks (Bebko & Luhaorg, 1998). Research also suggests that, in terms of information processing, people with mental disabilities are generally slower to automatize performance (Merrill et al., 1996), and as a consequence, these individuals may have less cognitive resources to allocate towards metacognition (planning, monitoring, etc.). However, once processes are automatized, individuals with mental disabilities may face another obstacle in that they may encounter difficulty when attempting to override these processes. This is particularly problematic in terms of academic performance if the automatized process is a frequently used but inappropriate learning strategy (Ellis et al., 1989; Short & Evans, 1990). In addition to these difficulties, individuals whose disabilities involve failure of inhibitory mechanisms (e.g., individuals with Attention Deficit Hyperactivity Disorder) may not be able to inhibit competing goals, which may lead these individuals to become distracted (van Haneghan & Turner, 2001) and generally impair their ability to self-regulate their cognition (Barkely, 1997).

Given the description above, it becomes quite obvious that many LD and mentally retarded students fall into the category of "poor self-regulators" and thus stand to benefit from interventions designed to improve their ability to plan, monitor, and control their cognitive processes. Research in the field of self-regulation and metacognition generally confirms this position. Strategic interventions in the domain of metacognition have been found to have moderate effect sizes (see Swanson, 2000, for a meta-analysis) and frequently raise the performance of LD students to the level attained by normally achieving peers (see Pressley & Levin, 1987, for review; Johnson et al., 1997; McGivern & Levin, 1983; Torgesen, 1980). The utilization of self-monitoring strategies has also been shown to improve mentally retarded students attention to tasks, task completion, and task accuracy (see Hughes et al., 1991, for review).

While training in self-regulation may decrease performance differences among LD or mentally retarded students and their normally achieving peers, it would be misleading to state that such interventions are likely to eliminate the discrepancy. Wong (1986) notes that poor performance among LD students is unlikely to be solely caused by a lack of appropriate metacognitive strategies and that metacognition cannot account for the cognitive deficiencies such as decoding problems, which are widespread among LD students. Furthermore, "because of the interdependence between knowledge and strategy, we cannot afford to overlook (the importance of) increasing the students' content knowledge in the domain upon which the inculcated metacognitive strategy is to be applied" (Wong, 1986, p. 23). In addition, Borkowski et al. (1987) warn that while some LD students profit considerably from training, generalization of strategies and skills is not readily achieved by most LD students. As mentioned earlier, due to individual differences among LD students, it is unlikely that a single approach or intervention will be maximally effective for all students within this diagnostic category (Butler, 1998).

These caveats are reflected in recent interventions that frequently combine remediation of domain knowledge with strategy instruction that is individually tailored to the processing strengths and weaknesses of the student (Bos & Anders, 1990; Butler, 1995; Graham & Harris, 1993). The Swanson et al. (1996) synthesis of intervention research (Swanson, 2000) indicates that this combined approach of direct content instruction and strategy instruction is, indeed, an effective procedure for remediating LD students when compared to other instructional models. They found that the effect sizes for cognitive processes (e.g., attribution and metacognition) were higher when coupled with academic domains than when isolated for intervention (Swanson et al., 1996).

B. Regulation of Motivation and Affect

In the same manner that learners can regulate their cognition, they can regulate their motivation and affect. However, there is not as much research on how students can regulate their motivation and affect as there has been on regulation of cognition, given all the research on metacognition and academic learning by cognitive and educational psychologists. The area of motivational regulation has been discussed more by personality, motivational, and social psychologists (e.g., Kuhl, 1984, 1985), not educational psychologists (see Boekaerts, 1993; Corno, 1989, 1993; Garcia et al., 1998, for exceptions), but this trend is changing as research on learning and self-regulation recognizes the importance of motivation in general and attempts to regulate motivation in the classroom (Wolters, 1998).

Regulation of motivation and affect would include attempts to regulate various motivational beliefs that have been discussed in the achievement motivation literature (see Pintrich & Schunk, 1996; Wolters, 1998) such as goal orientation (purposes for doing task) and self-efficacy (judgments of competence to perform a task) as well as task value beliefs (beliefs about the importance, utility, and relevance of the task) and personal interest in the task (liking of content area, domain). Kuhl (1984, 1985) as well as Corno (1989, 1993) discuss, under the label of volitional control, various strategies that individuals might use to control their motivation. They also include in their more global construct of volitional control, strategies for emotion control, as does Boekaerts (1993), that include coping strategies for adapting to negative affect and emotions such as anxiety and fear.

Accordingly, some of the volitional control strategies discussed by these researchers are included in the motivation/affect column in Table I. However, rather than introduce another term, volition or volitional control, it seems more parsimonious to just discuss regulation of motivation and affect, paralleling the discussion of the regulation of cognition. In the same manner, there is literature on metacognition which is fairly well-established on the awareness of and control of cognition, but there is little on "metamotivation" (but see Boekaerts, 1995), which would include students' awareness of and attempts to control their motivation. Again, in the interests of parsimony, the term metamotivation will not be used, but the model does include motivational self-awareness and control. Finally, although goal orientation is listed in Table I in the cell for activation of motivation, it will not be discussed in the current section, as it is the central focus of the second half of this chapter.

1. MOTIVATIONAL PLANNING AND ACTIVATION

In terms of the phases in Table I, planning and activation of motivation would involve judgments of efficacy as well as the activation of various motivational beliefs about value and interest. In terms of self-efficacy judgments, Bandura (1997) and Schunk (1989, 1991, 1994) have shown that individuals' judgments of their capabilities to perform a task have consequences for affect, effort, persistence, performance, and learning. Of course, once a learner begins a task, self-efficacy judgments can be adjusted based on actual performance and feedback as well as individual attempts to actively regulate or change one's efficacy judgments (Bandura, 1997).

In the cognitive research on memory, individuals can make determinations of the difficulty level of the task, such as how hard it will be to remember or learn the material, or in the Nelson and Narens (1990) framework what they call ease of learning judgments (EOL). These EOL judgments draw on both metacognitive knowledge of the task and metacognitive knowledge of the self in terms of past performance of the task. In the classroom context, students could make these EOL judgments as the teacher introduces a lesson or assigns a worksheet, project, or paper. These EOL judgments are similar to self-efficacy judgments although the emphasis is on the task, rather than on the self. In this sense, EOL judgments and self-efficacy judgments reflect the task difficulty perceptions and self-competence perceptions from expectancy-value models (e.g., Eccles, 1983).

Along with judgments of competence, learners also have perceptions of the value and interest the task or content area has for them. In expectancy-value models (Eccles, 1983; Wigfield, 1994; Wigfield & Eccles, 1992), task value beliefs include perceptions of the relevance, utility, and importance of the task. If students believe that the task is relevant or important for their future goals or generally useful for them (e.g., "Chemistry is important because I want to be a doctor"; "Math is useful because I need it to be a good consumer"), then they are more likely to be engaged in the task as well as choose to engage in the task in the future (Wigfield, 1994; Wigfield & Eccles, 1992). In terms of a model of self-regulated learning, it seems likely that these beliefs can be activated early on, either consciously or automatically and unconsciously, as the student approaches or is introduced to the task by teachers or others. In addition, in the current model of self-regulated learning, it is assumed that students can attempt to regulate or control these value beliefs (e.g., Wolters, 1998).

Beside value beliefs, learners also have perceptions of their personal interest in the task or in the content domain of the task (e.g., liking and positive affect towards math, history, science, etc.). The research on personal interest suggests that personal interest is a stable, enduring characteristic of an individual, but that the level of interest can be activated and vary according to situational and contextual features, which is labeled the psychological state of interest (Krapp et al., 1992; Schiefele, 1991). In addition, this research has shown that interest is related to increased learning, persistence, and effort. Although the research on interest has been pursued from both an expectancy-value framework (Wigfield, 1994; Wigfield & Eccles, 1992) as well as from intrinsic motivation or needs-based models (see Deci & Ryan, 1985; Renninger et al., 1992), it seems clear that interest can be activated by task and contextual features and that learners also can try to control and regulate it (Sansone et al., 1992; Wolters, 1998).

Finally, just as interest can be a positive anticipatory affect, learners also can anticipate other more negative affects such as anxiety or fear. In the academic learning domain, test anxiety would be the most common form of anxiety and the most researched in terms of its links with learning, performance, and achievement (Hembree, 1988; Hill & Wigfield, 1984; Wigfield & Eccles, 1989; Zeidner, 1998). Students who anticipate being anxious on tests and worry about performing poorly even before they begin the test can set in motion a downward spiral of maladaptive cognitions, emotions, and behaviors that lead them to do poorly on the exam (Bandura, 1997; Zeidner, 1998). In this way, these anticipatory affects such as anxiety or fear can influence the subsequent learning process and certainly establish conditions that require active and adaptive self-regulation of cognition, motivation, and behavior.

2. MOTIVATIONAL MONITORING

There is not as much research on how individuals become aware of their motivation and affect as there has been on metacognitive awareness and monitoring, but it is implied in the research on individuals attempts to control and regulate their motivation and affect. That is, as in the cognitive research, it can be assumed that in order for individuals to try to control their efficacy, value, interest, or anxiety, they would have to be aware of these beliefs and affects and monitor them at some level. In fact, paralleling the cognitive strategy intervention research (Pressley & Woloshyn, 1995), research on interventions to improve motivation often focuses on helping students become aware of their own motivation and adapting it to the task and contextual demands. For example, in the research on self-efficacy, the focus is on having individuals become aware of their own efficacy levels and self-doubts and then change their efficacy judgments to make them more realistic and adaptive (Bandura, 1997). Research on attributional retraining attempts to help individuals become aware of their maladaptive attributional patterns and then change them (Foersterling, 1985; Peterson et al., 1993). In the test anxiety research, besides attempts to change the environmental conditions that increase anxiety, there are a host of suggested coping strategies that individuals can adopt that include monitoring both the emotionality (negative affect) and cognitive (negative self-thoughts and doubts) components of anxiety (Hill & Wigfield, 1984; Tryon, 1980; Zeidner, 1998). In all of these cases, the monitoring of motivation and affect is an important prelude to attempts to control and regulate motivation and affect.

3. MOTIVATIONAL CONTROL AND REGULATION

There are many different strategies that individuals can use to control motivation and affect however, not as many perhaps as have been discussed by cognitive researchers investigating strategies to control cognition, but still there are a fair number of different motivation and emotion control strategies. Kuhl (1984, 1985), Corno (1989, 1993), Boekaerts (1993), and Boekaerts and Niemivirta (2000) have all discussed various strategies for motivation and emotion control.

These strategies include attempts to control self-efficacy through the use of positive self-talk (e.g., "I know I can do this task;" see Bandura, 1997). Students also can attempt to increase their extrinsic motivation for the task by promising themselves extrinsic rewards or making certain positive activities (taking a nap, watching television, talking with friends, etc.) contingent on completing an academic task (Wolters, 1998) (called self-consequenting in Zimmerman and Martinez-Pons, 1986; and incentive escalation in Kuhl, 1984). Wolters (1998) also found that college students would intentionally try to evoke extrinsic goals such as getting good grades to help them maintain their motivation. Students also can try to increase their intrinsic motivation for a task by trying to make it more interesting (e.g., "make it into a game," Sansone et al., 1992; Wolters, 1998) or to maintain a more mastery-oriented focus on learning (Wolters, 1998). Finally, Wolters (1998) also found that students would try to increase the task value of an academic task by attempting to make it more relevant or useful to them or their careers, experiences, or lives. In all of these cases, students are attempting to change or control their motivation in order to complete a task that might be boring or difficult.

In other cases, students may use a self-affirmation strategy whereby they decrease the value of a task in order to protect their self-worth, especially if they have done poorly on the task (Garcia & Pintrich, 1994). For example students who fail on an academic task might try to affirm their self-worth by saying it does not matter to them and that school is not that important compared to other aspects of their lives that they value more. Steele (1988, 1997) has suggested that self-affirmation and disidentification with school (devaluing of school in comparison to other domains) might help explain the discrepancy between African-American students' achievement and their self-esteem.

In addition, there are strategies students can use to try to control their emotions that might differ from those that they use to control their efficacy or value (Boekaerts, 1993; Boekaerts & Niemivirta, 2000; Corno, 1989, 1993; Kuhl, 1984, 1985; Wolters, 1998). Self-talk strategies to control negative affect and anxiety (e.g., "don't worry about grades now," "don't think about that last question, move on to the next question") have been noted by anxiety researchers (Hill & Wigfield, 1984; Zeidner, 1998). Students also may invoke negative affects, such as shame or guilt, to motivate them to persist at a task (Corno, 1989; Wolters, 1998). Defensive pessimism is another motivational strategy that students can use to actually harness negative affect and anxiety about doing poorly in order to motivate them to increase their effort and perform better (Garcia & Pintrich, 1994; Norem & Cantor, 1986). Self-handicapping, in contrast to defensive pessimism, involves the decrease of effort (little or no studying) or procrastination (only cramming for an exam, writing a paper at very end of deadline) in order to protect self-worth by attributing the likely poor outcome to low effort, not low ability (Baumeister & Scher, 1988; Berglas, 1985; Garcia & Pintrich, 1994; Midgley et al., 1996).

4. MOTIVATIONAL REACTION AND REFLECTION

After the students have completed a task, they may have emotional reactions to the outcome (e.g., happiness at success, sadness at failure) as well as reflect on the reasons for the outcome, that is, to make attributions for the outcome (Weiner, 1986). Following the attribution theory, the types of attributions that students make for their success and failure can lead to the experience of more complicated emotions like pride, anger, shame, and guilt (Weiner, 1986, 1995). As students reflect on the reasons for their performance, both the quality of the attributions and the quality of the emotions experienced are important outcomes of the self-regulation process. Individuals can actively control the types of attributions they make in order to protect their self-worth and motivation for future tasks. Many of the common attributional biases identified by social psychologists (Fiske & Taylor, 1991) may be used rather automatically (e.g., the fundamental attribution error, the actor-observer bias), but they could also be more intentional strategies used to protect self-worth (e.g., the self-serving or hedonic bias, the self-centered bias; see Fiske & Taylor, 1991; Pintrich & Schunk, 1996).

In fact, much of the attributional retraining literature is focused on helping individuals change their attributions or attributional style in order to have more adaptive cognitive, motivational, affective, and behavioral reactions to life events (Foersterling, 1985; Peterson et al., 1993). Finally, these reflections and reactions can lead to changes in the future levels of self-efficacy, expectancy for future success, as well as value and interest (Pintrich & Schunk, 1996; Weiner, 1986, 1995). In this manner, these potential changes in efficacy, value, and interest from phase four flow back into phase one and become the "entry" level motivational beliefs that students bring with them to new tasks.

5. APPLICATIONS TO STUDENTS WITH LEARNING PROBLEMS

Similar to the area of cognitive regulation, there is some variability in the motivational beliefs and attributions of students with learning disabilities and other learning problems. As before, it is important to note that LD or mentally retarded children are not the only ones who may at times lack motivation, experience negative affect, or make maladaptive attributions for their successes or failures. Even high achieving students, for example, experience negative affect, such as test anxiety, in certain circumstances. Unfortunately, motivational problems are believed to be somewhat more pervasive among students with learning disabilities and mental retardation than among "non-disabled" students (Butkowski & Willows, 1980; Licht, 1983; Torgesen & Licht, 1983). As such, the self-regulation of maladaptive motivational beliefs may be an important component in interventions designed to improve the performance of these individuals.

Research indicates, for example, that students with learning disabilities or with mild-to-moderate mental retardation are more likely than other students to causally attribute poor performance to insufficient ability and are less likely to view success as a result of their ability (Butkowski & Willows, 1980; Koestner et al., 1995; Turner, 1996; see Weisz, 1999 for review). This attributional pattern is generally maladaptive and may lead to a cycle of failure and the formation of a learned helpless belief system (Licht, 1983). An additional problem related to attributions is that children with mental retardation tend to hold more external locus of control orientations than their same-age peers without disabilities or LD peers (Wehmeyer, 1992; Wehmeyer & Palmer, 1997). Specifically, their perceptions of causality are unrealistic in that they reflect an over-reliance on luck, fate, chance, or powerful others (Wehmeyer, 2001).

The formation of a learned helpless belief system can be influenced by the behavior, expectations, and affect of teachers, parents, and caregivers. For example, particular patterns of teacher affect and response to LD or mentally retarded students' failures (e.g., pity coupled with little punishment) can send messages that may be interpreted as low-ability cues which may fuel a student's learned helpless beliefs. That is, a student may feel that a teacher's expression of pity indicates that they were not really expected to do well; if they were, the teacher would have likely responded with disappointment and anger for failure to perform up to one's potential (Clark, 1997; Weisz, 1999). Accordingly, interventions that focus on self-regulation of attributions and/or attributional retraining may need to be coupled with interventions at the contextual level.

It is important to note that there is some inconsistency in the research as to whether or not a "learned helplessness profile" best describes the attributional pattern of LD students. Friedman and Medway (1987) found that students with learning disabilities did not consistently display learned helpless behaviors. In addition, they found that the LD students did not show lower performance expectancies or show greater expectancy shifts following failure than those without learning disabilities. Pintrich et al. (1994) also found that

LD students do not necessarily fit a "helpless" profile. Instead of attributing failure to internal causes such as lack of ability (as would be predicted by a learned helplessness theory), the LD students in this study tended to attribute their failures to external causes.

Pintrich et al. (1994) also noted that the LD students did not differ from normally achieving students in terms of intrinsic orientation. These findings are in contrast to some research that suggests that students with learning disabilities and mental retardation tend to be more extrinsically motivated (Ellis, 1986; Haywood & Switzky, 1986; Wilson & David, 1994). The extent to which students are intrinsically or extrinsically motivated may have important implications in terms of their self-regulation. For example, Switzky (2001) argues that self-regulation might be difficult to produce in students who are predominately extrinsically motivated. He suggests that these individuals are primarily under the control of a strongly developed external reinforcement system and needs external direction in order to perform, which makes them less likely to engage in internally generated self-regulated activities (Switzky, 2001).

C. Regulation of Behavior

Regulation of behavior is an aspect of self-regulation that involves individuals' attempts to control their own overt behavior. Some models of regulation would not include this as an aspect of "self" regulation since it does not explicitly involve attempts to control and regulate the personal self and would just label it behavioral control. In contrast, the framework in Table I follows the triadic model of social cognition (Bandura, 1986; Zimmerman, 1989), where behavior is an aspect of the person, albeit not the internal "self" that is represented by cognition, motivation, and affect. Nevertheless, individuals can observe their own behavior, monitor it, and attempt to control and regulate it, and as such, these activities can be considered self-regulatory for the individual.

At the same time, as signaled by the brackets for the cell that represents the intersection of the row for phase 1 forethought, planning, and activation and the column for behavior, this cell for time and effort planning really represents "cognitions." In this sense, it could be placed in the cell that reflects the intersection of forethought and cognition. That is, there may not really be any "behavioral" planning that is not also "cognitive." However, there are models of intentions and intentional planning (e.g., Gollwitzer, 1996) that do conceptualize behavioral intentions as an aspect of volitional and regulatory control. Accordingly, in terms of the structure of the taxonomy in Table I, it seems reasonable to place students' attempts to intentionally plan their behavior in this cell and to discuss them as part of the column for behavioral regulation.

1. BEHAVIORAL FORETHOUGHT, PLANNING, AND ACTIVATION

Models of intentions, intentional planning, and planned behavior (e.g., Ajzen, 1988, 1991; Gollwitzer, 1996) have shown that the formation of intentions are linked to subsequent behavior in a number of different domains. In the academic learning domain, time and effort planning or management would be the kinds of activities that could be placed in this cell in Table I. Time management involves the making of schedules for studying and allocating time for different activities, which is a classic aspect of most learning and study skills courses (see Hofer et al., 1998; McKeachie et al., 1985; Pintrich et al., 1987; Simpson et al., 1997). Zimmerman and Martinez-Pons (1986) have shown that self-regulating learners and high achievers do engage in time management activities. In addition, Zimmerman (1998a) has discussed how expert writers, musicians, and athletes not just students, engage in time management activities. As part of time management, students also may make decisions and form intentions about how they will allocate their effort and the intensity of their work. For example, students might plan to study regularly one or two hours a night during the semester, but during mid-terms or finals intend to increase their effort and time spent studying.

Zimmerman (1998a, 2000) also has discussed how individuals can observe their own behavior through various methods and then use this information to control and regulate their behavior. For example, writers can record how many pages of text they produce in a day and record this information over weeks, months, and years (Zimmerman, 1998b). In order to enact these self-observational methods, some planning must be involved in order to organize the behavioral record-keeping. Many learning strategy programs also suggest some form of behavioral observation and record-keeping in terms of studying in order to provide useful information for future attempts to change learning and study habits. Again, the implementation of these self-observational methods requires some planning and the intention to actually implement them during learning activities.

2. BEHAVIORAL MONITORING AND AWARENESS

In phase 2, students can monitor their time-management and effort levels and attempt to adjust their effort to fit the task. For example, in phase 1, students may plan to spend only two hours reading two textbook chapters for the course, but once they begin reading, they realize that it is more difficult than they foresaw and that it will take either more time or more concentrated effort to understand the chapter. They could also realize that although they set aside two hours for reading the chapters in the library, they spent one hour of that time talking with friends who were studying with them. Of course, this type of monitoring should lead to an attempt to control or regulate their effort (e.g., set aside more time, do not study with friends, the next cell in Table I). This type of monitoring behavior is often assisted by formal procedures for self-observation (e.g., keeping logs of study time, diaries of activities, record-keeping, etc.) or self-experimentation (Zimmerman, 1998a, 2000). All of these activities will help students become aware of and monitor their own behavior, which provides information that can be used to actually control or regulate behavior.

3. BEHAVIORAL CONTROL AND REGULATION

Strategies for actual behavioral control and regulation address issues of behavioral control of physical health, mental health, work behaviors, and social relations with others, as well as behavioral control of activities for academic learning. As noted in the previous section, students may regulate the time and effort they spend studying two textbook chapters based on their monitoring of their behavior and the difficulty of the task. If the task is harder than they originally thought, they may increase their effort, depending on their goals, or they may decrease effort if the task is perceived as too difficult. Another aspect of behavioral control includes general persistence, which is also a classic measure used in achievement motivation studies as an indicator of motivation. Students may exhort themselves to persist through self-talk ("keep trying, you'll get it") or they may give up if the task is too difficult, again depending on their goals and monitoring activities.

The motivational strategies mentioned earlier, such as defensive pessimism and self-handicapping, included attempts to control anxiety and self-worth but also had direct implications for an increase in effort (defensive pessimism) or decrease in effort (self-handicapping). As such, these strategies are also relevant to behavioral control efforts. One aspect of self-handicapping is procrastination, which is certainly behavioral in nature in terms of delaying studying for an exam or writing a paper until the last minute. Of course, since effort and persistence are two of the most common indicators of motivation, most of the motivational strategies mentioned in the earlier section will have direct implications for the behaviors of effort and persistence.

Another behavioral strategy that can be very helpful for learning is help-seeking. It appears that good students and good self-regulators know when, why, and from whom to seek help (Karabenick & Sharma, 1994;

Nelson Le-Gall, 1981, 1985; Newman, 1991, 1994, 1998a,b, 2000; Ryan & Pintrich, 1997). Help-seeking is listed here as a behavioral strategy because it involves the person's own behavior as well as contextual control since it necessarily involves the procurement of help from others in the environment and as such is also a social interaction (Ryan & Pintrich, 1997). Help-seeking can be a dependent strategy for students who are seeking the correct answer without much work or who wish to complete the task quickly without much understanding or learning. In terms of this goal of learning and understanding, dependent help-seeking would be a generally maladaptive strategy, in contrast to adaptive help-seeking where the individual is focused on learning and is only seeking help in order to overcome a particularly difficult aspect of the task.

4. BEHAVIORAL REACTION AND REFLECTION

Reflection is a more cognitive process and so there may be no "behavioral" reflection, but just as with forethought, the cognitions an individual has about behavior can be classified in this cell. For example, reflections on actual behavior in terms of effort expended or time spent on a task can be important aspects of self-regulated learning. Just as students can make judgments or reflect on their cognitive processing or motivation, they can make judgments about their behaviors. They may decide that procrastinating in studying for an exam may not be the most adaptive behavior for academic achievement. In the future, they may decide to make a different choice in terms of their effort and time management. Certainly, in terms of reaction, the main behavior is choice. Students cannot only decide to change their future time and effort management efforts, but they also may make choices about what classes to pursue in the future (at least for high school and college students), or more generally, what general course of study they will follow. This kind of choice behavior results in the selection of different contexts and leads us into the last column in Table I. We discuss the applications of behavioral regulation to students with learning problems at the end of the next section on contextual regulation.

D. Regulation of Context

As noted above, Table I includes the individual's attempts to monitor, control, and regulate the context as an important aspect of self-regulated learning because the focus is on the personal self or individual that is engaged in these activities. Given that it is the active, personal self who is attempting to monitor, control, and regulate the context, it seems important to include these activities in a model of self-regulated learning.

1. CONTEXTUAL FORETHOUGHT, PLANNING, AND ACTIVATION

This cell in Table I includes individuals' perceptions of the task and context. As in the behavioral column, this cell is in brackets because these perceptions are really cognitions, not aspects of the context, but the focus of the perceptions is "outward" away from the individual's own cognition or motivation and towards the tasks and context. In a classroom context, these perceptions can be about the nature of the tasks in terms of the classroom norms for completing the task (e.g., the format to be used, the procedures to be used to do the task such as working with others is permitted or is considered cheating, etc.) as well as general knowledge about the types of tasks and classroom practices for grading in the classroom (Blumenfeld et al., 1987; Doyle, 1983).

In addition, perceptions of the classroom norms and climate are important aspects of students' knowledge activation of contextual information. For example, when students enter a classroom, they may activate knowledge about general norms or perceive certain norms (talking is not allowed, working with others is cheating, the teacher always has the correct answer, students are not allowed much autonomy or control, etc.), which can influence their approach to the classroom and their general learning. Students with learning problems may have particular difficulties in learning and understanding these norms.

2. CONTEXTUAL MONITORING

Just as students can and should monitor their cognition, motivation, and behavior, they also can and should monitor the task and contextual features of the classroom. In classrooms, just as in work and social situations, individuals are not free to do as they please, they are involved in a social system with various opportunities and constraints operating that shape and influence their behavior. If students are unaware of the opportunities and constraints that are operating, then they will be less likely to be able to function well in the classroom. Awareness and monitoring of the classroom rules, grading practices, task requirements, reward structures and general teacher behavior are all important for students to do well in the classroom. For example, students need to be aware of the different grading practices and how different tasks will be evaluated and scored for grades. If they are not aware that format can count (e.g., good penmanship in early grades) or that "original" thinking is important in a report, not just summarizing other material from books or encyclopedias, then they will be less likely to adjust their behavior to be in line with these requirements. In college classrooms, entering freshmen often have difficulty in their first courses because they are not monitoring or adjusting their perceptions of the course requirements to the levels expected by the faculty. Many college learning strategy or study skill courses attempt to help students become aware of these differences and adjust their strategy use and behavior accordingly (Hofer et al., 1998; Simpson et al., 1997).

3. CONTEXTUAL CONTROL AND REGULATION

Of course, as with cognition, motivation, and behavior, contextual monitoring processes are intimately linked to efforts to control and regulate the tasks and context. In comparison to control and regulation of cognition, motivation, and behavior, control of the tasks or context may be more difficult because they are not always under direct control of the individual learner. However, even models of general intelligence (e.g., the contextual subtheory; see Sternberg, 1985), often include attempts to shape, adapt, or control the environment as one aspect of intelligent behavior. Models of volitional control usually include a term labeled environmental control which refers to attempts to control or structure the environment in ways that will facilitate goals and task completion (Corno, 1989, 1993; Kuhl, 1984, 1985). In terms of self-regulated learning, most models include strategies to shape, control, or structure the learning environment as important strategies for self-regulation (Zimmerman, 1998a).

In the traditional classroom context, the teacher controls most of the aspects of the tasks and context and, therefore, there may be little opportunity for students to engage in contextual control and regulation. However, students often may attempt to negotiate the task requirements "downward" ("can we write 5 pages instead of 10?," "can we use our books and notes on the exam?," etc.) to make them simpler and easier for them to perform (Doyle, 1983). This kind of task negotiation has probably been experienced by all teachers from elementary through graduate school faculty and does represent one attempt by students to control and regulate the task and contextual environment even in classrooms with high levels of teacher control.

In more student-centered classrooms such as communities of learners classrooms and project-based instruction (e.g., Blumenfeld et al., 1991; Brown, 1997), students are asked to perform much more actual control and regulation of the academic tasks and classroom climate and structure. They often are asked to design their own projects and experiments, design how their groups will collect data or perform the task, develop classroom norms for discourse and thinking, and even work together with the teacher to determine how they will be evaluated on the tasks. These types of classrooms obviously offer a great deal more autonomy and responsibility to the students, and they provide multiple opportunities for contextual control and regulation. Of course, this does not mean that developmentally all students, especially those in the early elementary years, are able to regulate the academic tasks, classroom context, and themselves, but these types of classrooms do highlight the potential types of contextual regulation that is possible in the classroom context.

4. CONTEXTUAL REACTION AND REFLECTION

Finally, in terms of contextual reaction and reflection, students can make general evaluations of the task or classroom environment. These evaluations can be made on the basis of general enjoyment and comfort as well as more cognitive criteria regarding learning and achievement. In some of the more student-centered classrooms, there is time set aside for occasional reflection on what is working in the classroom and what is not working in terms of both student and teacher reactions (Brown, 1997). As with cognition and motivation, these evaluations can feed back into the phase 1 components when the student approaches a new task.

5. APPLICATIONS OF BEHAVIORAL AND CONTEXTUAL REGULATION TO STUDENTS WITH LEARNING PROBLEMS

There has not been as much research on behavioral and contextual regulation in general, so the applications to students with learning problems are more speculative. The LD students have been found to differ in a number of ways from other students in terms of their ability to self-regulate their behavior. The LD students are frequently described as lacking concentration and persistence in the face of difficulty. These difficulties are often attributed to maladaptive motivational belief systems. For example, the learned helplessness profile used to describe many LD students is associated with low effort/persistence (Butkowsky & Willows, 1980; Dweck & Wortman, 1982). However, as previously noted, learned helpless behaviors are not always evident among LD students. Further, Friedman and Medway (1987) found that LD boys actually showed greater persistence than non-LD boys. They argued that by staying with a hard task, the causes of failure rest clearly on task characteristics. In contrast, changing to an easier task and still experiencing failure would imply that the failure is more than likely due to one's own inability.

Difficulties in behavioral regulation among LD students may also be attributed in part to problems these students often have attending to relevant stimulus in the presence of irrelevant proximal stimuli (Hallahan & Bryan, 1981) or distracting internal stimuli such as anxiety, fear, or frustration (Westman, 1990). Medication is often used as an intervention to help LD students (attention deficit disorder [ADD]/ADHD students in particular) deal with these concentration problems. It is important to note, however, that interventions that encourage the self-regulation of behavior may have motivational advantages over medical interventions. Whalen

(1991) argues that the act of taking medication for behavioral control implies that the solution to a child's problems is outside of his/her volition. As mentioned earlier, attributing success to an internal locus of control (effort) rather than external locus of control (luck, or in this case, medication) is more adaptive from a motivational perspective.

Other aspects of behavioral regulation with which students with learning problems may struggle are monitoring and controlling time use when studying. According to Wong and Wong (1986), skilled readers tend to monitor and control their use of time and effort more efficiently than readers with learning disabilities. For example, skilled readers are more likely to focus their study efforts on parts of the text they have not mastered or have found to be more difficult (Wong & Wong, 1986). While interventions designed improve LD students' ability to self-monitor their attention or performance have been successful in increasing on-task behavior, there may be relatively little opportunity for LD students to put these self-regulatory strategies to use in the actual classroom. Ellis (1986) notes that resource room classroom structures, in particular, rarely allow for student input/control. Feedback is often heavily teacher-oriented ("let me check your answers ... "), and an overly helpful teacher may encourage the student to be more dependent on others for metacognitive processes such as goal setting and reinforcement ("I think you did a good job ... now I want you to ... " Ellis, 1986, p. 67).

In the context described above, opportunities for contextual regulation would likely be few and far between (e.g., negotiation of task requirements, choosing seating arrangements), therefore, a discussion of contextual regulation for individuals with mental retardation who are placed in such learning environments is probably not appropriate. However, for students with learning disabilities who are in regular education classrooms, issues highlighted in the general review of contextual regulation presented earlier should be relevant. Future research should, of course, specifically explore the applicability to this population.

II. GOAL ORIENTATION AND SELF-REGULATED LEARNING

As noted above, a key assumption of all models of regulation is that some goal, standard, criterion, or reference value exists that can serve as a gauge against which to assess the operation of the system and then guide regulatory processes. In self-regulated learning research, there have been two general classes of goals that have been discussed under various names such as target and purpose goals (e.g., Harackiewicz et al., 1998; Harackiewicz & Sansone, 1991) or task-specific goals and goal orientations (e.g., Garcia & Pintrich, 1994; Pintrich & Schunk, 1996; Wolters et al., 1996;

Zimmerman & Kitsantas, 1997). The general distinction between these two classes of goals is that target and task-specific goals represent the specific outcome the individual is attempting to accomplish. In academic learning contexts, it would be represented by goals such as "wanting to get 8 out of 10 correct on a quiz" or "trying to get an A on a mid-term exam."

In contrast, purpose goals or goal orientations reflect the more general reasons individuals perform a task and are related more to the research on achievement motivation (Elliot, 1997; Urdan, 1997). It is an individual's general orientation (or "schema" or "theory") for approaching the task, performing the task, and evaluating their performance on the task (Ames, 1992; Dweck & Leggett, 1988; Pintrich, 2000). In this case, purpose goals or goal orientations refer to *why* individuals want to get 8 out of 10 correct and *why* they want to get an A, as well as the standards or criteria (8 out of 10 correct, an A) they will use to evaluate their progress towards the goal. The inclusion of the reasons why an individual is pursuing a task allows for an integration of the achievement motivation literature into our models of self-regulated learning, since the achievement motivation literature is concerned with what, why, and how individuals are motivated to achieve in different settings (Pintrich & Schunk, 1996).

There are a number of different models of goal orientation that have been advanced by different achievement motivation researchers (refer to, Ames, 1992; Dweck & Leggett, 1988; Harackiewicz et al., 1998; Maehr & Midgley, 1991; Nicholls, 1984; Pintrich, 1989, 2000; Wolters et al., 1996). These models vary somewhat in their definition of goal orientation and the use of different labels for similar constructs. They also differ on the proposed number of goal orientations and the role of approach and avoidance forms of the different goals. Finally, they also differ on the degree to which an individual's goal orientations are more personal, based in somewhat stable individual differences, or the degree to which an individual's goal orientations are more situated or sensitive to the context and a function of the contextual features of the environment. Most of the models assume that goal orientations are a function of both individual differences and contextual factors, but the relative emphasis along this continuum does vary between the different models. Much of this research also assumes that classrooms and other contexts (e.g., business or work settings, laboratory conditions in an experiment) can be characterized in terms of their goal orientations, but for the purposes of this chapter the focus will be on individuals' personal goal orientation.

Most models propose two general goal orientations that concern the reasons or purposes individuals are pursuing when approaching and engaging in a task. These two general goal orientations go by a number of different labels and there are a number of different variations of these goals, but in this chapter we will use the labels of mastery and performance goals. Pintrich (2000) organized the different goals into a simple taxonomy of four goals. Table II displays this taxonomy. The columns in Table II reflect the general approach-avoidance distinction that has been a hallmark of achievement motivation research (Atkinson, 1957; Elliot, 1997; McClelland et al., 1953) since its inception, as well as more recent social cognitive perspectives on approaching and avoiding a task (e.g., Covington & Roberts, 1994; Harackiewicz et al., 1998; Higgins, 1997). In particular, recent social cognitive models of self-regulation, such as Higgins (1997), explicitly use this distinction of approach-avoidance (or promotion-prevention focus in his terms) to discuss different self-regulatory processes. An approach or promotion focus leads individuals to move towards positive or desired end states, to try to promote them to occur, while an avoidance or prevention focus leads individuals to move away from negative or undesired end states, to prevent them from occurring (Higgins, 1997). As such, there should be some important distinctions between approaching and avoiding certain goals with concomitant influences on self-regulated learning. For example, a promotion or approach orientation might be expected to have some generally positive relations with cognition, motivation, and behavior, while a prevention or avoidance orientation should be negatively related to these aspects of self-regulated learning.

TABLE II
Two Goal Orientations and Their Approach and Avoidance Forms

	Approach focus	Avoidance focus
Mastery orientation	–Focus on mastering task, learning, understanding	–Focus on avoiding misunderstanding, avoiding not learning or not mastering task
	–Use of standards of self-improvement, progress, deep understanding of task (learning goal, task goal, task-involved goal)	–Use of standards of not being wrong, not doing it incorrectly relative to task
Performance orientation	–Focus on being superior, besting others, being the smartest, best at task in comparison to others	–Focus on avoiding inferiority, not looking stupid or dumb in comparison to others
	–Use of normative standards such as getting best or highest grades, being top or best performer in class (performance goal, ego-involved goal, self-enhancing ego orientation, relative ability goal)	–Use of normative standards of not getting the worst grades, being lowest performer in class (performance goal, ego-involved goal, self-defeating ego orientation)

The rows in Table II reflect two general goals that students might be striving for and represent the general goals of mastery and performance that have been proposed by every one of the different models discussed here. The cells in Table II include in parentheses some of the different labels that have been proposed for the two main goal orientations in the different models. All the models agree that mastery goals (learning, task, task-involved) are represented by attempts to improve or promote competence, knowledge, skills, and learning, and that standards are self-set or self-referential with a focus on progress and understanding. In all of the models discussed, mastery goals have only been discussed and researched in terms of an approach orientation, that is, that students were trying to approach or attain this goal, not avoid it. As such, most models have only proposed the first cell in the first row in Table II, it is not clear if there is a "mastery avoidance" goal theoretically, and there has been little explicit empirical research on a mastery avoidance goal (but see Elliot & McGregor, 2001, and Zusho & Pintrich, 2000).

On the other hand, there may be occasions when students are focused on avoiding misunderstanding or avoiding not mastering the task. Some students that are more "perfectionistic" may use standards of not getting it wrong or doing it incorrectly relative to the task. These students would not be concerned about doing it wrong because of comparisons with others (a performance-avoidance goal), but rather in terms of their own high standards for themselves. Future empirical research will have to be done to determine if mastery avoidance goals exist or if adopting mastery avoidance goals leads to differential predictive relations with other motivational, cognitive, and affective outcomes (such as those outlined in Table I) in comparison to performance avoidance goals.

The second row in Table II reflects the general performance goal orientation that all of the models propose, but the approach and avoidance columns allow for the separation of the goal from trying to outperform or best others using normative standards from the goal of avoiding looking stupid, dumb, or incompetent relative to others. This distinction has been formally made in the work of Elliot, Midgley, Skaalvik and their colleagues, and all the studies have shown that there are differential relations between other motivational and cognitive outcomes and a performance approach goal and a performance avoidance goal (Harackiewicz et al., 1998; Middleton & Midgley, 1997; Midgley et al., 1998; Skaalvik, 1997; Skaalvik, Valas, & Sletta, 1994). In Dweck and Elliott (1988) model, the performance orientation included both trying to gain positive judgments of the self as well as trying to avoid negative judgments. In the Nicholls (1984) model, ego-involved or ego orientation also included both feeling successful when doing better than others and avoiding looking incompetent (Thorkildsen & Nicholls, 1998). Accordingly, most of the models did recognize the possibility that students could be seeking to gain positive judgments of the self by besting or outperforming others as well as trying to avoid looking stupid, dumb, or incompetent, although Dweck and Nicholls did not separate them conceptually as did Elliot, Midgley, and Skaalvik. In this case, within this performance row in Table II, in contrast to the mastery row in Table II, there is no doubt that both approach and avoidance goal orientations are possible, that students can adopt them, and that they can have differential relations to other motivational or cognitive outcomes.

Research on goal orientation also has revealed a number of other goals that students might adopt in classroom settings. For example, Pintrich and his colleagues (Pintrich 1989; Pintrich & De Groot, 1990; Pintrich & Garcia, 1991; Pintrich et al., 1994; Pintrich, Smith, Garcia, & McKeachie, 1993; Wolters et al., 1996) as well as others (e.g., Urdan, 1997) have discussed an extrinsic orientation to the classroom where the focus is on getting good grades, seeking approval, or avoiding punishment from teachers or other adults. This extrinsic orientation would be most similar to extrinsic motivation as discussed in the self-determination theory (Deci & Ryan, 1985). Nicholls and his colleagues have found two other goals, beyond ego- and task-involved goals, which they labeled work avoidance and academic alienation (Nicholls, 1989; Nicholls et al., 1989). Work avoidant goals concerned feeling successful when work or tasks were easy, while academic alienation goals were defined in terms of feeling successful when the students felt they could misbehave, not do their school work, and get away with it. Meece et al. (1988) also discussed work avoidant goals in terms of a desire to complete schoolwork without putting forth much effort, a goal of reducing effort. Urdan (1997), Urdan & Maehr (1995) as well as Wentzel (1991a,b) have discussed the role of social goals, where the focus is on seeking friendships or being socially responsible, and how these goals are linked to self-regulation and achievement.

Given all of these different goals and orientations which share some similar and some different features, future research needs to clarify the relations among these goals and their links to self-regulated learning. At the same time, given space considerations in this chapter, the remaining discussion will focus on the role of mastery and performance goals and their approach and avoidance forms, which seems appropriate given that most of the research has addressed these two general goals. There is clearly a role for extrinsic, work avoidant, and social goals in self-regulated learning given some of the extant research, but that discussion will not be the focus of the current chapter.

The remainder of this section of the chapter applies the goals in Table II to the various areas for regulation from Table I. The purpose is to discuss how the different types of goal orientations may be differentially related to aspects of self-regulation. If the proposed four cells of the taxonomy in Table II are to be theoretically productive and useful, they should result in differential predictions for how they are linked to motivation, cognition, and behavior.

A. Mastery Goals and Self-Regulated Learning

Given that all the different models of goal orientation have included mastery approach goals in their empirical research, there is a good deal of converging evidence on the positive influence mastery goals have on the different components of self-regulated learning. As all models of self-regulated learning have some goal construct included in them, a general goal or focus on mastery, improvement and learning should be propaedeutic for learning. That is, if individuals set their general criterion or standard for academic tasks to be learning and improving, then as they monitor their performance and attempt to control and regulate it, this standard should guide them towards the use of more self-regulatory processes. In fact, the vast majority of the empirical evidence from both experimental laboratory studies and correlational classroom studies suggest just such a stable generalization. Students that adopt or endorse a mastery approach goal orientation do engage in more self-regulated learning than those who do not adopt or endorse to a lesser extent a mastery goal (Ames, 1992; Pintrich & Schrauben, 1992; Pintrich & Schunk, 1996).

1. MASTERY GOALS AND COGNITIVE REGULATION

The studies have found that students who endorse a mastery goal are more likely to report attempts to self-monitor their cognition and to seek ways to become aware of their understanding and learning such as checking for understanding and comprehension monitoring (e.g., Ames & Archer, 1988; Dweck & Leggett, 1988; Meece et al., 1988; Meece & Holt, 1993; Middleton & Midgley, 1997; Nolen, 1988; Pintrich & De Groot, 1990; Pintrich & Garcia, 1991; Pintrich et al., 1994; Pintrich & Schrauben, 1992; Wolters et al., 1996). In addition, this research has consistently shown that students' use of various cognitive strategies is positively related to mastery goals. In particular, this research has shown that students' reported use of deeper processing strategies, such as the use of elaboration strategies (i.e., paraphrasing, summarizing) and organizational strategies (i.e., networking, outlining), is positively correlated with the endorsement of mastery goals (Ames & Archer, 1988; Bouffard et al., 1995; Graham &

Golen, 1991; Kaplan & Midgley, 1997; Meece et al., 1998; Pintrich et al., 1990; Pintrich & Garcia, 1991; Pintrich et al., 1993; Pintrich et al., 1994; Wolters et al., 1996). Switzky (1999) has found similar results for mentally retarded students who are intrinsically motivated, a construct that is similar, although not identical to mastery goals. In this work, mentally retarded students who are more interested in the work and intrinsically motivated learn better, learn more effectively, and are more cognitively engaged than extrinsically motivated students (Switzky, 1999).

Although there has been no research on mastery avoidance goals formally, it would be predicted that they would be less helpful in self-regulated learning than mastery approach goals. It could be that mastery avoidance goals would lead to less adaptive monitoring processes as the student would focus on not making mistakes, rather than on learning and progress. This might lead to the use of less deep processing strategies and perhaps more memorization of the material as the student tries to not be incorrect and relies on the text or content material to define what is correct. Mastery avoidance goals also would seem to lead to less risk-taking or less willingness to explore the material using different types of cognitive or thinking strategies. These are predictions that need to be tested in empirical research, but they do suggest that mastery approach and avoidance goals could establish different ways of approaching and engaging in an academic task in terms of cognition.

2. MASTERY GOALS AND MOTIVATIONAL REGULATION

There has been a great deal of research on how mastery goals are linked to other motivational beliefs such as efficacy, value, interest, attributions, and affect. Much of this research is not necessarily in a paradigm of research on self-regulated learning and has not explicitly conceptualized motivational beliefs as components that can be controlled and regulated. Rather, the research has been generated from a general achievement motivation paradigm and investigated how goal orientations can give rise to different patterns of motivation, attributions, interest, and affect. Nevertheless, within the framework of this chapter, this research is relevant for building theoretical linkages between goals and motivational regulation.

Again, as in the cognitive domain, summarizing the research on mastery approach goals and how they are related to other motivational constructs is fairly straightforward. Generally, the research shows that adopting a mastery goal has positive implications for self-efficacy, task value, interest, attributions, and affect. In one of the original formulations of mastery goals, Dweck and Leggett (1988) summarized mainly laboratory research that showed that students who were oriented to mastery and learning were able to maintain positive and adaptive efficacy beliefs and perceptions of competence in the face of difficult tasks. Other more correlational classroom research also has shown the same general pattern (e.g., Ames, 1992; Kaplan & Midgley, 1997; Middleton & Midgley, 1997; Pintrich & De Groot, 1990; Pintrich & Garcia, 1991; Pintrich et al., 1993; Thorkildsen & Nicholls, 1998; Wolters et al., 1996). Students who are focused on improving and learning would be more likely to interpret performance feedback in terms of the progress they have made, thereby supporting their efficacy beliefs.

Dweck and Leggett (1988) also showed that students who adopted a mastery goal were much more likely to make adaptive attributions for their performance. In fact, it was the search for factors that predicted why some individuals seemed to make adaptive attributions for failure and did not show a pattern of learned helplessness that generated some of the original goal theory research. In some of the early research, making certain kinds of attributions was seen as part of a general mastery goal orientation. Although it seems theoretically useful to separate goal orientations, which can be adopted at the start of a task, from attributions, which are reactive cognitions after task performance, the linkages between goals and attributions are strong. Most of the research repeatedly shows that students who adopt a mastery goal orientation are more likely to believe that effort will lead to success (positive effort-outcome covariation), that effort does not necessarily mean low ability (positive effort-ability covariation rather than inverse covariation), and that failure can be attributed to low effort or poor strategy selection (Ames, 1992; Dweck & Leggett, 1988; Nicholls, 1984; Pintrich & Schunk, 1996). This is an adaptive pattern of attributions for students who will often confront difficult tasks or tasks that they will fail, but with attributions to effort or strategy use, their future expectancies will not necessarily drop and their affect will remain positive, following the general findings in the attributional literature (Weiner, 1986).

In terms of the links between interest, task value, and mastery goals, the empirical research shows strong positive relations. In some cases, mastery goals have been measured in ways that are similar to personal interest or the mastery scales include items that reflect interest, but it is important for future research to separate these constructs conceptually. In general, the research shows that students who adopt a mastery approach goal report more personal interest, intrinsic interest, or enjoyment in the task (e.g., Butler, 1987; Harackiewicz et al., 1998; Meece et al., 1988) as well as higher levels of task value in terms of ratings of the utility and importance of school work (e.g., Wolters et al., 1996). Future research needs to examine the causal ordering of these constructs as it may just as well be that high levels of personal interest or task value for a domain or task may be part of the personal characteristics that give rise to mastery goals as would be suggested by interest and intrinsic motivation theories (Deci & Ryan, 1985; Renninger et al., 1992), rather than vice versa as goal theory assumes.

The research on mastery goals and the use of motivational strategies is not as voluminous as that on mastery goals and cognitive strategy use. Studies of self-handicapping (e.g., Midgley et al., 1996) show little relation of mastery goals to self-handicapping, although it is positively related to performance goals. Wolters (1998) found that college students' adoption of a mastery goal was positively related to their attempts to regulate their efficacy, interest, and value, what he labeled regulation of intrinsic motivation. He also found that mastery goals were negatively related to the use of extrinsic regulation strategies such as the use of rewards for regulating effort and motivation.

The general positive influence of mastery goals also appears in studies that have examined affective reactions. Given that mastery goals seem to be tied closely to an adaptive attributional pattern as noted above, it is not surprising, following the general principles and findings of attribution theory (Weiner, 1986), that mastery goals are linked to more positive affective reactions. Studies have found that mastery goals are associated with less anxiety and more pride and satisfaction (Ames, 1992; Dweck & Leggett, 1988; Jagacinski & Nicholls, 1984, 1987).

All of this research on mastery goals and motivation has only examined mastery approach goals, not mastery avoidance goals. Accordingly, research on the role of mastery avoidance goals is needed. However, given the general predictions of goal theory and avoidance forms of motivation (Higgins, 1997), it would be hypothesized that mastery avoidance goals would give rise to some negative motivational beliefs and affect. First, given the focus on not being wrong, it would be predicted that anxiety would be higher under a mastery avoidance goal than a mastery approach goal. In addition, interest and self-efficacy might be lower. Again, these predictions need to be tested in future empirical research, but they seem to follow the general model and may be more likely than the hypotheses offered for cognitive self-regulation in the previous section. It may be that mastery avoidance goals may not interfere greatly with cognition, but have their costs in terms of student motivation and affect. The important issue is that the separation of these goals into approach and avoidance forms allows for the clarification of these potential differential relations.

3. MASTERY GOALS AND BEHAVIORAL AND CONTEXTUAL REGULATION

There has not been as much research on goals and how individuals regulate their own behavior or attempt to shape or control their environment. There is a clear need for more research on how both mastery approach and avoidance goals are related to behavioral and contextual regulation. Studies have shown that mastery approach goals are more positively related to college students' attempts to manage their time and effort (Pintrich, 1989; Pintrich & Garcia, 1991; Pintrich et al., 1993), an important aspect of behavioral self-regulation. Research on help-seeking has consistently shown that adopting a personal mastery goal is positively associated with adaptive help-seeking (Newman, 1994, 1998a,b; Ryan & Pintrich, 1997, 1998). Students that approach a task with a mastery orientation focused on learning would not see help-seeking as reflecting negatively on their ability (e.g., showing others that they are unable). They would be more likely to see help-seeking as a strategy to help them learn (Newman, 1994, 1998a). Classroom research also shows that contexts that foster a mastery orientation in the classroom climate and structure lead to more adaptive help-seeking (Newman, 1998b, 2000; Ryan et al., in press). In contrast, mastery avoidance goals may lead to less adaptive help-seeking and more dependent help-seeking as the student is only concerned with not being incorrect, not with actual mastery.

In summary, mastery approach goals are generally related to positive outcomes including the use of more self-regulatory strategies for cognition, positive motivational beliefs and strategies, and behavior. There is a need for research on how mastery goals are linked to the activation of knowledge about cognition as well as self-knowledge and the clarification of the causal relations between goals and other motivational constructs (i.e., interest). It seems likely that these relations are reciprocal with mastery goals leading to interest and interest leading to mastery goals, but further specification of the dynamics of these reciprocal processes would be helpful for both theory and practice. For example, in terms of practice, goal theorists would concentrate on making classrooms more mastery and learning focused by changing the structural characteristics of the classrooms (feedback, opportunities for social comparison, reward structures, etc.), while interest theorists would focus on making the tasks more personally interesting to students. Of course, these intervention strategies are not mutually exclusive, but the example does highlight how practice might vary depending on the causal relations expected by the different theories. Finally, there is a need for more research on the meaning and operation of a mastery avoidance goal and if there are differential and more negative relations with self-regulation outcomes in comparison to a mastery approach goal.

B. Performance Goals and Self-Regulated Learning

The research on performance goals and self-regulated learning is not as easily summarized as the results for mastery goals. The original goal theory research generally found negative relations between performance goals and various cognitive, motivational, and behavioral outcomes (Ames, 1992; Dweck & Leggett, 1988; Pintrich & Schunk, 1996), although it did not discriminate empirically between performance approach and avoidance goals. The more recent research that has made the distinction between performance approach and avoidance goals does show some differential relations between approaching a task focusing on besting others and approaching a task focused on trying not to look stupid or incompetent. In particular, the general distinction between an approach and an avoidance orientation suggests that there could be some positive aspects of a performance approach orientation. If students are approaching a task trying to promote certain goals and strategies this might lead them to be more involved in the task than students who are trying to avoid certain goals, which could lead to more withdrawal and less engagement in the task (Harackiewicz et al., 1998; Higgins, 1997).

1. PERFORMANCE GOALS AND COGNITIVE REGULATION

Most of the research on performance goals that did *not* distinguish between approach and avoidance versions finds that performance goals are negatively related to students' use of deeper cognitive strategies (e.g. Meece et al., 1988; Nolen, 1988; however, refer to Bouffard et al., 1995). This would be expected given that performance goals that include items about besting others as well as avoiding looking incompetent would guide students away from the use of deeper strategies. Students focused on besting others may be less likely to exert the time and effort needed to use deeper processing strategies because the effort needed to use these strategies could show to others that they lack the ability, given that the inverse relation between effort-ability is usually operative under performance goals, and trying hard in terms of strategy use may signify low ability. For students who want to avoid looking incompetent, the same self-worth protection mechanism (Covington, 1992) may be operating, whereby students do not exert effort in terms of strategy use in order to have an excuse for doing poorly, which can be attributed to lack of effort or poor strategy use.

However, more recent research with measures that reflect only a performance approach or avoidance goal suggests that there may be differential relations between these two versions of performance goals. For example, Wolters et al. (1996) in a correlational study of junior high students found that, independent of the positive main effect of mastery goals, a performance approach goal focused on besting others was positively related to the use of deeper cognitive strategies and more regulatory strategy use. However, Kaplan and Midgley (1997) in a correlational study of junior high students found no relation between a performance approach goal and adaptive learning strategies, but performance approach goals were positively related to more surface processing or maladaptive learning strategies. These two studies did not include separate measures of performance avoidance goals. In contrast, Middleton and Midgley (1997) in a correlational study of junior high students found no relation between either performance approach or avoidance goals and cognitive self-regulation. Some of the differences in the results of these studies stem from the use of different measures, classroom contexts, and participants, making it difficult to synthesize the results. Clearly, there is a need for more theoretical development in this area and empirical work that goes beyond correlational self-report survey studies to clarify these relations.

Nevertheless, it may be that performance approach goals could lead to deeper strategy use and cognitive self-regulation, as suggested by Wolters et al. (1996) when students are confronted with overlearned classroom tasks which do not challenge them, interest them, or offer opportunities for much self-improvement. In this case, the focus on an external criterion of "besting others" or being the best in the class could lead them to be more involved in these boring tasks and try to use more self-regulatory cognitive strategies to accomplish this goal. On the other hand, it may be that performance approach goals are not that strongly related to cognitive self-regulation in either a positive or negative way as suggested by the results of Kaplan and Midgley (1997) and Middleton and Midgley (1997). Taken together, the conflicting results suggest that performance approach goals do not have to be negatively related to cognitive self-regulatory activities in comparison to performance avoidance goals. This conclusion suggests that there may be multiple pathways between performance approach and avoidance goals, cognitive strategy use and self-regulation, and eventual achievement. Future research should attempt to map out these multiple pathways and determine how performance approach and avoidance goals may differentially relate to cognitive self-regulation activities.

2. PERFORMANCE GOALS AND MOTIVATIONAL REGULATION

One factor that adds to the complexity of the results in discussing performance approach and avoidance goals is that in the Dweck and Leggett (1988) original model the links between performance goals and other cognitive, motivational, and achievement outcomes were assumed to be moderated by efficacy beliefs. That is, if students had high perceptions of their competence to do the task, then performance goals should not be detrimental for cognition, motivation, and achievement, and these students should show the same basic pattern as mastery oriented students. Performance goals were assumed to have negative effects only when efficacy was low. Students who believed they were unable and who were concerned with besting others or wanted to avoid looking incompetent did seem to show the maladaptive pattern of cognition, motivation, and behavior (Dweck & Leggett, 1988).

Other more correlational research that followed this work did not always explicitly test for the predicted interaction between performance goals and efficacy or did not replicate the predicted moderator effect. For example, both Kaplan and Midgley (1997) and Miller et al. (1993) did not find an interaction between performance approach goals and efficacy on cognitive outcomes such as strategy use. Harackiewicz et al. (1998), using both experimental and correlational designs, did not find moderator or mediator effects of efficacy in relation to the effects of mastery approach or performance approach goals on other outcomes such as actual performance or intrinsic motivation.

Correlational studies also have revealed a mixture of findings with regard to the linear relations between performance goals and efficacy. For example, Anderman and Midgley (1997) showed that performance approach goals were positively related to perceptions of competence for sixth graders, but unrelated to perceptions of competence for fifth graders. Wolters et al. (1996) found that performance approach goals were positively related to self-efficacy for junior high students, but Middleton and Midgley (1997) found in another sample of junior high students that performance approach goals were unrelated to efficacy, but performance avoidance goals were negatively related to efficacy. In two studies of junior high students, Skaalvik (1997) showed that performance approach goals were positively related to efficacy and performance avoidance goals were negatively related to efficacy.

It seems possible that students who are focused on performance approach goals would have higher perceptions of efficacy as long as they are relatively successful in besting others and demonstrating their high ability. Some of the conflicting findings might be due to differences in the samples and who is represented in the performance approach groups (e.g., actual high versus low achievers). In contrast, students oriented to avoiding looking incompetent or stupid would seem likely to have lower perceptions of self-efficacy. In fact, for these students, they seem to have some consistent self-doubts or concerns about their own competence, reflecting a schema that should generate low efficacy judgments. In addition, it may be that this relation may be moderated by the classroom context. In many of the studies the positive relations are found in junior high classrooms, but not in elementary classrooms. The literature suggests that junior high classrooms are more performance oriented than elementary classrooms that are generally more mastery oriented (see review by Midgley, 1993). In this case, then in junior high classrooms, there may be good reasons for efficacy to be positively related to performance approach goals, but not in elementary classrooms which are generally more mastery-oriented (Anderman & Midgley, 1997).

In terms of other motivational outcomes like interest or value, the results for performance goals are also mixed. Harackiewicz et al. (1998) have shown in both experimental and correlational studies that performance approach goals do not necessarily lead to less interest, intrinsic motivation, or task involvement, in comparison to mastery goals. In their experimental studies of college students playing pinball games or solving puzzles, a performance approach orientation did increase intrinsic motivation and task involvement, especially for students high in achievement motivation (a traditional personality measure of need for achievement) or in more competitive contexts (a situational variable). They suggest that both mastery and performance approach goals can draw students into an activity, depending on their personal characteristics and the context in which they are doing the task. At the same time, they do note that performance avoidance goals generally have negative effects on intrinsic motivation and performance (e.g., Elliot, 1997).

Some of the correlational studies generally support this view of the positive relations between performance approach goals and interest, intrinsic motivation, and task value and the negative relations between performance avoidance goals and these outcomes (e.g., Skaalvik, 1997; Wolters et al., 1996). In addition, work that has examined affective reactions shows that students who are oriented to avoiding negative judgments of their competence are clearly more anxious about tests and their performance (Middleton & Midgley, 1997; Skaalvik, 1997), in line with the original research on a general performance orientation (Ames, 1992; Dweck & Leggett, 1988). In contrast, performance approach goals are either uncorrelated with anxiety (Wolters, 1996), or show relatively low negative relations with anxiety (Middleton & Midgley, 1997; Skaalvik, 1997).

4. PERFORMANCE GOALS AND BEHAVIORAL AND CONTEXTUAL REGULATION

There has not been as much research on aspects of behavioral and contextual regulation activities as on cognition and motivation. However, the studies on self-handicapping show that students who are concerned with performance approach goals are more likely to report using self-handicapping strategies such as procrastination and low levels of effort (Midgley et al., 1996). Studies of help-seeking also suggest that students who are concerned with besting others or with not looking incompetent are less likely to seek help (Newman, 1991, 1994, 1998b; Ryan and Pintrich, 1997).

These are more public displays of behavior in the classroom in contrast to the use of cognitive strategies (which are generally covert), so it is not surprising that students who are concerned about either performance approach or avoidance issues are less likely to engage in behavior that can reflect poorly on their ability.

In summary, the results for performance approach and avoidance goals cannot be easily summarized in a simple generalization as for mastery approach goals. It does seem clear that a performance avoidance orientation is not an adaptive approach to academic tasks in the classroom, as would be predicted by both goal theory as well as the general framework proposed here. Students who are concerned about looking dumb or incompetent generally show a maladaptive pattern of cognition, motivation, affect, and behavior. However, it appears that a performance approach goal can have some positive relations with cognition and motivation, contrary to normative goal theory predictions, but in line with the general approach-avoidance framework presented here and by others (e.g., Harackiewicz et al., 1998; Higgins, 1997). Students who are somewhat more competitive and trying to best others can engage in tasks in a manner that involves some adaptive aspects of cognition (more use of strategies) and motivation (increased interest and value). At the same time, this focus on besting others can have some costs in terms of increases in anxiety and negative affect as well as decreases in the use of some adaptive strategies such as help-seeking. These results for performance approach goals may be moderated by both personal characteristics (need for achievement, efficacy level, actual achievement level, or success) as well as situational features (the competition level of the classroom or context). There is a need for more research on the various factors that might moderate and mediate the relations between performance approach goals and achievement.

III. CONCLUSIONS AND FUTURE DIRECTIONS FOR THEORY AND RESEARCH

The framework presented in this chapter and represented most explicitly in Tables I and II attempts to show how different self-regulatory processes and goal orientations can be categorized and then linked together to provide a comprehensive picture of the role of goal orientation in self-regulated learning. The review of the research suggests that self-regulated learning is a complex and multi-faceted phenomena and that the links to goal orientation are not simple. The taxonomy of goal orientations in Table II attempts to develop a framework for conceptualizing goals that allows for a more refined perspective on their role in self-regulated learning. The general proposal is that approach versions of goals can have some positive features, while avoidance versions are generally negative. Within this general principle, the exact type of goal orientation, mastery, or performance may have differential relations to adaptive or maladaptive cognition, motivation, or behavior. This framework suggests that different goal orientations are not simply "good" or "bad" or that they always have the same costs and benefits. Instead, the proposal is that by tracing the linkages between the different types of goals and different cognitive, motivational, and behavioral mediators and outcomes, we will be able to develop a more complex, sophisticated, but realistic, view of goals and self-regulated learning.

For example, the research clearly suggests that mastery approach goals are related to very adaptive patterns of cognition, motivation, and behavior. There is very little disagreement with this generalization in the literature. As the cell involving mastery avoidance goals is a new proposal, there is a clear need for research on the existence and operation of this form of a mastery goal and how it may be related to self-regulated learning. In contrast, the distinctions between performance approach and avoidance goals suggest that they can have both costs and benefits for students' self-regulated learning. It may be that adopting one kind of performance approach goal may result in some benefit for cognition and motivation, but it also may come at a cost of increased anxiety or negative affect. We need more carefully designed research that builds upon the existing analysis and attempts to determine when these different performance goals are adaptive and when they are maladaptive for self-regulated learning. The research needs to move beyond simplistic "good-bad" distinctions and investigate when these goals are adaptive, for what kinds of cognitive, motivational, or behavioral mediators and outcomes, for whom (different types of individuals, ages, genders, ethnic groups, cultures), and where and under what contextual conditions (types of tasks, classrooms, schools, other settings). This will help to clarify our theories and models, but it also will help to develop better applications and interventions to improve schooling.

The model, taxonomy, and review of research presented here have been developed to understand student motivation and learning in academic contexts. For the most part, the research has not included students with learning problems like LD or mentally retarded individuals. It is clear that there is a great deal of research needed in order to apply this general model to students with learning problems. The related research on students with learning problems that was cited in this chapter does suggest that some of the constructs of self-regulation and motivation are readily applicable to students with learning problems (e.g., strategy use, metacognition, attributions). Nevertheless, there is a need for the comprehensive testing of all facets of the model with different populations of students. The model will only have utility if it helps us understand how different groups of students learn to cope with and regulate their own cognition, motivation, and behavior in different contexts. At the same time, the model stresses the importance of integrating motivational and cognitive components of learning which should be useful in understanding the learning problems of all students. Students need not only the cognitive "skills" to perform academic tasks, but also the motivational and regulatory "will" to cope with the academic and contextual demands placed on them. This type of integrated model should be helpful in understanding student learning in classroom contexts.

REFERENCES

Ajzen, I. (1988). *Attitudes, personality, and behavior.* Chicago: Dorsey Press.
Ajzen, I. (1991). A theory of planned behavior. *Organizational Behavior and Human Decision Processes, 50,* 179–211.
Alexander, P., Schallert, D., & Hare, V. (1991). Coming to terms: How researchers in learning and literacy talk about knowledge. *Review of Educational Research, 61,* 315–343.
Ames, C. (1992). Classrooms: Goals, structures, and student motivation. *Journal of Educational Psychology, 84,* 261–271.
Ames, C., & Archer, J. (1988). Achievement goals in the classroom: Students' learning strategies and motivation processes. *Journal of Educational Psychology, 80,* 260–267.
Anderman, E., & Midgley, C. (1997). Changes in achievement goal orientations, perceived academic competence, and grades across the transition to middle-level schools. *Contemporary Educational Psychology, 22,* 269–298.
Atkinson, J. (1957). Motivational determinants of risk-taking behavior. *Psychological Review, 64,* 359–372.
Bandura, A. (1986). *Social foundations of thought and action: A social cognitive theory.* Englewood Cliffs, NJ: Prentice Hall.
Bandura, A. (1997). *Self-efficacy: The exercise of control.* New York: W.H. Freeman.
Barkely, R. (1997). Behavioral inhibition, sustained attention, and executive functions: Constructing unifying theory of ADHD. *Psychological Bulletin, 121,* 65–94.
Baron, J. (1994). *Thinking and deciding.* New York: Cambridge University Press.
Baumeister, R. F., & Scher, S. J. (1988). Self-defeating behavior patterns among normal individuals: Review and analysis of common self-destructive tendencies. *Psychological Bulletin, 104,* 3–22.
Bebko, J., & Luhaorg, H. (1998). The development of strategy use and metacognitive processing in mental retardation: Some sources of difficulty. In J. Burack, R. Hodapp, & E. Zigler (Eds.), *Handbook of mental retardation and development* (pp. 382–407). New York: Cambridge University Press.
Bereiter, C., & Scardamalia, M. (1987). *The psychology of written composition.* Hillsdale, NJ: Lawrence Erlbaum Associates.

Berglas, S. (1985). Self-handicapping and self-handicappers: A cognitive/attributional model of interpersonal self-protective behavior. In R. Hogan & W. H. Jones (Eds.), *Perspectives in personality: Theory, measurement, and interpersonal dynamics* (pp. 235–270). Greenwich, CT: JAI Press.

Blumenfeld, P., Mergendoller, J., & Swarthout, D. (1987). Task as a heuristic for understanding student learning and motivation. *Journal of Curriculum Studies, 19*, 135–148.

Blumenfeld, P., Soloway, E., Marx, R., Krajcik, J., Guzdial, M., & Palincsar, A. (1991). Motivating project-based learning: Sustaining the doing, supporting the learning. *Educational Psychologist, 26*, 369–398.

Boekaerts, M. (1993). Being concerned with well-being and with learning. *Educational Psychologist, 28*, 148–167.

Boekaerts, M. (1995). Self-regulated learning: Bridging the gap between metacognitive and metamotivation theories. *Educational Psychologist, 30*, 195–200.

Boekaerts, M., & Niemivirta, M. (2000). Self-regulated learning: Finding a balance between learning goals and ego-protective goals. In M. Boekaerts, P. R. Pintrich, & M. Zeidner (Eds.), *Handbook of self-regulation: Theory, research, and applications* (pp. 417–450). San Diego, CA: Academic Press.

Borkowski, J., Johnston, M., & Reid, M. (1987). Metacognition, motivation, and controlled performance. In S. Ceci (Ed.), *Handbook of cognitive, social and neuropsychological aspects of learning disabilities* (pp. 147–173). Hillsdale, NJ: Lawrence Erlbaum Associates Publishers.

Borkowski, J., Weyhing, R., & Carr, M. (1988). Effects of attributional retraining on strategy-based reading comprehension in learning-disabled students. *Journal of Educational Psychology, 80*, 46–53.

Bos, C., & Anders, P. (1990). Interactive teaching and learning: Instructional practices for teaching content and strategic knowledge. In M. Scruggs & B. Wong (Eds.), *Intervention research in learning disabilities* (pp. 166–185). New York: Springer-Verlag.

Bouffard, T., Boisvert, J., Vezeau, C., & Larouche, C. (1995). The impact of goal orientation on self-regulation and performance among college students. *British Journal of Educational Psychology, 65*, 317–329.

Brown, A. L. (1997). Transforming schools into communities of thinking and learning about serious matters. *American Psychologist, 52*, 399–413.

Brown, A. L., Bransford, J. D., Ferrara, R. A., & Campione, J. C. (1983). Learning, remembering, and understanding. In J. H. Flavell & E. M. Markman (Eds.), *Handbook of child psychology: Cognitive development* (Vol. 3, pp. 77–166). New York: Wiley.

Butkowsky, I., & Willows, D. (1980). Cognitive-motivational characteristics of children varying in reading ability: Evidence for learned helplessness in poor readers. *Journal of Educational Psychology, 72*, No. 3, 408–422.

Butler, D. (1995). Promoting strategic learning by postsecondary students with learning disabilities. *Journal of Learning Disabilities, 28*, No. 3, 170–190.

Butler, D. (1998). In search of the architect of learning: A commentary on scaffolding as a metaphor for instructional interactions. *Journal of Learning Disabilities, 31*, No. 4, 374–385.

Butler, R. (1987). Task-involving and ego-involving properties of evaluation: Effects of different feedback conditions on motivational perceptions, interest, and performance. *Journal of Educational Psychology, 79*, 474–482.

Butler, D. L., & Winne, P. H. (1995). Feedback and self-regulated learning: A theoretical synthesis. *Review of Educational Research, 65*, 245–281.

Chi, M., Feltovich, P., & Glaser, R. (1981). Categorization and representation of physics problems by experts and novices. *Cognitive Science, 5*, 121–152.

Clark, M. (1997). Teacher response to learning disability: A test of attributional principles. *Journal of Learning Disabilities, 30*, No. 1, 69–79.

Corno, L. (1989). Self-regulated learning: A volitional analysis. In B. J. Zimmerman & D. H. Schunk (Eds.), *Self-regulated learning and academic achievement: Theory, research and practice* (pp. 111–141). New York: Springer-Verlag.

Corno, L. (1993). The best-laid plans: Modern conceptions of volition and educational research. *Educational Researcher, 22*, 14–22.

Covington, M. V. (1992). *Making the grade: A self-worth perspective on motivation and school reform.* Cambridge: Cambridge University Press.

Covington, M. V., & Roberts, B. (1994). Self-worth and college achievement: Motivational and personality correlates. In P. R. Pintrich, D. R. Brown, & C. E. Weinstein (Eds.), *Student motivation, cognition and learning: Essays in honor of Wilbert J. McKeachie* (pp. 157–187). Hillsdale, NJ: Lawrence Erlbaum Associates.

Deci, E. L., & Ryan, R. M. (1985). *Intrinsic motivation and self-determination in human behavior.* New York: Plenum.

Doyle, W. (1983). Academic work. *Review of Educational Research, 53*, 159–199.

Dweck, C. S., & Leggett, E. L. (1988). A social-cognitive approach to motivation and personality. *Psychological Review, 95*, 256–273.

Dweck, C., & Wortman, C. (1982). Neglected parallels in cognitive, affective and coping responses. In H. W. Krohne & L. Laux (Eds.), *Achievement, stress, and anxiety* (pp. 93–125). Washington, DC: Hemisphere.

Eccles, J. S. (1983). Expectancies, values, and academic behaviors. In J. T. Spence (Ed.), *Achievement and achievement motives* (pp. 75–146). San Francisco: Freeman.

Elliot, A. J. (1997). Integrating the "classic" and "contemporary" approaches to achievement motivation: A hierarchical model of approach and avoidance achievement motivation. In M. L. Maehr & P. R. Pintrich (Eds.), *Advances in motivation and achievement* (Vol. 10, pp. 143–179). Greenwich, CT: JAI Press.

Elliot, A. J., & McGregor, H. A. (2001). A 2 × 2 achievement goal framework. *Journal of Personality of Social Psychology, 80*, 501–519.

Ellis, E. (1986). The role of motivation and pedagogy on the generalization of cognitive strategy training. *Journal of Learning Disabilities, 19*, No. 2, 66–70.

Ellis, N., Woodley-Zanthos, P., Dulaney, C., & Palmer, R. (1989). Automatic and effortful processing and cognitive inertia in persons with mental retardation. *American Journal on Mental Retardation, 93*, 412–423.

Fiske, S., & Taylor, S. (1991). *Social cognition.* New York: McGraw-Hill.

Flavell, J. H. (1979). Metacognition and cognitive monitoring: A new area of cognitive-developmental inquiry. *American Psychologist, 34*, 906–911.

Foersterling, F. (1985). Attributional retraining: A review. *Psychological Bulletin, 98*, 495–512.

Friedman, D., & Medway, F. (1987). Effects of varying performance sets and outcome on the expectations, attributions, and persistence of boys with learning disabilities. *Journal of Learning Disabilities, 20*, No. 5, 312–316.

Garcia, T., McCann, E., Turner, J., & Roska, L. (1998). Modeling the mediating role of volition in the learning process. *Contemporary Educational Psychology, 23*, 392–418.

Garcia, T., & Pintrich, P. R. (1994). Regulating motivation and cognition in the classroom: The role of self-schemas and self-regulatory strategies. In D. H. Schunk & B. J. Zimmerman (Eds.), *Self-regulation of learning and performance: Issues and educational applications* (pp. 127–153). Hillsdale, NJ: Lawrence Erlbaum Associates.

Gelzheiser, L. (1984). Generalization from categorical memory tasks to prose by learning disabled adolescents. *Journal of Educational Psychology, 76*, 1128–1138.

Goldstein, D., & Dundon, W. (1987). Affect and cognition in learning disabilities. In S. Ceci (Ed.), *Handbook of cognitive, social and neuropsychological aspects of learning disabilities* (pp. 233–250). Hillsdale, NJ: Lawrence Erlbaum Associates Publishers.

Gollwitzer, P. (1996). The volitional benefits of planning. In P. Gollwitzer & J. Bargh (Eds.), *The psychology of action: Linking cognition and motivation to behavior* (pp. 287–312). New York: Guilford Press.

Graham, S., & Golan, S. (1991). Motivational influences on cognition: Task involvement, ego involvement, and depth of information processing. *Journal of Educational Psychology, 83,* 187–194.

Graham, S., & Harris, K. (1993). Self-regulated strategy development: Helping students with learning problems develop as writers. *The Elementary School Journal, 94,* No. 2, 169–181.

Hagan, J., Barclay, C., & Newman, R. (1982). Metacognition, self-knowledge, and learning disabilities: Some thoughts on knowing and doing. *Metacognition and Learning, 2,* 19–26.

Hallahan, D., & Bryan, T. (1981). Learning disabilities. In J. Kauffman & D. Hallahan (Eds.), *Handbook of special education* (pp. 141–164). Englewood Cliffs, NJ: Prentice-Hall.

Hallahan, D., & Kauffman, J. (1982). *Exceptional children* (2nd ed.). Englewood Cliffs, NJ: Prentice-Hall.

Harackiewicz, J. M., Barron, K. E., & Elliot, A. J. (1998). Rethinking achievement goals: When are they adaptive for college students and why? *Educational Psychologist, 33,* 1–21.

Harackiewicz, J. M., & Sansone, C. (1991). Goals and intrinsic motivation: You can get there from here. In M. L. Maehr & P. R. Pintrich (Eds.), *Advances in motivation and achievement: Goals and self-regulation* (Vol. 7, pp. 21–49). Greenwich, CT: JAI Press.

Haywood, H., & Switzky, H. (1986). Intrinsic motivation and behavioral effectiveness in retarded persons. In N. Ellis (Ed.), *International review of research in mental retardation* (Vol. 14, pp. 1–46). NY: Academic Press.

Hembree, R. (1988). Correlates, causes, effects and treatment of test anxiety. *Review of Educational Research, 58,* 47–77.

Higgins, E. T. (1997). Beyond pleasure and pain. *American Psychologist, 52,* 1280–1300.

Hill, K., & Wigfield, A. (1984). Test anxiety: A major educational problem and what can be done about it. *Elementary School Journal, 85,* 105–126.

Hodapp, R., Burack, J., & Zigler, E. (1998). Developmental approaches to mental retardation: A short introduction. In J. Burack, R. Hodapp, & E. Zigler (Eds.), *Handbook of mental retardation and development* (pp. 3–19). New York: Cambridge University Press.

Hofer, B., Yu, S., & Pintrich, P. R. (1998). Teaching college students to be self-regulated learners. In D. H. Schunk & B. J. Zimmerman (Eds.), *Self-regulated learning: From teaching to self-reflective practice* (pp. 57–85). New York: Guilford Press.

Hughes, C., Korinek, L., & Gorman, J. (1991). Self-management for students with mental retardation in public school settings: A research review. *Education and Training in Mental Retardation, 26,* 271–291.

Jagacinski, C., & Nicholls, J. (1984). Conceptions of ability and related affects in task involvement and ego involvement. *Journal of Educational Psychology, 76,* 909–919.

Jagacinski, C., & Nicholls, J. (1987). Competence and affect in task involvement and ego involvement: The impact of social comparison information. *Journal of Educational Psychology, 79,* 107–114.

Johnson, L., Graham, S., & Harris, K. (1997). The effects of goal setting and self-instruction on learning a reading comprehension strategy: A study of students with learning disabilities. *Journal of Learning Disabilities, 30,* No. 1, 80–91.

Kaplan, A., & Midgley, C. (1997). The effect of achievement goals: Does level of perceived academic competence make a difference? *Contemporary Educational Psychology, 22,* 415–435.

Karabenick, S., & Sharma, R. (1994). Seeking academic assistance as a strategic learning resource. In P. R. Pintrich, D. R. Brown, & C. E. Weinstein (Eds.), *Student motivation, cognition, and learning: Essays in honor of Wilbert J. McKeachie* (pp. 189–211). Hillsdale, NJ: Lawrence Erlbaum Associates.

Koestner, R., Aube, J., Ruttner, J., & Breed (1995). Theories of ability and the pursuit of challenge among adolescents with mild mental retardation. *Journal of Intellectual Disability Research, 39*, 57–65.

Koriat, A. (1993). How do we know that we know? The accessibility model of the feeling of knowing. *Psychological Review, 100*, 609–639.

Koriat, A., & Goldsmith, M. (1996). Monitoring and control processes in the strategic regulation of memory accuracy. *Psychological Review, 103*, 490–517.

Krapp, A., Hidi, S., & Renninger, K. A. (1992). Interest, learning and development. In K. A. Renninger, S. Hidi, & A. Krapp (Eds.), *The role of interest in learning and development* (pp. 3–25). Hillsdale, NJ: Lawrence Erlbaum Associates.

Kuhl, J. (1984). Volitional aspects of achievement motivation and learned helplessness: Toward a comprehensive theory of action control. In B. Maher & W. Maher (Eds.), *Progress in experimental personality research* (Vol. 13, pp. 99–171). New York: Academic Press.

Kuhl, J. (1985). Volitional mediators of cognition-behavior consistency: Self-regulatory processes and action versus state orientation. In J. Kuhl & J. Beckman (Eds.), *Action control: From cognition to behavior* (pp. 101–128). Berlin: Springer-Verlag.

Larkin, J., McDermott, J., Simon, D., & Simon, H. (1980). Expert and novice performance in solving physics problems. *Science, 208*, 1335–1442.

Licht, B. (1983). Cognitive-motivational factors that contribute to the achievement of learning-disabled children. *Journal of Learning Disabilities, 16*, 483–490.

Maehr, M. L., & Midgley, C. (1991). Enhancing student motivation: A school-wide approach. *Educational Psychologist, 26*, 399–427.

McClelland, D., Atkinson, J. W., Clark, R. A., & Lowell, E. L. (1953). *The achievement motive.* New York: Appleton-Century-Crofts.

McGivern, J., & Levin, J. (1983). The keyword method and children's vocabulary learning: An interaction with vocabulary knowledge. *Contemporary Educational Psychology, 8*, 46–54.

McKeachie, W. J., Pintrich, P. R., & Lin, Y. G. (1985). Teaching learning strategies. *Educational Psychologist, 20*, 153–160.

Meece, J., Blumenfeld, P., & Hoyle, R. (1988). Students' goal orientation and cognitive engagement in classroom activities. *Journal of Educational Psychology, 80*, 514–523.

Meece, J., & Holt, K. (1993). A pattern analysis of students' achievement goals. *Journal of Educational Psychology, 85*, 582–590.

Merrill, E., Goodwyn, E., & Gooding, H. (1996). Mental retardation and the acquisition of automatic processing. *American Journal on Mental Retardation, 101*, 49–62.

Middleton, M., & Midgley, C. (1997). Avoiding the demonstration of lack of ability: An underexplored aspect of goal theory. *Journal of Educational Psychology, 89*, 710–718.

Midgley, C. (1993). Motivation and middle level schools. In M. L. Maehr & P. R. Pintrich (Eds.), *Advances in motivation and achievement: Motivation and adolescence* (Vol. 8, pp. 217–274). Greenwich, CT: JAI Press.

Midgley, C., Arunkumar, R., & Urdan, T. (1996). "If I don't do well tomorrow, there's a reason": Predictors of adolescents' use of academic self-handicapping strategies. *Journal of Educational Psychology, 88*, 423–434.

Midgley, C., Kaplan, A., Middleton, M., Maehr, M. L., Urdan, T., Anderman, L., Anderman, E., & Roeser, R. (1998). The development and validation of scales assessing students' achievement goal orientations. *Contemporary Educational Psychology, 23*, 113–131.

Miller, R., Behrens, J., Greene, B., & Newman, D. (1993). Goals and perceived ability: Impact on student valuing, self-regulation, and persistence. *Contemporary Educational Psychology, 18*, 2–14.

Miller, G., Galanter, E., & Pribram, K. (1960). *Plans and the structure of behavior.* New York: Holt.

Nelson, T., & Narens, L. (1990). Metamemory: A theoretical framework and new findings. In G. Bower (Ed.), *The psychology of learning and motivation* (Vol. 26, pp. 125–141). New York: Academic Press.

Nelson-Le Gall, S. (1981). Help-seeking: An understudied problem solving skill in children. *Developmental Review, 1*, 224–246.

Nelson-Le Gall, S. (1985). Help-seeking behavior in learning. *Review of research in education* (Vol. 12, pp. 55–90). Washington DC: American Educational Research Association.

Newman, R. (1991). Goals and self-regulated learning: What motivates children to seek academic help? In M. L. Maehr & P. R. Pintrich (Eds.), *Advances in motivation and achievement: Goals and self-regulatory processes* (Vol. 7, pp. 151–183). Greenwich, CT: JAI Press.

Newman, R. (1994). Adaptive help-seeking: A strategy of self-regulated learning. In D. H. Schunk & B. J. Zimmerman (Eds.), *Self-regulation of learning and performance: Issues and educational applications* (pp. 283–301). Hillsdale, NJ: Lawrence Erlbaum Associates.

Newman, R. (1998a). Adaptive help-seeking: A role of social interaction in self-regulated learning. In S. Karabenick (Ed.), *Strategic help-seeking: Implications for learning and teaching* (pp. 13–37). Hillsdale, NJ: Lawrence Erlbaum Associates.

Newman, R. (1998b). Students' help-seeking during problem solving: Influences of personal and contextual goals. *Journal of Educational Psychology, 90*, 644–658.

Newman, R. (2000). Social influences on the development of children's adaptive help seeking: The role of parents, teachers, and peers. *Developmental Review, 20*, 350–404.

Nicholls, J. (1984). Achievement motivation: Conceptions of ability, subjective experience, task choice, and performance. *Psychological Review, 91*, 328–346.

Nicholls, J. (1989). *The competitive ethos and democratic education.* Cambridge, MA: Harvard University Press.

Nicholls, J., Cheung, P., Lauer, J., & Patashnick, M. (1989). Individual differences in academic motivation: Perceived ability, goals, beliefs, and values. *Learning and Individual Differences, 1*, 63–84.

Nisbett, R. (1993). *Rules for reasoning.* Hillsdale, NJ: Lawrence Erlbaum Associates.

Nolen, S. (1988). Reasons for studying: Motivational orientations and study strategies. *Cognition and Instruction, 5*, 269–287.

Norem, J. K., & Cantor, N. (1986). Defensive pessimism: Harnessing anxiety as motivation. *Journal of Personality and Social Psychology, 51*, 1208–1217.

Paris, S. G., Lipson, M. Y., & Wixson, K. K. (1983). Becoming a strategic reader. *Contemporary Educational Psychology, 8*, 293–316.

Paris, S., & Myers, M. (1981). Comprehension monitoring, memory and study strategies of good and poor readers. *Journal of Reading Behavior, 8*, 6–22.

Peterson, C., Maier, S., & Seligman, M. (1993). *Learned helplessness: A theory for the age of personal control.* New York: Oxford University Press.

Pintrich, P. R. (1989). The dynamic interplay of student motivation and cognition in the college classroom. In C. Ames & M. L. Maehr (Eds.), *Advances in motivation and achievement: Motivation-enhancing environments* (Vol. 6, pp. 117–160). Greenwich, CT: JAI Press.

Pintrich, P., Anderman, E., & Klobucar, C. (1994). Intraindividual differences in motivation and cognition in students with and without learning disabilities. *Journal of Learning Disabilities, 27*, 360–370.

Pintrich, P. R., & De Groot, E. V. (1990). Motivational and self-regulated learning components of classroom academic performance. *Journal of Educational Psychology, 82,* 33–40.
Pintrich, P. R., & Garcia, T. (1991). Student goal orientation and self-regulation in the college classroom. In M. L. Maehr & P. R. Pintrich (Eds.), *Advances in motivation and achievement: Goals and self-regulatory processes* (Vol. 7, pp. 371–402). Greenwich, CT: JAI Press.
Pintrich, P. R., Marx, R., & Boyle, R. (1993). Beyond cold conceptual change: The role of motivational beliefs and classroom contextual factors in the process of conceptual change. *Review of Educational Research, 63*(2), 167–199.
Pintrich, P. R., McKeachie, W., & Lin, Y.-G. (1987). Teaching a course in learning to learn. *Teaching of Psychology, 14,* 81–86.
Pintrich, P. R., Roeser, R., & De Groot, E. (1994). Classroom and individual differences in early adolescents' motivation and self-regulated learning. *Journal of Early Adolescence, 14,* 139–161.
Pintrich, P. R., Smith, D., Garcia, T., & McKeachie, W. (1993). Predictive validity and reliability of the Motivated Strategies for Learning Questionnaire (MSLQ). *Educational and Psychological Measurement, 53,* 801–813.
Pintrich, P. R., & Schrauben, B. (1992). Students' motivational beliefs and their cognitive engagement in classroom tasks. In D. Schunk & J. Meece (Eds.), *Student perceptions in the classroom: Causes and consequences* (pp. 149–183). Hillsdale, NJ: Erlbaum.
Pintrich, P. R., & Schunk, D. H. (1996). *Motivation in education: Theory, research and applications.* Englewood Cliffs, NJ: Prentice Hall Merrill.
Pintrich, P. R., Wolters, C., & Baxter, G. (2000). Assessing metacognition and self-regulated learning. In G. Schraw & J. Impara (Eds.), *Issues in the measurement of metacognition* (pp. 43–97). Lincoln, NE: Buros Institute of Mental Measurements.
Pintrich, P. R. (2000). The role of goal orientation in self-regulated learning. In M. Boekaerts, P. R. Pintrich, & M. Zeidner (Eds.), *Handbook of self-regulation* (pp. 451–502). San Diego, CA: Academic Press.
Pressley, M., & Afflerbach, P. (1995). *Verbal protocols of reading: The nature of constructively responsive reading.* Hillsdale, NJ: Lawrence Erlbaum Associates.
Pressley, M., & Levin, J. (1987). Elaborative learning strategies for the inefficient learner. In S. Ceci (Ed.), *Handbook of cognitive social and neuropsychological aspects of learning disabilities* (pp. 175–212). Hillsdale, NJ: Lawrence Erlbaum Associates Publishers.
Pressley, M., & Woloshyn, V. (1995). *Cognitive strategy instruction that really improves children's academic performance.* Cambridge, MA: Brookline Books.
Renninger, K. A., Hidi, S., & Krapp, A. (1992). *The role of interest in learning and development.* Hillsdale, NJ: Erlbaum.
Ryan, A., & Pintrich, P. R. (1997). "Should I ask for help?" The role of motivation and attitudes in adolescents' help seeking in math class. *Journal of Educational Psychology, 89,* 329–341.
Ryan, A., & Pintrich, P. R. (1998). Achievement and social motivational influences on help-seeking in the classroom. In S. Karabenick (Ed.), *New directions in research on help-seeking* (pp. 103–123). Mahwah, NJ: Lawrence Erlbaum Associates.
Ryan, A., Gheen, M., & Midgley, C. (1998). Why do some students avoid asking for help? An examination of the interplay among students' academic efficacy, teachers' social–emotional role, and the classroom goal structure. *Journal of Educational Psychology, 90,* 528–535.
Sansone, C., Weir, C., Harpster, L., & Morgan, C. (1992). Once a boring task, always a boring task? The role of interest as a self-regulatory mechanism. *Journal of Personality and Social Psychology, 63,* 379–390.

Schiefele, U. (1991). Interest, learning, and motivation. *Educational Psychologist, 26*, 299–323.
Schneider, W., & Pressley, M. (1997). *Memory development between 2 and 20*. Mahweh, NJ: Lawrence Erlbaum Associates.
Schoenfeld, A. (1992). Learning to think mathematically: Problem solving, metacognition, and sense making in mathematics. In D. Grouws (Ed.), *Handbook of research on mathematics teaching and learning* (pp. 334–370). New York: Macmillan.
Schraw, G., & Moshman, D. (1995). Metacognitive theories. *Educational Psychology Review, 7*, 351–371.
Schunk, D. (1985). Participation in goal setting: Effects on self-efficacy and skills of learning-disabled children. *The Journal of Special Education, 19*, 307–317.
Schunk, D. H. (1989). Social cognitive theory and self-regulated learning. In B. J. Zimmerman & D. H. Schunk (Eds.), *Self-regulated learning and academic achievement: Theory, research, and practice* (pp. 83–110). New York: Springer-Verlag.
Schunk, D. H. (1991). Self-efficacy and academic motivation. *Educational Psychologist, 26*, 207–231.
Schunk, D. H. (1994). Self-regulation of self-efficacy and attributions in academic settings. In D. H. Schunk & B. J. Zimmerman (Eds.), *Self-regulation of learning and performance: Issues and educational applications* (pp. 75–99). Hillsdale, NJ: Lawrence Erlbaum Associates.
Short, F., & Evans, S. (1990). Individual differences in cognitive and social problem-solving skills as a function of intelligence. In N. W. Bray (Ed.), *International review of research in mental retardation* (Vol. 16, pp. 89–123). San Diego, CA: Academic Press.
Simpson, M., Hynd, C., Nist, S., & Burrell, K. (1997). College academic assistance programs and practices. *Educational Psychology Review, 9*, 39–87.
Skaalvik, E. (1997). Self-enhancing and self-defeating ego orientation: Relations with task avoidance orientation, achievement, self-perceptions, and anxiety. *Journal of Educational Psychology, 89*, 71–81.
Skaalvik, E., Valas, H., & Sletta, O. (1994). Task involvement and ego involvement: Relations with academic achievement, academic self-concept and self-esteem. *Scandinavian Journal of Educational Research, 38*, 231–243.
Snow, R., Corno, L., & Jackson, D. (1996). Individual differences in affective and conative functions. In D. Berliner & R. Calfee (Eds.), *Handbook of Educational Psychology* (pp. 243–310). New York: Macmillan.
Steele, C. M. (1998). The psychology of self-affirmation: Sustaining the integrity of the self. *Advances in Experimental Social Psychology, 21*, 261–302.
Steele, C. M. (1997). A threat in the air: How stereotypes shape intellectual identity and performance. *American Psychologist, 52*, 613–629.
Sternberg, R. (1985). *Beyond IQ: A triarchic theory of intelligence*. New York: Cambridge University Press.
Swanson, H. L. (1990). Instruction derived from the strategy deficit model: Overview of principles and procedures. In T. Scruggs & B. Wong (Eds.), *Intervention research in learning disabilities* (pp. 34–65). New York: Springer-Verlag.
Swanson, H. L. (2000). What instruction works for students with learning disabilities? Summarizing the results from a meta-analysis of intervention studies. In R. Gersten, E. Schiller, & S. Vaughn (Eds.), *Contemporary special education research: Syntheses of the knowledge base on critical instructional issues* (pp. 1–30). Mahwah, NJ: Lawrence Erlbaum Associates Publishers.
Swanson, H. L., Carson, C., & Saches-Lee, C. (1996). A selective synthesis of intervention research for students with learning disabilities. *School Psychology Review, 25*, No. 3, 370–391.

Switzky, H. (1999). Intrinsic motivation and motivational self-system processes in persons with mental retardation: A theory of motivational orientation. In E. Zigler & D. Bennett-Gates (Eds.), *Personality development in individuals with mental retardation* (pp. 70–106). New York: Cambridge University Press.

Switzky, H. (2001). Personality and motivational self-system processes in persons with mental retardation: Old memories and new perspectives. In H. N. Switzky (Ed.), *Personality and motivational differences in persons with mental retardation* (pp. 57–145). Mahweh, NJ: Lawrence Erlbaum Associates.

Thorkildsen, T., & Nicholls, J. (1998). Fifth graders' achievement orientations and beliefs: Individual and classroom differences. *Journal of Educational Psychology, 90,* 179–201.

Torgesen, J. (1980). Conceptual and educational implications of the use of efficient task strategies by learning disabled children. *Journal of Learning Disabilities, 13,* 364–371.

Torgesen, J., & Licht, B. (1983). The learning disabled child as an inactive learner: Retrospects and prospects. In J. McKinney & L. Feagans (Eds.), *Current topics in learning disabilities* (Vol. 1, pp. 3–31). Norwood, NJ: Ablex.

Tryon, G. (1980). The measurement and treatment of test anxiety. *Review of Educational Research, 50,* 343–372.

Turner, L. (1996). Attributional beliefs of persons with mild mental retardation. In M. Lewis & M. Sullivan (Eds.), *Emotional development in atypical children* (pp. 149–159). Mahweh, NJ: Lawrence Erlbaum Associates.

Urdan, T. (1997). Achievement goal theory: Past results, future directions. In M. L. Maehr & P. R. Pintrich (Eds.), *Advances in motivation and achievement* (Vol. 10, pp. 99–141). Greenwich, CT: JAI Press.

Urdan, T., & Maehr, M. L. (1995). Beyond a two-goal theory of motivation: A case for social goals. *Review of Educational Research, 65,* 213–244.

van Haneghan, J., & Turner, L. (2001). Information processing and motivation in people with mental retardation. In H. N. Switzky (Ed.), *Personality and motivational differences in persons with mental retardation* (pp. 319–371). Mahweh, NJ: Lawrence Erlbaum Associates.

Wehmeyer, M. (2001). Self-determination and mental retardation: Assembling the puzzle pieces. In H. N. Switzky (Ed.), *Personality and motivational differences in persons with mental retardation* (pp. 147–198). Mahweh, NJ: Lawrence Erlbaum Associates.

Wehmeyer, M. (1992). Self-determination and the education of students with mental retardation. *Education and Training in Mental Retardation, 27,* 302–314.

Wehmeyer, M., & Palmer, S. (1997). Perceptions of control of students with and without cognitive disabilities. *Psychological Reports, 81,* 195–206.

Weiner, B. (1986). *An attributional theory of motivation and emotion.* New York: Springer-Verlag.

Weiner, B. (1995). *Judgments of responsibility: A foundation for a theory of social conduct.* New York: Guilford Press.

Weinstein, C. E., & Mayer, R. (1986). The teaching of learning strategies. In M. Wittrock (Ed.), *Handbook of research on teaching and learning* (pp. 315–327). New York: Macmillan.

Weisz, J. (1999). Cognitive performance and learned helplessness in mentally retarded persons. In E. Zigler & D. Bennett-Gates (Eds.), *Personality development in individuals with mental retardation* (pp. 17–46). New York: Cambridge University Press.

Wentzel, K. (1991a). Social and academic goals at school: Motivation and achievement in context. In M. L. Maehr & P. R. Pintrich (Eds.), *Advances in motivation and achievement: Goals and self-regulatory processes* (Vol. 7, pp. 185–212). Greenwich, CT: JAI Press.

Wentzel, K. (1991b). Social competence at school: Relation between social responsibility and academic achievement. *Review of Educational Research, 61,* 1–24.

Westman, J. (1990). *Handbook of learning disabilities: A multisystem approach.* Needham Heights, MA: Allyn and Bacon.

Wigfield, A. (1994). Expectancy-value theory of achievement motivation: A developmental perspective. *Educational Psychology Review, 6,* 49–78.

Wigfield, A., & Eccles, J. (1989). Test anxiety in elementary and secondary school students. *Educational Psychologist, 24,* 159–183.

Wigfield, A., & Eccles, J. (1992). The development of achievement task values: A theoretical analysis. *Developmental Review, 12,* 265–310.

Wilson, D., & David, W. (1994). Academic intrinsic motivation and attitudes toward school and learning of learning disabled students. *Learning Disabilities Research and Practice, 9,* 148–156.

Wolters, C. (1998). Self-regulated learning and college students' regulation of motivation. *Journal of Educational Psychology, 90,* 224–235.

Wolters, C., Yu, S., & Pintrich, P. R. (1996). The relation between goal orientation and students' motivational beliefs and self-regulated learning. *Learning and Individual Differences, 8,* 211–238.

Wong, B. (1982). Strategic behaviors in selecting retrieval cues in gifted, normal achieving and learning-disabled children. *Journal of Learning Disabilities, 15,* No. 1, 33–37.

Wong, B. (1985). Metacognition and learning disabilities. In T. Waller, D. Forrest-Pressley, & E. MacKinnon (Eds.), *Metacognition, cognition and human performance* (pp. 137–180). New York: Academic Press.

Wong, B. (1986). Metacognition and special education: A review of a view. *Journal of Special Education, 20,* No. 1, 9–29.

Wong, B., & Wong, R. (1986). Study behavior as a function of metacognitive knowledge about critical task variables: An investigation of above average, average and learning disabled readers. *Learning Disabilities Research, 1,* 101–111.

Zeidner, M. (1998). *Test anxiety: The state of the art.* New York: Plenum.

Zigler, E. (1999). The individual with mental retardation as a whole person. In E. Zigler & D. Bennett-Gates (Eds.), *Personality development in individuals with mental retardation* (pp. 1–16). New York: Cambridge University Press.

Zimmerman, B. J. (1989). A social cognitive view of self-regulated learning and academic learning. *Journal of Educational Psychology, 81*(3), 329–339.

Zimmerman, B. J. (1994). Dimensions of academic self-regulation: A conceptual framework for education. In D. H. Schunk & B. J. Zimmerman (Eds.), *Self-regulation of learning and performance: Issues and educational applications* (pp. 3–21). Hillsdale, NJ: Lawrence Erlbaum Associates.

Zimmerman, B. J. (1998a). Academic studying and the development of personal skill: A self-regulatory perspective. *Educational Psychologist, 33,* 73–86.

Zimmerman, B. J. (1998b). Developing self-fulfilling cycles of academic regulation: An analysis of exemplary instructional models. In D. H. Schunk & B. J. Zimmerman (Eds.), *Self-regulated learning: From teaching to self-reflective practice* (pp. 1–19). New York: Guilford Press.

Zimmerman, B. J. (2000). Attaining self-regulation: A social cognitive perspective. In M. Boekaerts, P. R. Pintrich, & M. Zeidner (Eds.), *Handbook of self-regulation* (pp. 13–39). San Diego, CA: Academic Press.

Zimmerman, B. J., & Kitsantas, A. (1997). Developmental phases in self-regulation: Shifting from process to outcome goals. *Journal of Educational Psychology, 89,* 29–36.

Zimmerman, B. J., & Martinez-Pons, M. (1986). Development of a structured interview for assessing student use of self-regulated learning strategies. *American Educational Research Journal, 23,* 614–628.

Zimmerman, B. J., & Martinez-Pons, M. (1988). Construct validation of a strategy model of student self-regulated learning. *Journal of Educational Psychology, 80*(3), 284–290.

Zusho, A., & Pintrich, P. R. (2000). Fear of not learning? The role of mastery avoidance goals in Asian American & European Amercian college students. Paper presented in a symposium on "Gender and ethnic differences in motivation and self-regulated learning," American Educational Research Association convention. New Orleans.

Learner-Centered Principles and Practices: Enhancing Motivation and Achievement for Children with Learning Challenges and Disabilities

BARBARA L. McCOMBS

UNIVERSITY OF DENVER RESEARCH INSTITUTE

This chapter begins with an introduction of issues regarding children with special needs, followed by a description of the *learner-centered psychological principles* (LCPs) currently disseminated by the American Psychological Association (APA, 1997). The implications of the LCPs for instructional practices are then discussed, with a particular focus on practices that meet the motivational and learning needs of children with learning challenges and disabilities. The chapter concludes with specific recommendations for practice, policy, and research that would be expected to enhance the motivation and achievement of special needs children.

Throughout the history of education, educators have been concerned with finding ways to meet the diverse needs of learners. At this point in our history not only are our nation's schools attempting to help all students achieve at higher levels, but they are attempting to find ways to address the needs of a growing number of school-age children with education-related learning challenges and disabilities, such as attention deficit disorders and behavioral problems. Many of the children placed in special education programs come from particular ethnic and racial backgrounds, notably African American and American Indian (SEDL & NiDRR, 1999). In 1998, 8.6% of all public school children were identified as having disabilities that qualified them for special education services (U.S. Department of Education, 1998). However, the percentages were 20 and 21.9 for African-American and American-Indian students, respectively. Regardless of the children's type of disability and racial/ethnic or academic background, there are a number of common elements in successful programs. These include the following elements identified by Leone and Drakeford (1999) and the Office of Special Education Programs (2000):

- High expectations, challenging standards, relevant curriculum, and a clear focus on academic learning.
- Meaningful participation of all children in all aspects of the schools, including academic and non-academic, extra-curricular, and assessments.
- Good leadership and organizational vitality, including a strong level of autonomy and professional decision-making.
- Quality ongoing professional development, including opportunities for teacher input and observations of teaching in other settings.
- Sense of community, including parents as an integral part of the school community.

The foregoing list is similar to the one created from a study of nine high-performing, high-poverty urban elementary schools (Johnson & Asera, 1999). Despite geographic, demographic, and programmatic differences among the nine schools, there were several common strategies that were used to improve academic achievement in all nine schools. These included:

- Identifying an important, visible, yet attainable first goal and achieving success on this goal before moving toward more ambitious goals.
- Directing time and energy to be of service to children rather than on conflicts among adults in the school.
- Fostering a sense of responsibility for appropriate behavior and an environment in which students were likely to behave well.
- Creating a collective sense of responsibility for school improvement.
- Sharing leadership and increasing the quantity and quality of time spent on instructional leadership activities.
- Aligning instruction to state standards and assessments.
- Making sure school leaders and teachers had the resources, materials, equipment, and professional development to help students achieve at high levels.

When studying these points, it becomes clear that success with all students requires addressing personal, technical, and organizational needs in the educational system. The solutions are a balance of these three domains that influence outcomes in any living system. The purpose of this chapter is to focus on what we know about learning and learners that can help provide a foundation for designing the kinds of instructional practices and contexts that can enhance motivation, learning, and achievement for all learners. Particular attention will be given to identifying those practices that would be particularly beneficial for students with special learning needs. We begin by observing the knowledge base represented by the research-validated *learner-centered psychological principles* (LCPs) (APA, 1997).

I. THE LCPs AS A FOUNDATIONAL KNOWLEDGE BASE

What is the foundational knowledge base needed to define the learning experiences and conditions that create quality learning and meet social, emotional, and cognitive learning needs for students with a variety of learning needs? To address this question, it is instructive to look first at the working definition of a disability. This will allow for a deeper look at the knowledge base, which may provide a foundation for designing effective instructional practices and learning contexts for children with special learning needs.

A. Defining Disability

The following definition is given in the Individuals With Disabilities Education Act (IDEA, 1997, p. 9):
In general—the term 'child with a disability' means a child—

1. with mental retardation, hearing impairments (including deafness), speech or language impairments, visual impairments (including blindness), serious emotional disturbance (hereafter referred to as 'emotional disturbance'), orthopedic impairments, autism, traumatic brain injury, other health impairment, or specific learning disabilities; and
2. who, by reason thereof, needs special education and related services.

For younger children, ages 3 through 9 years, this also includes those experiencing developmental delays in physical, cognitive, communication, social, emotional, or adaptive development.

The foregoing definition, combined with research on practices that work for students with disabilities, confirms that a focus on personal and motivational outcomes balanced with a focus on high achievement and challenging standards is vital. This balance is also essential in reducing negative trends for students with disabilities such as school dropout, delinquency, and violence (e.g., Burrell & Warboys, 2000). There is growing recognition that schooling must prepare all children to behave in moral and ethical ways. For example, many educators are calling for caring, democratic schooling and instructional methods that build on each student's background, experience of reality, and perspective (e.g., Bartolome, 1994; McWhorter et al., 1996; Noddings, 1995; Rudduck et al., 1997). These practices address personal domain concerns of educational systems that focus on *human processes* and on personal and interpersonal *relationships, beliefs, and perceptions* that are affected by the educational system as a whole. This domain must be balanced with technical domain concerns that focus on curriculum and content mastery, and organizational domain concerns that focus on management structures and decision-making processes.

To apply such practices, research-validated principles are needed to guide their design, including the design of comprehensive, integrated, and inclusive programs for students with disabilities. The knowledge base underlying the principles of learners and learning becomes a research-validated foundation for comprehensive school reform that focuses on meeting cognitive, social, and emotional human needs and fostering positive teacher/student relationships. The principles lead to understanding students as knowledge generators, active participants in their own learning, and co-creators of learning experiences and curricula.

B. The LCPs as a Foundational Framework

Education is one of many complex living systems that function to support particular human needs (refer to Wheatley, 1999). Such systems are by their nature unpredictable, but can be understood in terms of principles that define human needs, cognitive and motivational processes, and development and individual differences. The research-validated LCPs (APA, 1993, 1997) provide a knowledge base for understanding learning and motivation as natural processes that occur when the *conditions and context* of learning are supportive of individual learner needs, capacities, experiences, and interests. The foundation of the research-validated LCPs is essential to designing programs and practices that attend holistically and systemically to the needs of all learners—including students, their teachers, administrators, family, and community members.

1. THE LCPs

In 1990, the American Psychological Association (APA) appointed a special Task Force on Psychology in Education, one of whose purposes was to integrate research and theory from psychology and education in order to surface general principles that have stood the test of time and can provide a framework for school redesign and reform. The result was a document that specified 12 fundamental principles about learners and learning that, taken together, provide an integrated perspective on factors influencing learning for *all* learners (APA, 1993). This document was revised in 1997 and now includes 14 principles that are essentially the same as the original 12 except that attention is now given to principles dealing with diversity and standards (APA, 1997). (Note: Research and theory reviewed in developing the LCPs are described in McCombs and Whisler (1997). Further research support is also provided in Alexander and Murphy (1998), Lambert and McCombs (1998), and Weinstein (1998)).

The 14 LCPs are categorized into four domains as shown in Table I. These categories group the principles into research-validated domains important to learning: metacognitive and cognitive factors, motivational and affective factors, developmental and social factors, and individual difference factors. An understanding of these domains and the principles within them establishes a framework for designing learner-centered practices at all levels of schooling. It also defines what "learner-centered" means from a research-validated perspective.

2. DEFINING "LEARNER-CENTERED"

From an integrated and holistic look at the LCPs, the following definition emerges:

> "Learner centered" is the perspective that couples a focus on individual learners—their heredity, experiences, perspectives, backgrounds, talents, interests, capacities, and needs—with a focus on learning—the best available knowledge about learning and how it occurs and about teaching practices that are most effective in promoting the highest levels of motivation, learning, and achievement for all learners. This dual focus then informs and drives educational decision making. Learner-centered is a reflection in practice of the LCPs—in the programs, practices, policies, and people that support learning for all (McCombs & Whisler, 1997).

This definition of learner-centered is based on an understanding of the LCPs as a representation of current knowledge about learners and learning. The LCPs apply to *all* learners, in and outside of school, young and old. Learner-centered is also related to the beliefs, characteristics, dispositions, and practices of teachers—practices primarily created by the teacher. When teachers derive their practices from an understanding of the LCPs, they (1) include learners in decisions about how and what they learn and how that learning is assessed; (2) value each learner's unique perspectives; (3) respect and accommodate individual differences in learners' backgrounds, interests, abilities, and experiences; and (4) treat learners as co-creators and partners in the teaching and learning process.

TABLE I
THE LEARNER-CENTERED PSYCHOLOGICAL PRINCIPLES

Cognitive and Metacognitive Factors

Principle 1: Nature of the learning process
The learning of complex subject matter is most effective when it is an intentional process of constructing meaning from information and experience.

Principle 2: Goals of the learning process
The successful learner, over time and with support and instructional guidance, can create meaningful, coherent representations of knowledge.

Principle 3: Construction of knowledge
The successful learner can link new information with existing knowledge in meaningful ways.

Principle 4: Strategic thinking
The successful learner can create and use a repertoire of thinking and reasoning strategies to achieve complex learning goals.

Principle 5: Thinking about thinking
Higher order strategies for selecting and monitoring mental operations facilitate creative and critical thinking.

Principle 6: Context of learning
Learning is influenced by environmental factors, including culture, technology, and instructional practices.

Motivational and Affective Factors

Principle 7: Motivational and emotional influences on learning
What and how much is learned is influenced by the learner's motivation. Motivation to learn, in turn, is influenced by the individual's emotional states, beliefs, interests, goals, and habits of thinking.

Principle 8: Intrinsic motivation to learn
The learner's creativity, higher-order thinking, and natural curiosity all contribute to motivation to learn. Intrinsic motivation is stimulated by tasks of optimal novelty and difficulty, relevant to personal interests, and providing for personal choice and control.

Principle 9: Effects of motivation on effort
Acquisition of complex knowledge and skills requires extended learner effort and guided practice. Without learners' motivation to learn, the willingness to exert this effort is unlikely without coercion.

Developmental and Social Factors

Principle 10: Developmental influence on learning
As individuals develop, they encounter different opportunities and experience different constraints for learning. Learning is most effective when differential development within and across physical, intellectual, emotional, and social domains is taken into account.

Principle 11: Social influences on learning
Learning is influenced by social interactions, interpersonal relations, and communication with others.

Individual Differences Factors

Principle 12: Individual differences in learning
Learners have different strategies, approaches, and capabilities for learning that are a function of prior experience and heredity.

TABLE I (Continued)

Principle 13: Learning and diversity
Learning is most effective when differences in learners' linguistic, cultural, and social backgrounds are taken into account.

Principle 14: Standards and assessment
Setting appropriately high and challenging standards and assessing the learner and learning progress—including diagnostic, process, and outcome assessment—are integral parts of the learning process.

Others who have used the term "learner-centered" (e.g., Darling-Hammond, 1996; Sparks & Hirsh, 1997) refer to learning new beliefs and visions of practice that are responsive to and respectful of the diverse needs of students and teachers as learners. All learning, for students and teachers, must support diverse learners, provide time for reflection, and offer opportunities for teachers and students to co-create practices that enhance learning, motivation, and achievement. This view of "learner-centered" is a research-validated paradigm shift that transforms education—including how best to use programs to support the new vision (refer to Sparks & Hirsh, 1997).

Our work with kindergarten-through college-age students over the past eight years has revealed that learner-centered practices consistent with educational psychology's knowledge base and the LCPs enhance learner motivation and achievement (McCombs, 2000, 2001; McCombs & Whisler, 1997; Weinberger & McCombs, 2001). Of particular significance in this work is that student perceptions of their teachers' instructional practices account for between 45% to 60% of the variance in student motivation and achievement, whereas teacher beliefs and perceptions only account for 4% to 15% of this variance. The single most important domain of practice for students in all age ranges is the domain of practice that promotes a positive climate for learning and interpersonal relationships between and among students and teachers. Also important are practices that provide academic challenge and give students choice and control, that encourage the development of critical thinking and learning skills, and that adapt to a variety of individual developmental differences.

Using teacher and student surveys based on the LCPs, called the Assessment of Learner-Centered Practices (ALCP), teachers can be assisted in reflecting on individual and class discrepancies in perceptions of classroom practice and in changing practices to meet student needs (McCombs, 2001). Results of our research with the ALCP teacher and student surveys at both the secondary and post-secondary levels have confirmed that at all levels of our educational system, teachers and instructors can be helped to improve instructional practices and change toward more learner-centered practices by attending to what students are perceiving and spending more time creating positive climates and relationships—critical connections so important to personal and system learning and change.

Of additional significance in my own work with learner-centered practices and self-assessment tools based on the LCPs for teachers and students in K–12 and college classrooms is the finding that what defines "learner-centeredness" is not solely a function of particular instructional practices or programs (McCombs, 2001, 2003a,b; McCombs & Lauer, 1997; McCombs & Whisler, 1997). Rather, it is a complex interaction of qualities of the teacher in combination with characteristics of instructional practices—as perceived by individual learners. That is, "learner-centeredness" is in "the eye of the beholder" and varies as a function of learner perceptions which, in turn, are the result of each learner's prior experiences, self-beliefs, and attitudes about schools and learning as well as their current interests, values, and goals. Thus, the quality of "learner-centeredness does not reside in programs or practices by themselves—no matter how well designed the program may be."

When learner-centered is defined from a research perspective that includes the knowledge base on both learning and learners, it also clarifies what is needed to create positive learning contexts and communities. When this occurs at the classroom and school levels, it increases the likelihood of success for more students and their teachers. In addition, a research-validated foundation that focuses on both learners and learning can lead to increased clarity about the requisite dispositions and characteristics of school personnel who are in service to learners and learning—particularly teachers. From this perspective, the LCPs can become a foundational framework for determining how to use and assess the efficacy of programs in providing instruction, curricula, and personnel to enhance the teaching and learning process. The voice and perceptions of the learner regarding the degree to which programs and practices meet individual cognitive, social, and emotional needs are part of the assessment of ongoing learning, change, and improvement. This component is particularly critical in meeting the needs of students with disabilities and learning challenges.

II. WHAT ARE PRACTICE AND POLICY IMPLICATIONS OF THE LEARNER-CENTERED FRAMEWORK FOR SERVING THE NEEDS OF STUDENTS WITH DISABILITIES AND LEARNING CHALLENGES?

With the research-validated LCPs as a foundation, important practice and policy implications of the learner-centered framework for implementing and integrating programs and concepts into comprehensive school reform efforts can be derived. Some concrete suggestions for children with special needs are provided in the sections that follow.

A. Implications for Practice

In the areas of *practice*, a key implication is that the larger context of education must support and value individual learners as well as diverse learning outcomes. As Burnette (1996) has said in support of including students with disabilities in general education classrooms, appropriate practices meet the needs and enhance the education of *all* students. She goes on to describe characteristics of effective inclusive schools (also recommended by the Office of Special Education and Rehabilitative Services [OSERS] (2000), and present in schools where IDEA is well implemented). These characteristics of successful schools include:

- a sense of community based on a philosophy and vision that all children belong and are part of the learning community;
- strong leadership that actively involves all school staff in planning and implementing successful learning and community building strategies;
- high standards that provide all children with the opportunity to reach high educational outcomes through programs and practices that reflect individual needs;
- collaboration and cooperation among students and staff via strategies such as cooperative learning, peer tutoring, team and co-teaching, buddy systems, and teacher-student assistance teams;
- changing roles and responsibilities that include teachers and psychologists working more closely together and everyone being actively involved in the learning process;
- an array of services that meet students' health, mental health, and social services needs within coordinated educational models used by the entire staff;
- partnership with parents such that they are embraced as equal and essential partners in their children's education;
- flexible learning environments that follow individual learning paths, with flexible groupings and practices that emphasize participation by all students;
- strategies based on research on how people learn that are systematically applied to the education of all students;
- new forms of accountability that rely less on standardized tests and more on measuring each student's progress toward achieving individualized learning goals;

- access to all aspects of school life via building modifications or use of appropriate assistive technologies; and
- continuing professional development that allows all staff to receive training that continuously improves their knowledge and skills for educating all students.

When applying best practices as discussed in the previous sections, the culture and climate must acknowledge the purpose of education as going beyond academic competence and content knowledge alone. There must be a shared vision, value, and purpose of education. As Comer states (in O'Neil, 1997, pp. 9–10): "It is difficult to internalize a sense of well-being, high self-esteem, and a passion for achievement in an environment that is chaotic, abusive, or characterized by low expectations for students ... What children need more than anything is the chance to attach with and bond to adults who are meaningful and important to them." Restoring a sense of community is seen as the fundamental way to provide social and emotional support.

1. CHANGING PERSONAL CONCEPTIONS OF ABILITY AND MOTIVATION

In creating a new vision for education, research by Gardner (1993, 1995), Renzulli and Reis (1985), Renzulli et al. (1995), and Wang (1992, 1998) highlights the importance of broadening our view of abilities and educational achievement beyond the traditionally narrow view embedded in educational systems. Gardner's research informs us that everyone has multiple intelligences and talents—any of which may be present and/or develop during our life span. Renzulli's research in particular reminds us that our focus for increasing the motivation *of any low performing group* is to recognize and value individual interests. When learners of any age are allowed to pursue their natural interests, their natural motivation follows, and levels of achievement in these areas of highest interest are beyond what we might prejudge to be possible. Wang's research provides empirically based strategies and practices for engaging even the most disenfranchised and alienated students in learning through adaptive instructional environments.

The multiple intelligences theory of Gardner (1995) captures the essence of designing such environments. This theory is exemplified in school practices such as: approaching curriculum in a variety of ways and from a variety of perspectives; using assessment strategies that help students display their new understandings in a variety of ways; and personalizing approaches to education such that each student has the maximum opportunity to master those materials. Similarly, in my own work (McCombs, 1995, 1998, 2000, 2003a,b; McCombs & Lauer, 1997; McCombs & Quiat, 2002; McCombs & Whisler, 1997) I have argued that we need school models that see all children as "gifted" and that use students' interests and goals as the "sorting system" into enrichment clusters—not abilities, grade levels, or other categories that often negatively impact potential as perceived by both students and teachers.

To support this contention, we found in our research that teachers were not absolutely learner-centered or completely non–learner-centered in terms of their beliefs about student potential to learn (refer to McCombs, 2001). At the same time, however, specific *beliefs or teaching practices* could be classified as learner-centered (likely to enhance motivation, learning, and success) or non–learner-centered (likely to hinder motivation, learning, and success). Learner-centered teachers are defined as those who meet an empirically validated "learner-centered rubric" related to profiles of beliefs and practices. For example, *believing all students learn* is part of a learner-centered profile, while *believing that some students cannot learn* is part of a non–learner-centered profile. Learner-centered teachers view each student as unique and capable of learning, have a perspective that focuses on the learner knowing that this promotes learning, understand basic principles defining learners and learning, and honor and accept the student's point of view (McCombs & Lauer, 1997; McCombs & Quiat, 1999). As a result, the student's natural inclinations to learn, master the environment, and grow in positive ways are enhanced.

Developing student potential is underscored by the research of Renzulli et al. (1995). This research confirms that all youth, and learning challenged students in particular, benefit from an educational system that values and supports their gifts and diversity—that addresses the personal domain. Renzulli's Schoolwide Enrichment Model, which allows students to pursue curricula matched to their interests, has demonstrated that we need to broaden our limited stereotype of human potential (defined by achievement and intelligence test scores). When students are allowed to govern their own learning process by following their interests, they benefit from a motivation and achievement perspective. Students who would have been classified as low ability or special education have been shown to *outperform* their peers *in their areas of highest interest*. Of critical importance is helping these students to see their learning environments as rich, challenging, personally relevant, accepting, and supportive. The key is to relate to every student as being gifted in a unique way and to design learning experiences and environments that enhance the potential of each student.

The Community for Learning (CFL) program developed by Wang (1998) is a research-based, comprehensive K–12 school reform model that focuses on high standards of student achievement and positive student self-perceptions, particularly for poor minority students from urban and rural areas. The classroom instruction component helps teachers tailor learning experiences to the individual needs of each student in the classroom.

Therefore, the CFL program addresses both the academic and motivational needs of individual students. Based on 20 years of research (Wang, 1992, 1998; Wang et al., 1997), the classroom instruction component, Adaptive Learning Environments Model (ALEM), helps teachers tailor learning experiences to the individual needs of each student in the classroom. Teachers use a variety of strategies to assist students in learning to take responsibility and the initiative for planning and assessing their attainment of educational objectives and standards. Strategies include continually assessing the students to insure that the individually prescribed assignments are working for the learner and modifying the assignments as necessary. Constant individual attention by the teachers is available for students who require more classroom support. The CFL program also recognizes that students learn in environments other than those related to the classroom. To implement this concept as well as provide the organizational structure for program support, a site-based CFL facilitator is trained to connect the community, district, and schools to enhance student and family learning in all environments. These comprehensive features of the overall CFL model have been shown to be particularly beneficial to the special needs students with diverse learning challenges (Wang, 1998; Wang et al., 1997).

2. DEVELOPING PERSONAL AND SOCIAL RESPONSIBILITY

Not only can individualized programs that address the LCPs enhance motivation and academic learning for children with special needs, they can also be applied to areas that develop children's personal and social responsibility. These are the moral dimensions of school as described by Berreth and Berman (1997). Such dimensions attempt to nurture empathy and self-discipline and to help all students develop social skills and moral values. The practices of small schools, caring adults, community service, and parent involvement are recommended, along with processes and practices of modeling, direct instruction, real-world experience, and continual practice. With the framework of the dimensions of emotional intelligence, children with special needs can be assisted to learn and develop high levels of self-awareness, self-control, empathy, perspective taking, and social skills. An important guideline is for students be active partners in creating a caring classroom climate and community (Elias et al., 1997).

As shown by a number of researchers working in the area of self-regulated learning (e.g., Zimmerman, 1994; Zimmerman & Schunk, in press), responsibility begins with making choices. Without the opportunity to choose, make decisions, and face the consequences of those decisions, there is no sense of ownership. A sense of ownership, resulting from choices, is empowering. Without a sense of empowerment and ownership there is no responsibility or accountability—there is blaming and compliance. With ownership, learning is more fun and exciting for both students and teachers, and both share in the pleasures and responsibilities of control. Teachers and students share both responsibility and power—a key feature of learner-centered practices that address the personal domain.

In short, it is the nature of human beings to strive for control and autonomy, to feel they are masters of their own destinies. When learning opportunities are provided to meet this innate need through the inclusion of the personal domain in education, the natural response are feelings of empowerment, ownership, and responsibility. *We own what we create*—an important implication of the LCPs and framework that is increasingly being supported in new leadership and professional development models for special education.

3. A FOCUS ON STUDENT PERCEPTIONS AND VOICE

Another critical implication for practice is that attention be given to the role of student perceptions and input. Freiberg (1998) acknowledges that few climate measures use students as a source of feedback but believes each student's perspective is critical, particularly during transitions from one school level to the next. A concerns survey format (What Students Worry About) is used to collect feedback for reshaping school climates. For middle school students, Freiberg reports that their areas of highest concern were being sent to the principal, failure, drugs, taking tests, and giving a presentation in front of others. High school students reported their areas of highest concern were failure, keeping up with assignments, taking tests, giving a presentation in front of others, and hard class work. Given the importance of this feedback, Freiberg argues that using such measures should be part of all school reform efforts.

Research by Battistich et al. (1997) builds on Deci and Ryan's (1991) research as the theoretical rationale for developing caring school communities through the use of student perception data. They argue that all students have basic psychological needs for belonging, autonomy, and competence, on which their level of engagement/disengagement with school is largely dependent. "Sense of school as community" was assessed by the student perception measure. Items for this measure included: "students in this school work together to solve problems," "people care about each other in this school," and "I feel I can talk to the teachers in this school about things that are bothering me." Results of their research with middle school students indicated that their scores on this measure were consistently associated with a positive orientation toward school and learning, including attraction to school, task orientation toward learning, educational aspirations, and trust and respect for teachers. The data also indicated that students' perceptions of community were positively associated with pro-social attitudes, social skills, and sense of autonomy and efficacy; they were negatively related to students' drug use and involvement in delinquent behavior. The findings of Battistich et al. are consistent with other research showing that when schools are experienced as communities, they satisfy basic psychological needs, and students will become attached to such schools and accept their values.

Recent work by King (2000) directly relates to hearing the voices of students with a variety of emotional and learning challenges. She studied the effects of students' educational status (special education [SPED], non–special education [NSPED]) and type of classroom (learner-centered [LC], non–learner-centered [NLC]) in terms of how it affected students' perceptions of their teachers' practices, their motivation, and their achievement. Students studied were in grades 6 and 7 from five suburban middle schools, for a total of 657 students, 167 of whom were SPED and 490 of whom were NSPED. Students classified as SPED were those identified for participation in inclusion classrooms who had a variety of special learning needs. These learning needs ranged from mild learning disabilities, behavioral disorders, and mental retardation. Students with more severe learning needs who were in self-contained SPED classrooms or who had such poor reading or attentional issues that they could not complete the questionnaire were excluded from the study.

The gender mix for SPED/NSPED was 54/262 female and 113/228 male students; the LC/NLC breakdown for SPED/NSPED was 92/224 female and 102/239 male students. Using the ALCP (McCombs, 1999), surveys for students and teachers, primary findings were:

1. SPED students perceived significantly lower rates of LC teacher practices, had lower motivation, and have lower achievement than their NSPED peers.
2. SPED students in NLC classrooms had the lowest achievement of all student groups.
3. Both SPED and NSPED student perceptions were a better measure of LC versus NLC classrooms than either teacher perceptions or outside observations.
4. SPED students perceived LC teachers to be more caring than NLC teachers; however, even with LC teachers, SPED students did not perceive as much support for practices that encouraged their use of higher-order thinking and learning skills as NSPED students, indicating differential treatment from NSPED students.

Based on these findings, King concluded that although caring is an important attribute of LC classrooms, SPED students also need the same level of support for critical thinking and learning skills as their NSPED peers. She concludes that the challenge is to prepare teachers to give the kind of individual attention to diverse learning needs of SPED students via accommodations and adjustments while *not eliminating* the needs of these SPED students for a challenging learning experience that prepares them for meaningful and lifelong skill development.

4. A FOCUS ON CARING AND CRITICAL RELATIONSHIPS

A case can certainly be made for the importance of caring and positive development for all students. Elias et al. (1997, p. 6) state: "Caring is central to the shaping of relationships that are meaningful, supportive, rewarding, and productive. Caring happens when children sense that adults in their lives think they are important and accept and respect them, regardless of any particular talents they have. Caring is a product of a community that deems all of its members to be important, believes everyone has something to contribute, and acknowledges that everyone counts." Further, children considered at-risk for any number of reasons, including having some type of learning disability, are those most frequently growing up without caring. But can the importance of caring be acknowledged as a critical part of the reform agenda for children with special learning needs and challenges?

In describing issues involved, Palmer (1999) argues that we need to acknowledge that teaching and learning not only involve intellect and emotion, but also involve the human spirit. He underscores the point that teaching and learning are not either-or in the sense of being intellectual or spiritual. In his words (p. 10): "Teaching and learning, done well, are done not by disembodied intellects but by whole persons whose minds cannot be disconnected from feeling and spirit, from heart and soul. To teach as a whole person to the whole person is not to lose one's professionalism as a teacher but to take it to a deeper level." He contends that teachers—regardless of their subject matter and who their students are—end up teaching *who* they are. The biggest challenge is to provide teachers with adequate time and support to reflect on questions that are worth living. The time for self-reflection can renew and transform their practices and ways of relating to self and others. Teachers need opportunities to learn and change their minds.

Lipsitz (1995) also argues that to develop a caring culture in schools requires a change in attitude—not just a restructuring of policies, curricula, and systems. Caring is necessary for establishing an effective culture for learning. It does not replace high expectations and standards for learning, but represents a core set of beliefs about relating to other people. In describing benefits of caring school cultures, Chaskin and Rauner (1995) focus on the effect of the teacher/student relationship that is often overlooked: the ability of such relationships to offset students' feelings of frustration with or alienation from school. Caring was found to be what differentiated successful from unsuccessful programs in research funded by the Lily Endowment's Research Program on Youth and Caring. Caring works because it responds to the basic psychosocial needs, particularly for connection, belonging and membership, safety and support, and individual and social competency. It also creates a "context of possibilities" in which genuine education occurs through relationships, settings, and practices that encourage youth to value caring as a way to approach the self and others, including the larger community and society.

Research has shown that when youth with diverse backgrounds and capabilities have opportunities to care for others they have an increased sense of social responsibility, higher self-esteems, better school attendance, and decreases in depression. To accomplish lasting effects and true trusting relationships, strategies for promoting cultures of caring in schools need to be implemented gradually and incrementally by committed individuals. Chaskin and Rauner (1995) emphasize that there is no single best way to promote caring cultures, that caring has to be promoted by example and, to be successful, the particular caring culture that evolves needs to be relevant to particular interpersonal and academic needs of its clients, students, and teachers alike.

According to Noddings (1995), the technical and structural changes necessary to create cultures of caring in schools are relatively simple and inexpensive to accomplish. She identifies the larger issue of achieving a fundamental attitude shift among educators, policymakers, and the public. They must be convinced that in addition to responding to the pressure to produce high test scores, it is legitimate and even necessary to focus on the development of caring and competent people. School time spent developing trusting relationships, talking with students about personal problems, and guiding them to be more sensitive and competent across all domains of caring must also be deemed valuable. This type of intervention is particularly critical for helping students with special learning needs to feel like a valued part of the school community.

B. Concrete Suggestions for Applying the Learner-Centered Framework in Practice

Understanding the basic principles of learning and motivation provides a foundation for analyzing and designing interventions that enhance motivation and achievement for children with learning disabilities and challenges. One way in which learner-centered activities can be easily introduced into the learning context is through project-based instruction. McWhorter et al. (1996) offer the following suggestions to teachers for making project-based instruction learner-centered:

1. Solicit and encourage student input into the daily workings of the classroom. Negotiate classroom decisions between the teacher and students within acceptable parameters.
2. Provide students with a range of choices in activities, reading material, and subject matter—in all aspects of their learning.
3. Connect student learning to the outside world or integrate material into a meaningful context.
4. Encourage students to examine their own work, critique its strengths and weaknesses, and set goals for continued improvement.
5. Balance depth of learning and content coverage. Learning activities should serve multiple purposes and/or objectives in order to maximize instructional time.
6. Involve students in determining the standards and criteria for assessment within the framework of the instructional project and the larger context of the skills required.
7. Establish flexible parameters for projects that permit change for the purpose of increasing student interest and learning.

Designing learning contexts that are responsive to diverse learner needs can be simplified by asking the learners directly. McWhorter et al. (1996) summarize the following lessons learned by teachers who involved all of their students in generating learning experiences:

- *The classroom environment must be conducive to collaboration between the teacher and the students.* That is, teachers need to take time to get to know students and let students get to know each other. Projects need to grow out of student interests and concerns. To facilitate collaboration, teachers should provide the widest range of choices in reading material, presentation options, and assessment methods.
- *The teacher must be willing to share responsibility for learning with the students by developing and nurturing a sense of mutual trust.* Trust and respect are facilitated when there is tolerance for mistakes and opportunities to learn from mistakes. The strategy of negotiation must become common to all.
- *A strong emphasis on group dynamics, teamwork, and collaboration is essential in student-centered/student-generated learning experiences.* To support group and team working experiences, teachers need to help students understand the strengths and weaknesses of group members.

Teachers must also help students strengthen their commitment to work well with each other and respect diversity.

- *Teachers must allocate more instructional time during the initial development of student-centered learning contexts to permit talk about learning, negotiation, and decision-making.* To invite and use student input in structuring learning opportunities requires additional time.
- *Developing a teaching style that places students at the center of concern, that involves students in instructional decision-making, and visualizing one's new role as teacher is a gradual process.* Implementation of a student-centered learning environment involves changing how teachers regard their role. Teachers gradually become dissatisfied with the old way of doing things and evolve to being a facilitator or guide. Once the teacher feels comfortable with and accepts this new role, the energy of both students and teachers is increased, along with student motivation and personal engagement.
- *Students often have difficulty becoming active learners, particularly students who have been successful in teacher-centered classrooms.* Teachers need to understand that for students who have become accustomed to being "passive" learners, they may at first resist more active and responsible roles. Students need time in the context of carefully coordinated experiences to adjust to the new learning environment and responsibilities. Adjustment is facilitated when there is a sense of community in the classroom.

In my own work (McCombs, 1995, 1998, 2001, 2003a,b) I have outlined what I see as three primary areas of intervention for enhancing motivation to learn: (1) *learner-focused interventions*, (2) *interventions that focus on learning tasks and instructional materials*, and (3) *interventions that focus on instructional contexts and practices*. The basis of this work has emerged from those who see schools as "living systems"—systems that are in service to learners and serve the basic function of learning for the primary recipient (the learner) as well as the other humans who support learning (teachers, administrators, parents). Building on the living systems concept, proponents of this "learner-centered" perspective contend that education and schooling must concern itself with how to provide the most supportive learning context for diverse students—a context that is created primarily by the teacher and where that teacher "comes from" in terms of valuing and understanding the rich array of individual differences and needs that students present (e.g., Marshall, 1998; Sarason, 1995). From this perspective, curriculum and content are important but not the exclusive factors for achieving desired motivation, learning, and achievement. Attention to meeting individual learner needs and considering student perceptions of the degree to which these needs are being met are as important and fundamental to how well content is learned.

Those working within a living systems framework also contend that system change is the result of personal change and of critical connections (Wheatley & Kellner-Rogers, 1998). That is, personal change in one's perceptions, values, attitudes, and beliefs results from transformations in thinking. In turn, transformations in thinking most often result from critical connections that are made by the person in their understanding, knowledge, and ways of thinking, as well as critical connections or personal relationships that are made between the person and others of significance in the learning environment. For example, a teacher confronted with the awareness that prior instructional practices are not working with a new group of students is most likely to change those practices to more learner-centered approaches if: (1) he or she learns that this group of students has a higher level of prior knowledge about topics being covered than prior groups of students (new information component); and (2) a valued colleague has worked with similar students successfully with new instructional practices that give the students more choice and control over the instructional process (personal relationship component).

As people in living systems, such as education, are given more opportunities to be creatively involved in how their work is accomplished, Wheatley and Kellner-Rogers (1998) contend that not only will they create conditions that facilitate rapid change (new relationships, new insights, greater levels of commitment), but they also will increase their capacity for learning and growth. When individuals are engaged in designing the changes, they create more and better connections and relationships that can help the system change from within. Although the availability of new and richer information helps people change personal constructions of meaning and understanding, it is increasing the number, variety, and strengths of interpersonal connections and relationships that moves the system toward better functioning and health. Standards of functioning are not imposed or mandated from outside, but rather, these standards, measures, values, organizational structures, and plans need to come from within, through ongoing dialogue and conversations in which people share perceptions, seek out a diversity of interpretations, and agree on what needs to be done. Thus, the three primary areas of intervention for enhancing motivation to learn flow from this research base.

First, in *learner-focused interventions*, the goal is to help students develop their metacognitive self-awareness and understanding of the function of thought and self-as-agent. These interventions are particularly helpful for students with disabilities and learning challenges as it is frequently assumed that they are not capable of higher-order thinking processes. The focus is on helping students learn how to step outside their conditioned beliefs about their capabilities, see that they can control their thoughts, and access natural self-esteem and motivation to learn. Students are taught dispositions and strategies for developing various types of thinking found helpful to learning and achievement. These include teaching students the following kinds of thinking dispositions and strategies:

1. Thinking that establishes the personal meaning of learning (e.g., strategies for constructing meaning, such as personal stories, and strategies for establishing personal relevance, such as relating to personal interests and prior knowledge);
2. Thinking that facilitates self-regulation of learning (e.g., strategies for setting learning goals, managing and controlling learning, and monitoring and evaluating learning);
3. Thinking that encourages reflective self-awareness (e.g., strategies for reflecting and analyzing meaning or for examining choices in thinking and actions); and
4. Thinking that engages creativity and problem-solving (e.g., strategies for developing progressively deeper insight, such as brainstorming and imagination exercises).

Another area of thinking that can be taught is that of goal setting. Teachers who wish to develop a learning goal orientation among students should provide activities that are meaningful and interesting, minimize social comparisons, reward and recognize personal learning growth and improvement, provide opportunities for peer collaboration, and enable students to make decisions and choices.

In the second area of intervention, *learning tasks and instructional materials*, the objective is to increase the personal relevance and meaningfulness of learning tasks such that they approximate "authentic" thinking and learning experiences from the students' perspectives. Learning tasks support student choice and autonomy, while also helping students understand the responsibilities and benefits of their agency in the learning process. Current research has shown that it is critical—for enhancing and drawing on students' natural curiosity and motivation to learn—to relate learning tasks and materials to what students perceive as important (i.e., to personal interests and self-goals). Not only is it important that the *content* be perceived as personally meaningful, but it is also important that the process of learning new knowledge and skills is meaningful from the students' perspectives and related to how they think and learn. Thus, instructional materials and learning tasks are most personally meaningful and engaging to students if they:

1. Are interdisciplinary and integrative, with tasks meaningful from the students' perspectives and representative of real-world issues and complexities while providing for group learning experiences that recognize the social nature of learning and the need for students to apply what they have learned outside the classroom context;
2. Provide opportunities for individual and group learning, student choice and support for autonomy, cooperative versus competitive achievement opportunities, and facilitate the pursuit of learning as opposed to performance goals;
3. Provide challenges, stimulate curiosity, allow for creative and self-determining constructions and expressions of knowledge, and engage imagination; and
4. Teach basic skills, such as those involved in reading or mathematics, in the context of larger themes or topics that students perceive to be meaningful and that require the development of particular skills as a logical part of the process of exploring or learning about the topic area.

In the third area of interventions, *instructional contexts and practices*, the objective is to create climates of positive social and emotional support by attending to positive social relationships that operate reciprocally for students and teachers (McCombs, 1995, 1998). Interventions include creating opportunities for teachers and students to role-play and model effective behavior, and to participate in simulated listening and interpersonal activities. In essence, as teachers themselves experience the self-determining, self-constructive nature of learning and a positive climate of support and quality relationships, they can internalize new roles and metaphors of teaching that are consistent with the current knowledge base on learning and learners' needs. Functions of teaching that enhance teachers' roles as a motivator include:

1. Diagnosing and understanding students' unique needs, interests, and goals;
2. Helping students define their own personal goals and the relationship of these personal goals to learning goals;
3. Relating learning content/activities to students' personal needs, interests, and goals;
4. Challenging students to invest effort and energy in taking personal responsibility and to be actively involved in learning activities;
5. Providing students with opportunities to exercise personal control and choice over selected task variables such as the type of learning activity, ways of demonstrating personal mastery, and skills to master;

6. Creating a safe, trusting, and supportive climate by showing real interest, caring, and concern for each student;
7. Attending to classroom goal structures and goal orientations, with an emphasis on cooperative structures and learning goals;
8. Modeling both self-directed learning skills and personal qualities associated with positive interpersonal relationships;
9. Highlighting the value of student accomplishment, the value of students' unique skills and abilities, and the value of the learning process and the learning task; and
10. Rewarding students' accomplishments and encouraging them to reward themselves and develop pride in their accomplishments.

In *summary*, interventions that can promote motivation and engagement in educational settings include the following:

- Opportunities for taking personal responsibility for learning activities and outcomes;
- Participatory decision-making, goal-setting, alternative performance assessments;
- Individual goals and standards of learning and mastery versus grading and evaluation;
- Instructional practices that encourage initiative, self-expression, and imagination;
- Reciprocal empowerment of teachers and students through flexible structures and respectful relationships; and
- Quality interpersonal interactions with teachers who demonstrate genuine concern, caring, and interest in students.

Conditions need to be created that provide choice, challenge, control, collaboration, opportunities to construct meaning, and positive consequences in the learning context. From my own work (McCombs, 1995, 2000, 2001, 2003a,b; McCombs & Whisler, 1997), we have identified a number of additional conditions for addressing LCPs. These conditions were identified in research with over 20,000 students from kindergarten through high school. It was also verified that all four domains addressed by the LCPs (APA, 1997) must be present for maximum motivation and achievement. Attention must be provided to practices that enhance cognitive and metacognitive factors, affective and motivational factors, social and developmental factors, and other individual difference factors including developmental and ability differences in students. To addresses the LCPs in each of these domains, conditions present in the learning context must include opportunities to experience personal relevance, responsibility, respect, cooperation, competence, connections to personal interests/talents, and positive relationships with adults and peers. Strategies, such as peer tutoring and mentoring, are especially helpful for children with disabilities and learning challenges, but these approaches work best when a positive learning climate and community have first been established between and among students and their teachers.

C. Implications for Policy

In the area of *policy*, a number of recommendations can be given to help balance current reform efforts that emphasize punitive, high-stakes testing, and accountability sanctions. Practices, such as grading of schools, teachers, and administrators based on the quality of their students' learning and achievement, can misplace the responsibility for learning (refer to McCombs, 2000). Vatterott (1995) points out that although teachers are held responsible for student learning, *it is the student who makes the decision to learn*. Teachers *cannot make learning happen*; they can encourage and persuade with a variety of incentives. And teachers know well that many incentives (e.g., grades, fear of discipline) work only for some students. When teachers overly control the learning process or impose responsibility within the teacher's parameters and rules, they may get obedience or compliance, but they will not get responsibility.

Reliance on learning research has resulted in a growing emphasis on high standards, thematic and integrated curricula, instructional practices that help all learners—teachers and diverse students alike—take a more active and responsible role in directing their own learning. New assessment methods focus not only on what learners know but what they can do to demonstrate and apply that knowledge in real-life or life-like settings. These technical changes (i.e., domains of educational systems design that are concerned with standards, curriculum, instruction, and assessment) and organizational changes (management structures and policies) have occurred in response to what is known about optimal learning. However, the research demonstrates (refer to, Fullan, 1996; Joyce & Calhoun, 1995) that technical and organizational changes are not sufficient because they often downplay the role of the learner and learning environment. Similarly, they rarely focus on or provide effective strategies for off-setting the problems of alienation, lack of engagement, fear of failure, or stress and overwhelm. Without a focus on individual learners, those students who are "different" can be singled out for bullying and other problems. Thus, people, all of whom are learners, must be the focus—together with a focus on the learning process, which is innate and lifelong for all people.

1. FINDING THE RIGHT BALANCE

Policies governing educational systems design must balance the concerns with: (1) standards and learning outcomes; (2) how standards are implemented and assessed; and (3) assumptions about human nature, learning, and the capacities of individual learners. They must honor diverse talents and abilities, diverse interests and motivations, and seek to broaden rather than narrow the rich diversity of students that enter at preschool age and exit as young adults. These policies must take seriously research findings of Gardner (1993, 1995), Renzulli et al. (1995), and Goleman (1995) that show the value of programs based on new assumptions about intelligence and the powerful role of interest and emotions in learning and achievement.

All learners have a right to be responsible for helping to create the best climates and learning experiences that meet their special learning needs (Margalit, 2001). Margalit (2001) points out that international work on the rights of children receiving special education services is increasingly using an educational-preventive approach that can enhance the emotional resilience of all students, help them develop confidence in themselves and their surroundings, increase their willingness to perceive difficulties as challenges, and enhance their ability to cope with difficult situations. Special education policies are thus focusing on strength and resilience models that can increase the participation of all learners—with and without disabilities—to be active participants in their own learning and in the development of positive school cultures.

Policies must emphasize new leadership roles through the use of strategies that empower teachers and students alike to take increased control over their own learning and development. For example, increased attention is needed for programs such "Generation WHY" developed by Harper (1997, 1998) that are listening to what kids have to say. Students in grades 6 to 12 are involved as partners and leaders in collaboration with teachers, the local community, higher education, and corporate sponsors to assist in the restructuring of education through telecommunications. New positive relationships are formed between youth and teachers and new school cultures of mutual respect and caring have emerged. Students who would have dropped out of school are now making plans to attend college and/or enter high-tech careers.

2. THE IMPORTANCE OF A LIVING SYSTEMS FRAMEWORK

From a broad systems view, a growing body of educators, researchers, and policymakers are converging in their opinions that the current educational systems are not working (e.g., Nissen, 1999; Norris, 1999; Wheatley, 1999). They see them as not only unconnected but based on outdated thinking and old models of human learning, growth, and development. Further, these current systems are often based on principles applicable to non-living, mechanical systems and do not match the uncertainty and complexity of living, human systems. Thus, it is time to explore a new model that includes what is needed in living systems to bring the system into balance. It is time to support a cycle of positive teacher and youth development and learning.

Why and how does learner-centeredness address a balance in perspectives? Examples abound of schools that are implementing practices consistent with research on learning (e.g., Fullan, 1997). In some cases, these examples show high success and in others, they do not. What accounts for this difference? When successful efforts are analyzed, the critical difference is in *how* these practices are implemented and in whether there is explicit and shared attention given to individual learners and their unique cognitive as well as social and emotional learning needs. Thus, *the critical difference is whether or not they are learner-centered and have a focus on the personal domain—on learners as well as on learning.*

A focus on the learner and the personal domain emerges from those who see schools as "living systems" (Wheatley and Kellner-Rogers, 1998). People in living systems such as education thrive when they are given more opportunities to be creatively involved in how their work gets done, i.e., setting their own standards, measures, values, organizational structures, and plans from within. This is best accomplished through an ongoing dialogue in which people share perceptions, seek out a diversity of interpretations, and agree on what needs to be done. In this process of learning and change, research-validated principles that are agreed upon can be guides to determine what will work well in the current situation or context such that the system is designed to take care of the self, others, and the place (Wheatley & Kellner-Rogers, 1998).

3. REDUCING ISOLATION AND BARRIERS TO INCLUSION

In many K–12 institutions and particularly in secondary education settings, teachers and disciplines are isolated from each other. It is difficult to find examples of cross-department collaborations in course design, multidisciplinary learning opportunities, organizational structures, or physical facilities that allow interactions and dialogue among teachers or instructors. Content and people are isolated and fragmented. Change is often mandated from above or outside the system. Critical connections are not being made and thus change is difficult and often resisted because of personal fears or insecurities. Those fears and insecurities disappear when people participate together in creating how their work gets done. This includes all staff, parents, and the students themselves in creating positive learning and social experiences.

Work by Fullan (1995) on systemic educational reform highlights the importance of creating cultures in which people are free to share basic beliefs and values as well as the struggle to bring these into agreement in a mission and vision for the school. Weinstein (1998) further argues that to accomplish school-level changes, it is necessary to help both teachers and students "change their minds" or modify their current thinking. One example of such a change in thinking is teachers learning to value student perceptions of practice. They then use negotiation strategies, working together collaboratively with their students to define changes in practice and expectations. When beliefs change, teacher practices and school climate also change. Student outcomes then shift to more positive expectations, higher motivation, increased learning, and higher achievement. Critical in the context of enhancing the motivation and achievement of students with disabilities and learning challenges is the opportunity to form relationships among all students, teachers, administrators, parents, and the larger community. These relationships are central to "changing one's mind" and appreciating diverse perspectives. As Brendtro (1999) has argued, the broken bonds between and among at-risk students, teachers, and others are best healed through practices that help engender empathy and the ability to see other perspectives.

The spirit of vitality of learner-centered schools is that aspect of the culture committed to learning and change. Research shows that teachers' needs to be learners must be part of a culture that supports student motivation, learning, and achievement. The nature of the culture formed among teachers committed to high achievement for all learners is one that is also committed to ongoing learning, change, and improvement. Fullan (1993) suggests that the following characterize such a culture: (1) commitment to being agents of educational and social improvement; (2) commitment to continuous improvement through program innovation and evaluation; (3) valuing and practicing exemplary teaching; (4) engaging in constant inquiry; (5) modeling and developing life-long learning among staff and students; (6) modeling and developing collaboration among staff and students; (7) being respected and engaged as a vital part of the whole system; (8) forming partnerships with relevant groups and agencies; (9) being visible and valued in the local and global community; and (10) working collaboratively to build regional, national, and international networks.

4. BUILDING A NEW CULTURE

It is important to note that building a culture of learning, caring, and change must be *built from within* the organization. The process must be one that supports continuous examination and improvement of the education process at every level (Joyce & Calhoun, 1995). Critical inquiry into ways of helping students learn better must become a normal activity that involves the whole faculty and builds community. An outcome of facilitating this kind of change from within, as reported Joyce and Calhoun (1995), is that faculty realize that teaching and learning involves a *neverending process* of trying to reach all students in the best ways currently known. The vision is subject to change, and the whole system maintains flexibility and openness to new learning, transformation, and change.

Caine and Caine (1997) define a learning community as a community with shared values, a common agenda, and collegial connections with and among teachers and students. An addition for me is that communities have the further defining qualities of acceptance of, room for, and honoring of all diverse views. In healthy learner-centered learning communities, individuals welcome divergent perspectives because they understand that the underlying outcome is learning and change in a context of respect and caring. Individuals also understand that learning communities broaden their perspectives to make room for the learning that can occur to encompass all points of view without making anyone wrong. The healthy learning community works for everyone and encourages rather than eliminates diverse perspectives. When different world views and beliefs are held, inclusive dialogue becomes the process for learning and relationships become the vehicle for change. As Caine and Caine (1997) acknowledge, learning communities facilitate self-organization as a natural process in adaptive, living systems. They meet individual needs for safety and security, and they encourage new relationships and ways of generating new relationships. In the context of positive relationships and climate for learning, beliefs and assumptions about learning, learners, and teaching can be examined. Active listening, reflection, and critical questioning are tools of the learning dialogue.

Each learner's perspective is a valued and honored medium of learning and a catalyst for change and improvement in programs that value quality. These programs themselves must be a model of the very process and quality they want to engender in teachers as learners. To produce quality teaching and learning, learners must experience both quality content and processes. Systems that foster quality by fear-based or punitive measures engender fear, withdrawal, and half-hearted compliance. Unfortunately, this is coloring much of today's reform agenda. As Rudduck et al. (1997) have recognized, the successful change agenda creates time for dialogue and engages all learners in the process of exploring standards for judging quality. Principles of respect, fairness, autonomy, intellectual challenge, social support, and security guide the standard-setting and implementation process. Time for learning and change, to share successful practices, experiment, and continually improve are provided for and acknowledged.

For learner- and person-centered practices such as these to become realities, however, teachers need to become more aware of their relationship with students as knowledge generators and active participants in their own learning. When power is shared by students and teachers, teaching methods become a means to an end rather than an end in themselves. As Schaps and Lewis (1999) report in reflections on the "perils" of building school community, it is essential for schoolwide change to have a dual emphasis on: (1) a sense of community *and* on academic learning, and (2) student *and* teacher thinking and voice in shaping classroom lessons and decisions. To apply such practices, research-validated principles are needed to guide their design. The knowledge base underlying the principles of learners and learning becomes a research-validated foundation for comprehensive school reform that focuses on meeting cognitive, social, and emotional human needs and fostering positive teacher/student relationships. The principles lead to understanding students as knowledge generators, active participants in their own learning, and co-creators of learning experiences and curricula.

Even with attention to a research-validated and learner-centered perspective there is perhaps still a missing piece. This piece, called "the inner edge," was named by Holmes-Ponder et al. (1999). It more broadly addresses the personal domain and spiritual condition of school leaders and teachers. Holmes-Ponder et al. (1999) point out that to truly transform education and allow *all learners to live and work successfully* requires that people relate differently to themselves and to each other. It also requires deep self-knowledge and a strong connection to one's purpose for living. This requires an awareness of spiritual influences and conditions that support or erode a sense of self and the difference one is making in the mission to support learning for all. Educators, policymakers, and researchers must reconnect the nation's teachers with feelings of empowerment and spiritual joy that originally brought them to teaching and learning. From this perspective, collaboration adds *a spirit of community and success*—a process that recognizes teachers' collective and shared self.

III. IMPLICATIONS FOR RESEARCH

To advance the study of how best to enhance motivation and achievement for children with learning challenges and disabilities, it is essential that there be ongoing *research*. Part of this research must keep pace with new developments influencing our understanding of intelligence. These include interdisciplinary fields of research that can offer multiple perspectives on complex human phenomena. Ochsner and Lieberman (2001) describe the emergence of social cognitive neuroscience that allows three levels of analysis: (1) a social level concerned with motivational and social factors influencing behavior and experience; (2) a cognitive level concerned with information processing mechanisms that underlie social-level phenomena; and (3) a neural level concerned with brain mechanisms that instantiate cognitive processes. Although still in its infancy, this multidisciplinary field promises to provide new insights about human functioning that can be useful in studying learners and learning in complex living systems, such as schools. It also follows the trend toward more integrative and holistic research practices.

Consistent with this integrative trend is research by Robinson et al. (2000) on the similarities and differences between people at the two tails of the normal curve, the mentally retarded and the gifted. As operationalized in tests of intelligence, deviance from the norm by performance two standard deviations from the mean (IQ of 70–75 or lower, or IQ of 125–130 or higher) typically defines individuals who are mentally retarded or gifted, respectively. In looking at educational issues, Robinson et al. (2000) raise the following points:

- A one-size-fits-all paradigm for education does not accommodate individual differences in level and pace of learning, creating major problems for meeting the needs of diverse students in the current system designed for the average student.
- Strategies and approaches that work well for gifted children need to become models for improving the school experiences of all children.
- The basic philosophies and values of American schools are in keeping, at least theoretically, with the concept of adapting to individual differences in abilities, thereby providing an opportunity for our schools to become models of how best to deal with students in the two tails of the normal curve.
- More work is needed to solve the problems of economic and ethnic disadvantages that skew distributions of IQ scores leading to discrimination by gender, race, and ethnic origin in terms of over-placement of minority students in special services and under-representation of minority students in gifted services.
- Research agendas in areas such as neurodevelopmental science, brain function, and genetics need to look at both ends of longitudinal studies that can provide insight into how to design interventions that overcome current maladaptive approaches to learning and performance which can hinder retarded and gifted students.

1. BASIC RESEARCH DIRECTIONS

Taking these developments and my own learner-centered perspective into account, a number of suggestions can be made, including the following:

- Research that can further refine and elucidate alternative conceptions of ability and intelligence and broaden our understanding of the interplay between cognitive, affective, neurobiological, and social factors that influence the development of competencies.
- Research on effective uses of peer tutoring, problem-based learning, intersections of cooperative learning and curriculum, strategies for professional development and follow-up support for cooperative learning, and how well cooperative learning works for learning challenged students or other students at the margins.
- Research on promoting literacy for struggling readers, along with more research on how teaching word recognition or phonics also affects these readers, and how to develop teachers to deliver motivational reading and writing programs.
- Research on the cultural aspects of learning and contrasts between various theoretical perspectives in terms of their usefulness as alternative views for understanding the sociocultural context of the teaching and learning process for children with learning challenges and disabilities.
- Research that explores relations between self-regulation and volition, the development of self-regulation in children with different learning challenges and disabilities, appropriate strategies for teaching self-regulation within the curriculum, and how to promote self-regulation across the lifespan.

2. APPLIED RESEARCH DIRECTIONS

Along with these basic research directions, more applied research is needed on the contexts of learning environments best suited to the diverse needs of children with special learning needs. This research must consider the complex interactions between personal, organizational, and community levels of learning in schools as living systems. From my learner-centered perspective, attention is needed to applied research in the following areas:

- Research on teacher development including what teachers cite as the biggest challenge—the students themselves. Excellent teaching is called a complex balancing act and research that identifies excellent teachers already effectively reaching a range of special needs children is needed.
- Research on what can be learned about motivation, learning, and human adaptability in existing schools as they begin to increasingly use e-learning technologies in new ways. These new ways of learning promise to create a new paradigm for learning and assessment that can reduce barriers to learning and motivation for children with special learning needs.

- Research to better understand the comprehensive dimensions of successful schools as: (1) promoting a sense of belonging and agency, (2) engaging families in children's learning and education, (3) using a quality and integrated curriculum, (4) providing ongoing professional development in both content and child development areas (including pedagogy appropriate to a range of learning challenges and disabilities), (5) having high student expectations, and (6) providing opportunities for success for all students.
- Research to identify the best socialization experiences for positive adjustment with diverse student populations. This research needs to examine how different groups of children understand rules and norms, how these change, and how they are complementary or compatible with peer and adult norms. This research also needs to examine what differential impacts that teachers' reward structures have, depending on students' particular learning needs and family environment, and further examine student beliefs and perceptions of social support from teachers and peers for diverse groups of students.
- Research that identifies teacher preparation practices that can foster the development of metacognition in all groups of students. Teacher preparation programs that are successful in preparing teachers to teach metacognitive strategies to all groups of learning-challenged and special-need students must be identified, including the strategies for how teachers are prepared to apply metacognition to their own instruction.
- Research on school-based methodologies for studying the complex interrelationships between and among individual, organizational, and community levels of learning and functioning that can provide solid and credible evidence to support conclusions about the best approaches to build inclusive, caring, and learner-centered learning communities.

IV. CONCLUSIONS

In order to bring harmony and balance to conflicting views on how to promote high motivation and achievement for all students and particularly learning-inefficient children, it is necessary to acknowledge the *holistic needs of all people in the system*. Fullan (1997) speaks to the roles of emotion and hope during times of intense change and pressure. He suggests that in such times the barriers to learning and change must be reduced. These include isolation, lack of empathy, not giving intuition and emotion a respected role, and supporting hope as a healthy virtue. To be effective, educational reform must be constructive and build individual and group capacity to handle negative emotions, frustrations, and fears while maintaining hope and the commitment to future positive possibilities. For me, that means beginning with research-validated, LCPs.

These LCPs confirm the foundation for best practice and give permission to slow down, reflect on the needs of all learners, establish trust, and use our collective knowledge of best practices for supporting optimal learning and development for all learners. When this happens, we stop looking for the quick fix and begin seeing what defines quality learning, teaching, and continuing motivation for the life-long learning process. High learning standards and quality teaching are balanced with a concern for supporting *all learners*, including those teachers and administrators committed to the education of all children. School pressures and alienation are reduced rather than increased, while supporting high standards. In this context, programs and practices for students with a variety of learning challenges can be positively evaluated as a framework for defining quality programs.

In summary, LCPs and learner-centered practices suggest that the best way to enhance motivation and achievement in *all* learners is to understand the importance of students' beliefs in themselves as successful learners. The problem is that many learning-disabled and learning-challenged students do not believe this and/or do not understand how to be responsible for their own learning. The research-validated LCPs help us to understand how to help students know their worth, their competencies, their abilities to choose and be in control, and their own role in generating the will to learn.

An understanding of the research on learning and learners helps us to see that all children are gifted and talented—in different ways. We have a responsibility in the systems that serve the function of educating all school-age children to foster the kinds of beliefs, learning environments, and learning communities that benefit all learners and value their diversity. To do less is to perpetuate negative stereotyping and treatment of children with certain kinds of intellectual, emotional, social, or physical differences. We know that such negative thinking and practice for special-needs children leads to lower learning and achievement, to greater personal and interpersonal conflict, and to higher levels of despair and hopelessness for a growing number of children. We can do better than that. To guide our thinking and practice, there is a set of research-validated LCPs that can provide the foundation for new schooling designs. The new designs are those that develop and reward high levels of learning and academic achievement for all learners in diverse and individual areas and ways. Practices that emerge from these learner-centered designs are those that help all learners form valued attitudes, skills, and dispositions for learning and for life.

REFERENCES

Alexander, P. A., & Murphy, P. K. (1998). The research base for APA's learner-centered psychological principles. In N. Lambert & B. L. McCombs (Eds.), *How students learn: Reforming schools through learner-centered education*. Washington, DC: American Psychological Association.

APA Task Force on Psychology in Education (1993, January). *Learner-centered psychological principles: Guidelines for school redesign and reform*. Washington, DC: American Psychological Association and Mid-Continent Regional Educational Laboratory.

APA Work Group of the Board of Educational Affairs (1997, November). *Learner-centered psychological principles: A framework for school reform and redesign*. Washington, DC: American Psychological Association.

Bartolome, L. I. (1994). Beyond the methods fetish: Toward a humanizing pedagogy. *Harvard Educational Review, 64*(2), 173–194.

Battistich, V., Soloman, D., Watson, M., & Schaps, E. (1997). Caring school communities. *Educational Psychologist, 32*(3), 137–151.

Berreth, D., & Berman, S. (1997). The moral dimensions of schools. *Educational Leadership, 54*(8), 24–27.

Brendtro, L. K. (1999, June). *Tools for reclaiming at-risk youth*. Keynote presentation at the 8th Annual Rocky Mountain Regional Conference in Violence Prevention in Schools and Communities, Denver.

Burnette, J. (1996). Including students with disabilities in general education classrooms: From policy to practice. *ERIC Review: Inclusion, 4*(3), 1–13.

Burrell, S., & Warboys, L. (2000, July). Special education and the juvenile justice system. *Juvenile Justice Bulletin*. Office of Juvenile Justice and Delinquency Prevention.

Caine, R. N., & Caine, G. (1997). *Education on the edge of possibility*. Alexandria, VA: Association for Supervision and Curriculum Development.

Chaskin, R. J., & Rauner, D. M. (1995). Youth and caring: An introduction. *Phi Delta Kappan, 76*(9), 667–674.

Darling-Hammond, L. (1996). The quiet revolution: Rethinking teacher development. *Educational Leadership, 53*(6), 4–10.

Deci, E. L., & Ryan, R. M. (1991). A motivational approach to self: Integration in personality. In R. Dienstbier (Ed.), *Nebraska symposium on motivation: Perspectives on motivation* (Vol. 38). Lincoln, NE: University of Nebraska Press.

Elias, M. J., Zims, J. E., Weissberg, R. P., Frey, K. DS., Greenberg, M. T., Haynes, N. M., Kessler, R., Schwab-Stone, M. E., & Shriver, T. P. (1997). *Promoting social and emotional learning: Guidelines for educators*. Alexandria, VA: Association for Supervision and Curriculum Development.

Freiberg, H. J. (1998). Measuring school climate: Let me count the ways. *Educational Leadership, 56*(1), 22–26.

Fullan, M. G. (1993). Why teachers must become change agents. *Educational Leadership, 51*(7), 12–17.

Fullan, M. G. (1995). The limits and the potential of professional development. In T. R. Guskey & M. Huberman (Eds.), *Professional development in education: New paradigms and practices* (pp. 253–267). New York: Teachers College Press.

Fullan, M. G. (1996). Turning systemic thinking on its head. *Phi Delta Kappan, 77*(6), 420–423.

Fullan, M. (1997). Emotion and hope: Constructive concepts for complex times. In A. Hargreaves (Ed.), *Rethinking educational change with heart and mind* (pp. 216–223). Alexandria, VA: 1997 ASCD Yearbook.

Gardner, H. (1993). *Multiple intelligences*. New York: Basic Books.

Gardner, H. (1995). *Intelligence: Multiple perspectives.* Fort Worth, TX: Harcourt Brace College Publishers.

Goleman, D. (1995). *Emotional intelligence.* New York: Bantam Books.

Harper, D. (1997, May). *Generation www. Y: First annual report.* Washington, DC: U.S. Department of Education.

Harper, D. (1998, May). *Generation www. Y: Second annual report.* Washington, DC: U.S. Department of Education.

Holmes-Ponder, K., Ponder, G., & Bell, P. (1999). Giving school leaders the inner edge. *Professional Development Newsletter,* Spring, 1, 4, 6. Alexandria, VA, Association for Supervision and Curriculum Development.

Individuals with Disabilities Education Act (1997). Amendments H.R.5 made at the one hundred fifth congress of the United States of America. Signed into law by President Clinton. Archived at *http://www.ed.gov/policy/speced/leg/idea/idea.pdf* (retrieved 4/26/04).

Johnson, J. F. Jr., & Asera, R. (1999). *Hope for urban education: A study of nine high-performing, high-poverty, urban elementary schools.* Austin, TX: The Charles A. Dana Center, University of Texas.

Joyce, B., Calhoun, E. (1995). School renewal: An inquiry, not a formula. *Educational Leadership,* 52(&), 51–55.

King, I. C. (2000, August). *Learner-centered inclusion classrooms: The need for empowerment through caring.* Paper presented in the symposium, "Learner-Centered Principles in Practice: Addressing the Personal Domain," at the annual meeting of the American Psychological Association, Washington, DC.

Lambert, N., & McCombs, B. L. (1998). *How students learn: Reforming schools through learner-centered education.* Washington, DC: APA Books.

Leone, P. E., & Drakeford, W. (1999, December). Alternative education: From a "last chance" to a proactive model, *The Clearing House,* 3(2). Washington, DC: Heldref Publications.

Lipsitz, J. (1995). Prologue: Why we should care about caring. *Phi Delta Kappan,* 76(9), 665–666.

Margalit, M. (2001). Responses to questions regarding the work of Israel's Committee for Examining the Implementation of the Law of Special Education. *In Touch with Mofet, 8,* 7–10 (A publication of the Institute for Intercollegiate Professional Training, Support and Advocacy for Teacher Education, Department of Teacher Education of the Ministry of Education, State of Israel).

Marshall, H. H. (1998). Teaching educational psychology: Learner-centered and constructivist perspectives. In N. Lambert & B. L. McCombs (Eds.), *How students learn: Reforming schools through learner-centered education* (pp. 449–473). Washington, DC: APA Books.

McCombs, B. L. (1995). Commentary to Renzulli and Hebert's "The Plight of High-Ability Students in Urban Schools." In M. C. Wang & M. C. Reynolds (Eds.), *Making a difference for students at risk: Trends and alternatives.* Thousand Oaks, CA: Corwin Press, Inc.

McCombs, B. L. (1998). Integrating metacognition, affect, and motivation in improving teacher education. In B. L. McCombs & N. Lambert (Eds.), *Issues in school reform: Psychological perspectives on learner-centered schools.* Washington, DC: APA Books.

McCombs, B. L. (1999). What role does perceptual psychology play in educational reform today? In H. J. Freiberg (Ed.), *Perceiving, behaving, becoming: Lessons learned.* Alexandria, VA: Association for Supervision and Curriculum Development.

McCombs, B. L. (2000, August). *Addressing the personal domain: The need for a learner-centered framework.* Paper presented in the symposium, "Learner-Centered Principles in Practice: Addressing the Personal Domain," at the annual meeting of the American Psychological Association, Washington, DC.

McCombs, B. L. (2001). What do we know about learners and learning? The learner-centered framework: Bringing the educational system into balance *Educational Horizons, 79*(4), 182–193.

McCombs, B. L. (2003a). Applying educational psychology's knowledge base in educational reform: From research to application to policy. In W. M. Reynolds & G. E. Miller (Eds.), *Comprehensive Handbook of Psychology, Volume 7: Educational Psychology*. New York: John Wiley & Sons.

McCombs, B. L. (2003b). Providing a framework for the redesign of K-12 education in the context of current educational reform issues. *Theory Into Practice, 42(2), 93–101.* (Special Issue on Learner-Centered Principles — B. L. McCombs, Guest Editor).

McCombs, B. L., & Lauer, P. A. (1997). Development and validation of the learner-centered battery: Self-assessment tools for teacher reflection and professional development. *The Professional Educator, 20*(1), 1–21.

McCombs, B. L., & Quiat, M. A. (2002). What makes a comprehensive school reform model learner-centered? *Urban Education, 37*(4), 476–496.

McCombs, B. L., & Whisler, J. S. (1997). *The learner-centered classroom and school: Strategies for increasing student motivation and achievement*. San Francisco: Jossey-Bass.

McWhorter, P., Jarrard, B., Rhoades, B., & Wiltcher, B. (1996, Summer). *Student-generated curriculum: Lessons from our students.* (Instructional Resource No. 30). University of Georgia and University of Maryland: National Reading Research Center.

Nissen, L. B. (1999, June). *The power of the strength approach.* Keynote presentation at the 8th Annual Rocky Mountain Regional Conference in Violence Prevention in Schools and Communities, Denver.

Noddings, N. (1995). Teaching themes of care. *Phi Delta Kappan, 76*(9), 675–679.

Norris, T. (1999, June). *Healthy communities for healthy youth.* Keynote presentation at the 8th Annual Rocky Mountain Regional Conference in Violence Prevention in Schools and Communities, Denver.

Office of Special Education Programs (2000, March). *Schools with ideas that work.* Washington, DC: U.S. Department of Education.

O'Neil, J. (1997). Building schools as communities: A conversation with James Comer. *Educational Leadership, 54*(8), 6–10.

Ochsner, K. N., & Lieberman, M. D. (2001). The mergence of social cognitive neuroscience. *American Psychologist, 56*(9), 717–734.

Palmer, P. J. (1999). Evoking the spirit in public education. *Educational Leadership, 56*(4), 6–11.

Renzulli, J. S., & Reis, S. M. (1985). *The schoolwide enrichment model: A comprehensive plan for educational excellence.* Mansfield Center, CT: Creative Learning Press.

Renzulli, J. S., Reis, S. M., Hebert, T. P., & Diaz, E. I. (1995). The plight of high-ability students in urban schools. In M. C. Wang & M. C. Reynolds (Eds.), *Making a difference for students at risk* (pp. 61–98). Thousand Oaks, CA: Corwin Press, Inc.

Robinson, N. M., Zigler, E., & Gallagher, J. J. (2000). Two tails of the normal curve: Similarities and differences in the study of mental retardation and giftedness. *American Psychologist, 55*(12), 1413–1424.

Rudduck, J., Day, J., & Wallace, C. (1997). Student perspectives on school improvement. In A. Hargreaves (Ed.), *Rethinking educational change with heart and mind: 1997 ASCD Yearbook* (pp. 73–91). Alexandria, VA: Association for Supervision and Curriculum Development.

Ryan, R. M., & Powelson, C. L. (1991). Autonomy and relatedness as fundamental to motivation and education. *Journal of Experimental Education, 60*(1), 49–66.

Sarason, S. B. (1995). Some reactions to what we have learned. *Phi Delta Kappan, 77*(1), 84–85.

Schaps, E., & Lewis, C. (1991). Perils on an essential journey: Building school community. *Phi Delta Kappan, 81*(3), 215–218.

SEDL & NiDRR (1999, April). *A review of the literature on topics related to increasing the utilization of rehabilitation research outcomes among diverse consumer groups.* Southwet Educational Development Laboratory, SEDL, and National Institute on Disability and Rehabilitation Resources, NiDRR.

Sparks, D., & Hirsh, S. (1997). *A new vision for staff development.* Alexandria, VA: Association for Supervision and Curriculum Development.

U.S. Department of Education (1998). To assure the free appropriate public education of all children with disabilities: Twentieth annual report to Congress on the implementation of the Individuals with Disabilities Education Act. Washington, DC: U.S. Department of Education.

Vatterott, C. (1995). Student-focused instruction: Balancing limits with freedom. *Middle School Journal, 27*(11), 28–38.

Wang, M. C. (1992). *Adaptive education strategies: Building on diversity.* Baltimore: Paul H. Brookes Publishing Co.

Wang, M. C. (1998). *The community for learning program: A planning guide.* Philadelphia: Temple University Center for Research in Human Development and Education.

Wang, M. C., Haertel, G. D., & Walberg, H. J. (1997). *What do we know: Widely implemented school improvement programs.* Philadelphia, PA: Temple University Center for Research in Human Development and Education, Laboratory for Student Success.

Weinberger, E., & McCombs, B. L., (2001, April). *The impact of learner-centered practises on the academic and non-academic outcomes of upper elementary and middle school students.* Paper presented in the Symposium, "Integrating What We Know About Learners and Learning: A foundation for Transforming PreK-20 Practices," at the annual meeting of the American Educational Research Association, Seattle.

Weinstein, R. S. (1998). Promoting positive expectations in schooling. In N. Lambert & B. L. McCombs (Eds.), *How students learn: Reforming schools through learner-centered education.* New York: APA Books.

Wheatley, M. J. (1999). *Leadership and the new science: Discovering order in a chaotic world.* (2nd ed.). San Francisco: Berrett-Koehler Publishers.

Wheatley, M. J., & Kellner-Rogers, M. (1998, April–May). Bringing life to organizational change. *Journal of Strategic Performance Measurement,* 5–13.

Zimmerman, B. J., & Schunk, D. H. (in press). *Self-regulated learning and academic achievement: Theory, research, and practice* (2nd ed.). Mahwah, NJ: Erlbaum.

Zimmerman, B. J. (1994). Dimensions of academic self-regulation: A conceptual framework for education. In D. H. Schunk & B. J. Zimmerman (Eds.), *Self-regulation of learning and performance: Issues and educational applications* (pp. 3–21). Hillsdale, NJ: Erlbaum.

Why Pinocchio Was Victimized: Factors Contributing to Social Failure in People with Mental Retardation

STEPHEN GREENSPAN

UNIVERSITY OF COLORADO HEALTH SCIENCES CENTER

In the present book, as in the field of mental retardation (MR) generally (Switzky, 2001), scholars interested in motivation have mainly explored its contribution to various school learning-related outcomes. An example of this emphasis can be found in the many studies of Zigler and colleagues (Balla & Zigler, 1979; Zigler & Yando, 1972), who have used motivational constructs (such as an "external orientation") and social variables (such as one's history of "social deprivation") primarily as a means to understand why individuals with MR perform poorly on some learning tasks, even when one controls for mental age. Social competence has generally been studied less for its own sake than for the contribution it might make to academic goals, such as succeeding in school (as in the work of Siperstein & Leffert, 1997). This relative emphasis on academic rather than social outcomes suggests an underlying assumption that academic incompetence is the core problem for people with MR. But there is ample evidence, from literature over many decades, that social, rather than academic, incompetence is the defining characteristic of MR and the impairment most likely to interfere with successful integration into the community (Doll, 1936; Greenspan, 2003; Greenspan & Shoultz, 1981; Greenspan et al., 1996; Switzky et al., 2002; Tredgold, 1922; Wilson et al., 1996).

The most socially incompetent individuals among us are not socially incompetent all of the time. One disastrous incident a day, or even a year, may be enough to diminish all hopes for an integrated community placement (slashing a neighbor's tires or masturbating on the job are two actual examples). Disastrous social behavior is always motivated and often influenced by strong emotions such as anger, greed, or fear. Intelligence, in its various aspects, enters prominently into the mix as well. A contextualist, or developmental systems, perspective requires one to look at all behavior as resulting from the complex transaction of many personal inclinations and abilities, as they confront a specific micro-situation (Ford & Lerner, 1992). To appreciate the role of motivation in social functioning, it is thus necessary to approach social competence in contextualist terms, as a transaction with specific situational challenges, rather than as a global trait of which one possesses some finite amount (Greenspan, 1999; Switzky et al., 2003).

Spitz (1988) has argued that MR is a disorder of thinking rather than learning. By this, he meant that the true test of one's competence level is not how well one does in routine situations (such as getting to work on a bus) but in how well one does in challenging or novel situations (such as when the bus breaks down). People with MR can learn to deal remarkably well with routine situations, but it is a much different story when the challenge is a novel one, posing unique intellectual and/or affective challenges. Such challenges, more often than not, are interpersonal, as when one is confronted by a deceitful manipulator seeking to use one financially, sexually, or otherwise.

To illustrate my point and to explore the utility of a heuristic model for analyzing socially incompetent transactions, I shall use a case study, drawn from a widely loved children's book, about a socially incompetent—and, arguably, developmentally disabled—puppet: *Pinocchio*. The case presentation is followed by a discussion of a heuristic model, which is used to explain why Pinocchio was so socially incompetent and also why he eventually attained some degree of "normality." In the final section, I will address the question of whether, and how, socially incompetent people (or puppets), with or without disabilities, can develop the skills needed to survive in a world where predators, unfortunately, are eager to prey on the weak and the too-trusting.

I. A CASE STUDY DRAWN FROM CHILDREN'S LITERATURE

As noted by Cantor and Genero (1986), fictional prototypes can prove useful in illustrating issues in the classifying and understanding of real people. An advantage in using the Pinocchio story to illustrate an explanatory model of social ineffectiveness is that readers have a common experience of the character to draw upon, even if, as in this case, that experience is filtered through the "Disney treatment." Furthermore, there are enough tragic stories of exploitation and victimization of people with MR to suggest that the Pinocchio story may not be entirely invented.

Most of us know the Pinocchio tale mainly through the animated Walt Disney movie, first released in 1940 and re-released many times since. I have chosen to rely on the original 19th-century novel, by Italian children's book author Carlo Collodi. The book differs from the animated film in some notable respects. For example, the cricket makes a fleeting appearance in the book (before Pinocchio squashes him against a wall) but is a major figure in the film. The basic elements of the book and movie are quite similar, however, and proceed as follows: Pinocchio was a marionette made of wood who yearned to be a real boy, and who engaged in a long series of adventures seeking to reunite with his "father"/creator, the lonely old man Gepetto. As a result of a series of encounters with manipulators and deceivers, Pinocchio is repeatedly duped and sidetracked from attaining his goal. Finally, with the help and forgiveness of the "Fairy with Blue Hair," Pinocchio develops both the social intelligence and moral backbone to survive and prevail in a world of swindlers and con artists, and becomes reunited with Gepetto and turned by the fairy into a real boy.

This story, written in the land of Machiavelli, really has less to do with the importance of a conscience (despite the "always let your conscience be your guide" theme sung by the cricket in the film) than it has to do with attaining the skills to deal with fakers. A listing of Pinocchio's many mishaps shows his gradual movement from an extremely socially incompetent puppet to a more socially effective human being. The first social incompetence episode occurred after the puppet told Gepetto that he was willing to go to school. The old man sold his coat to buy Pinocchio a spelling book. On his way to school, Pinocchio is tempted to attend a puppet show, and sells the book for 5¢ so that he can procure a ticket (this scene is depicted in Figure 1). The theater owner feels sorry for Pinocchio and gives him five gold coins to buy Gepetto another coat. But Pinocchio is tricked by a fox and a cat into going with them to the "Wonder Field" in order to turn his 5 coins into 2,000 coins by planting them over night. (Pinocchio was quite guileless, as he quickly told them of his treasure.) A bird tells Pinocchio, "do not heed the advice of bad companions," but Pinocchio ignores him. When confronted by robbers (the fox and cat in obvious disguise), Pinocchio hides the coins in his mouth but reveals the hiding place when they threaten to kill Gepetto. Pinocchio escapes and is rescued by the Fairy with Blue Hair (this is where his nose grows as punishment for telling her a lie). He promises the fairy that he will wait for Gepetto to arrive but he is again duped by the fox and the cat into following them to a city called "Fools-Cap," in order to plant his remaining coins in the Wonder Field. Returning 20 minutes after planting the coins, Pinocchio finds them missing, while a parrot laughingly proclaims: "I laugh at those simpletons who believe every tomfoolery that is told them and who fall into every trap." Even then, it takes a while for Pinocchio to understand what has happened to the coins.

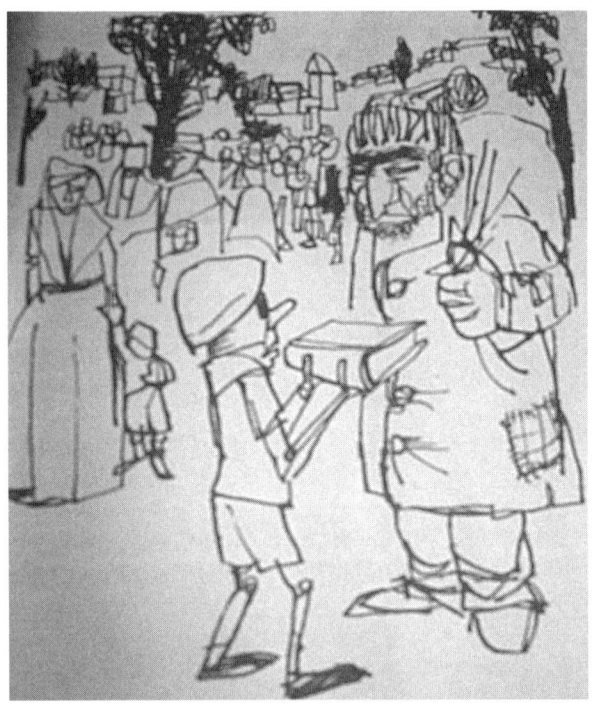

FIG. 1. Pinocchio sells his spelling book (illustration by William Dempster, in Collodi, 1968/1881).

The first glimmer of social competence and guile occurs when Pinocchio is chained to a doghouse by a farmer annoyed that he has eaten his grapes. Some weasels arrive and try to trick Pinocchio into letting them steal some chickens in exchange for giving him one (an arrangement they claim to have had with the farmer's late guard dog). But Pinocchio sees through this ruse, which earns him his freedom from the grateful farmer. Another sign of social intelligence occurs when he recognizes the Fairy with Blue Hair in disguise (previously, Pinocchio was always taken in by disguises). Pinocchio promises the fairy that he will attend school and be a responsible boy. Some boys trick him into skipping school, however, by telling Pinocchio that the dog-fish (a giant shark, not the whale of the movie) that ate Gepetto has been sighted. But Pinocchio quickly figures out the trick and becomes quite assertive, easily parrying the verbal ploys used by the boys. Pinocchio is chased by a mastiff and they jump into the ocean. The mastiff starts to drown and begs Pinocchio for help. The marionette understands that this may be a trick. He decides to risk helping the dog, but does it in a very careful manner, thus demonstrating both goodness and social caution. This combination of kindness and social shrewdness continues to mark Pinocchio's future behavior, promulgating Collodi's apparent message that what some have termed "social with-it-ness" does not require one to become selfish and unfeeling.

Before becoming fully human, however, Pinocchio suffers one major setback. The fairy, impressed with Pinocchio's improved school attendance, proposes to make him human at an evening ceremony at her house, to which she allows Pinocchio to invite all of his friends. Pinocchio promises to be home in time for the event, but is tempted by his best friend, Lampwick, into accompanying him to "Playtime Land," a reputed paradise where the residents are on perpetual vacation. At first, Pinocchio resists but Lampwick makes all sorts of promises and inducements (for example, that 100 other boys have already committed, they will be traveling in a nice coach, the Fairy will not really be mad at him, they will never have to work or go to school), and Pinocchio finally agrees. After a short time of merry-making in Playtime Land, Pinocchio turns into a donkey and is sold to a circus, where he becomes lame. Pinocchio is thrown into the ocean in order to drown him so he can be skinned, but he turns back into a marionette and is swallowed by the dog-fish, in whose stomach he has a tearful reunion with Gepetto. They escape and begin to walk home. Along the way, they encounter the fox and the cat, but this time Pinocchio resists them, saying "Good bye, cheats ... You tricked me once but you can't catch me again." Pinocchio returns home with Gepetto, and is rewarded for several months of hard work by being made human by the Fairy, who says: "My good Pinocchio! Because of your kind heart I forgive you for all of your misdeeds ... Always listen to good counsel, and you will be happy."

II. USE OF AN ACTION MODEL TO EXPLAIN PINOCCHIO'S INCOMPETENCE

Even with this relatively uni-dimensional fictional character, socially incompetent behavior appears multi-determined, arising out of a complex mix of situational and personal factors. To say that one is the sole cause makes no more sense than saying that "this loaf of bread is due to flour, while this one if due to yeast." Social incompetence can be discussed in outcome terms (getting in trouble) as well as in input terms (the particular skill deficits that get one in trouble). From an outcome standpoint, Pinocchio's incompetence is defined by his inability to attain his conscious goal, namely, to be reunited with his father and to live happily ever after in his father's home, hopefully as a real boy. He is unable to attain that goal because he cannot deal with the diverting tricks and traps set by a number of actors who use devious methods to hoodwink him. Among these were the fox and the cat, who stole his money and diverted him to the city of Fools Cap, and his friend Lampwick, in league with the donkey recruiter, who talked him into going to Playtime Land, where he was turned into a donkey. To understand how these disastrous social outcomes occurred, it is necessary to examine the particular challenging events in detail, in an effort to understand how Pinocchio's various impairments and personality tendencies make him a sitting duck for the ploys used by deceitful manipulators.

Figure 2 contains a multi-dimensional action model of social incompetence that is an adaptation of a more general model of human effectiveness devised by Martin Ford (1986, 1992) in his book *Motivating Humans*. The model (Also see Greenspan (1999) and Greenspan et al. (2001)) depicts the following equation: Social Ineffectiveness = Social Situation + Everyday intelligence + Motivational Factors (Goals × Personal Agency Beliefs × Affect × Morality) + Communication + Physical Ability. The four personal competence factors—everyday intelligence, motivation, communication, and physical ability—in the model are all borrowed from a static model of personal competence developed over a period of years (Greenspan, 1981; Greenspan & Driscoll, 1997). The model of motivation is exactly as devised by Ford, except for the addition of "morality."

The conversion of the earlier static model into the current dynamic action model reflects several influences. As a result of an increasing interest in the "gullibility" and "credulity" of persons with developmental disabilities (Greenspan et al., 2001) stimulated by my involvement in a notorious case of false confession (Greenspan, 1995), I began to realize that social competence/incompetence must be understood not as a general trait but as a failure to navigate specific difficult social situations. An additional influence was exposure to Ford and Lerner's (1992) "developmental systems theory," an exposure that triggered a personal paradigm shift, from "formism" (analogous to using a shoemaker's last or a toolmaker's die) to "developmental contextualism" (analogous to doing historical analysis). Interestingly, before I became interested in psychology I had earned a

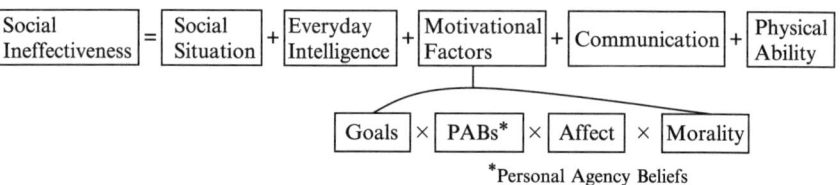

FIG. 2. Action model explaining social ineffectiveness.

graduate degree in history but, until recently, never thought that its methods might be useful in pursuing my current interests. I now recognize that any behavior must be understood as resulting from the complex historical interplay of numerous factors (internal and external, biological and functional, past and present) coming together at a given point in time. Finally, my discovery of the motivational model of Ford (1992)—and the urgings of Switzky—helped me to understand how motivation could be injected into an action model of social competence/incompetence.

Ford's influence is reflected in the various elements in my model (which are similar, but not identical, to his), in the way in which the situational and personal elements combine to explain a behavioral outcome and, most importantly, in the design of the box in Figure 2 labeled "Motivational Factors." In each sub-section below, I define these concepts and discuss how each can contribute, separately or in combination, to a socially incompetent outcome, using illustrations from the story of Pinocchio.

A. Situational Factors Contributing to Pinocchio's Ineffectiveness

Disastrous social behavior does not occur in a vacuum. Using Piaget's biological metaphor, a challenging situation serves as the "ailment" that triggers social failure, or growth, just as some conceptual challenge is needed to trigger academic failure or growth. Some social situations are, obviously, more problematic than others. As in the non-social realm, what makes a problem difficult to solve is when there are elements that are ambiguous, hidden, or incongruent, and when the most salient cues may be misleading. In the social realm, difficult social situations almost always involve people whose true motivations are different from what they appear to be. An extreme case of that would be someone—such as a scam artist or a sexual predator—who claims to have one's interests at heart but is actually using one for his or her own ends.

Situations can be characterized according to how much they influence an incompetent response, but also according to how much they may minimize the likelihood of such a response. Among the factors that influence an incompetent response are the use of various threat or scare tactics, the use of peer pressure and other forms of group pressure, and other forms of psychological manipulation and influence techniques. On the other end of the spectrum are interventions or arrangements that can strengthen the resolve of individuals or provide them with useful information. For those with MR, or who are otherwise vulnerable to victimization, it helps, for example, to have relationships with others who have good judgment and can intervene or provide useful advice when needed.

The characters who diverted Pinocchio from his desired goal of going home all used coercive methods that can be found in Cialdini's (1984) book *Influence: How and Why People Agree to Things*. One of the main tactics used on Pinocchio is what Cialdini termed "social proof," in which the observed or attributed behaviors of others provide normative evidence that a particular behavior is acceptable. For Pinocchio, as for any other wayward youth, peer pressure is very difficult to resist and lies at the root of most of his troubles. One form of social proof, used in most of the Pinocchio episodes, involves two or more influence agents working in tandem. This is seen in all of the fox and the cat episodes, in the school hooky episode where Pinocchio is tricked into visiting the dog-fish, and in the episode in which Lampwick (himself tricked) and the donkey trapper talk Pinocchio into making the trip to Playtime Land.

B. Contribution of Everyday Intelligence to Pinocchio's Incompetence

In Ford's model of human effectiveness, there is a general "competence" component. Such an element has obvious predictive power, as people who are relatively capable are more likely to be effective, assuming motivation and other factors to be equal, than people who are less capable. The competence component in Ford's model is not well-developed, however, and (because his model is not particularly focused on social effectiveness) its social components are not clearly defined. In Figure 2, the term "everyday intelligence" (Greenspan et al., 1996) is substituted for competence.

The term everyday intelligence has been borrowed from Sternberg (1984), who used this term to differentiate it from what he titled "academic intelligence" (i.e., IQ). In line with the tripartite content model of multiple intelligences devised over 80 years ago by Thornidke (and which has far more empirical support than Gardner's better-known, but highly idiosyncratic, model), everyday intelligence contains two important domains that are not recognized by standardized intelligence tests: "social intelligence" and "practical intelligence." The term social intelligence refers to understanding and cognitive processing of interpersonal phenomena, while the term practical intelligence refers to understanding and cognitive processing of mechanical and other material phenomena. It is safe to assume that social intelligence has greater utility in navigating social situations than practical intelligence, but one can imagine situations in which lack of practical knowledge (e.g., in knowing about the Hale-Bopp comet) might contribute to a socially ineffective outcome (e.g., in joining the Heaven's Gate mass suicide scheme based on naively believing the assurance that one would be picked up by a spaceship said to be waiting behind the comet).

As with academic intelligence, everyday intelligence (Jones & Day, 1997) involves both raw information processing power (something akin to "fluid" intelligence) as well as one's accumulated knowledge and wisdom about the everyday world (something akin to "crystallized intelligence"). The former ability contributes to social adaptation by enabling one to determine the true nature of the situation that they are facing. For example, a common ploy used by pyramid scheme salespeople is to invite you to what is labeled a social get-together. However, once there, it is in the individual's best interest to recognize as quickly as possible that the true intent of the inviter is not to offer friendship but rather to enroll one in a pyramid sales scheme.

Virtually all exploitation situations involve some form of deception, and survival in such situations depends to some extent on the ability to see through the deception so that one can activate the most relevant set of goals and behaviors (e.g., survival/escape as opposed to friendship). Such decoding ability may be considered "fluid" in that every complex social situation is somewhat different and one must be able to integrate various situation-specific cues (e.g., non-verbal behaviors of the exploiter) in order to cope successfully with specific features of the situation. Perspective-taking, so central to social intelligence research (Greenspan, 1979; Greenspan & Love, 1997), may be considered the paradigmatic process involved in fluid everyday intelligence, as the ability to see through deception requires one to recognize the deceiver's true intentions.

The crystallized aspect of everyday intelligence is less dependent on general information processing and is more dependent on one's actual experience in the world. For this reason, it is possible that people with MR, especially if they are adults who have experienced some independence, may have achieved somewhat greater crystallized everyday knowledge than might be inferred from their IQ scores or from the degree of their social "with-it-ness" (Yalon-Chamovitz, 2000). Nevertheless, people with MR generally also have significant deficits in crystallized aspects of everyday intelligence.

An aspect of crystallized everyday intelligence that has attracted virtually no scholarly attention involves what might be termed "credulity," i.e., the ease with which one can be convinced that unreal phenomena (e.g., professional wrestling, Santa Claus, stories in supermarket tabloids, and so on) are real. While credulity is, to some extent, affected by interpersonal trust (an aspect of personality rather than intelligence), it is to a large extent a sign of one's degree of accumulated cognitive sophistication and knowledge. Credulity has relevance to social adaptation in that deceptive communications often use misstatements that are quite obvious to someone with content wisdom. For example, if a magazine sweepstakes flyer suggests that you need to buy several magazines in order to win $1 million, someone with content wisdom might know that: (1) legitimate such events do not require one to purchase a subscription, and (2) these are long-odds lotteries that typically use misleading tactics (such as enclosing real-looking phony checks) to activate motivating affective schemas (e.g., greed).

Pinocchio had some real intellectual deficits which undoubtedly contributed to his social victimization. These deficits are not quite in the realm of academic intelligence (IQ) as reflected in the fact that he did well in school on occasions when he applied himself (his initial school problems probably reflected cultural disadvantage—his background as a stick of wood—or what Feuerstein et al. (1980), termed an absence of "mediated learning experiences"). His intellectual deficits are found mainly in the area of everyday intelligence, particularly in processing social information, and have central relevance to understanding why he gets into so much trouble.

Throughout the first two-thirds of the book, Pinocchio shows a complete inability to recognize deception clues, or even to see through obvious disguises. He has a relatively intact general information processing ability, as reflected by his above-average school performance (once he started applying himself). Social transactions (especially involving deception) have hidden and unique elements, however, and are more difficult to master, especially when one has a limited background of peer experiences.

Pinocchio arrived on the scene with no background knowledge, and this undoubtedly contributed to his over-reliance on others. An example would be when the fox and the cat told him that by planting four coins in the soil of the Field of Wonders for 20 minutes (in their first telling it was overnight) they would be turned into 2,000 coins (again, far less in the first telling). Had Pinocchio possessed greater fluid intelligence, he might have become suspicious about the constantly shifting nature of the promised returns and methods. His limitations in crystallized everyday intelligence are reflected in believing such a tall tale in the first place.

What physical mechanism, including alchemy, can explain the process by which coins can be multiplied through planting? Anyone with even the most rudimentary understanding of physics or chemistry, except perhaps for a very young child, would be suspicious of such magic. Then there is the matter of knowledge of the investment field. A promise to return 500 coins for every coin planted is Warren Buffett territory, and even he could not deliver such a profit in 20 minutes. What are the investment credentials of the fox and the cat to make such a promise? And if they had such a track record, why would they need Pinocchio's measly four coins? Had Pinocchio watched *Moneyline* on CNN, may be he would have been a little more careful about whom he trusted to provide investment advice.

C. Role of Motivation and Personality in Pinocchio's Victimization

Motivation obviously contributes to incompetence in interpersonal situations, just as it does to performance in academic situations. The motivational component in Figure 2 is derived from Ford's (1992) "motivational systems theory" (MST). This theory builds on the work of Bandura and other motivation theorists as well as on the "developmental systems" meta-model of Ford and Lerner (1992). A hallmark of Ford's contextualist theory is that "all of the component processes of the person ... are organized in complex patterns of unitary functioning in variable environments" (Ford, 1992, p. 245). As a consequence, a hallmark of MST is its anchoring in "the broader framework [that] makes it possible to describe how motivational processes interact with biological, environmental, and non-motivational psychological and behavioral processes to produce effective or ineffective functioning in the person as a whole" (p. 245).

In MST, motivation is defined as "the organized patterning of an individual's personal goals, emotions, and personal agency beliefs" (Ford, 1992, p. 78). By personal agency beliefs (or "PABs" in Ford's theory), he is referring to something close to Bandura's (1997) self-efficacy (i.e., the anticipatory expectancy that one can accomplish a particular task), although PABs are somewhat broader. Ford divides PABs into "capability beliefs" (expectancy that one has the ability to accomplish a goal) and "context beliefs" (expectancy that an environment will be responsive to and supportive of one's efforts). In this paper, I have added "morality" to Ford's triad, in part because it is not explicitly dealt with in his model, and because one cannot account for social behavior without taking it into account (especially when discussing Pinocchio, who is known to be somewhat "conscience-challenged").

Ford represents his definition of motivation with the formula: Motivation = Goals × Emotions × Personal Agency Beliefs. I have adapted it to read "Social Motivation" = Affect × Agency Beliefs × Goals × Morality. By using multiplication rather than addition signs, Ford meant to suggest that "the relationships among the components of human motivational patterns are often complex and nonlinear" (Ford, 1992, p. 79). This framework, which appears to have considerable utility for explaining the quality of adaptation to specific social situations by people with MR, will be described later in further detail.

1. GOALS

Goal selection and awareness plays a central role in Ford's constructivist motivation model. In contrast, older drive-oriented formulations emphasize physiological or unconscious motives. There is a definite cognitive component to this aspect of the model, as goal importance involves identification of relevant goals, and coordination of goals which may be in conflict. Effectiveness is influenced by goal selection, as one is likely to make an adequate effort to overcome a difficult obstacle only if one sees that as an important objective. Thus, if one does not care about being liked by peers, one is less likely to behave in a manner to make one popular than if one does hold peer approval as an important goal.

Ford notes that there are two ways in MST in which a "behavior episode" (a micro-situation, such as resisting a manipulative social interaction) will be prematurely terminated: (1) if the goal is evaluated as unattainable (i.e., the person does not think he/she can accomplish it in that context), or (2) if some other goal takes precedence over it. Ford notes several categories of goals (described briefly earlier in discussing his work on social intelligence), but indicates that the two goals most typically operative (and often conflicting) in social situations are "social relationship" (friendship) goals and "task" (survival) goals. Where these, and other, goals are in concert, motivation is quite strong. But it is often the case that one has difficulty in deciding which goal is applicable in a given situation.

This is certainly the case in many manipulative situations (such as being invited to what is labeled a social gathering only to discover that one is being given a sales pitch). Because people with MR have difficulty in coordinating multiple goals and are less likely to perceive the true nature of subtle situations (Leffert & Siperstein, in press), they are less likely to choose a goal which is in accord with their true desires or interests.

Ford notes that little recent attention has been paid in the motivation literature to the problem of goal selection. In contrast to an earlier period in motivation research in which much attention was paid to categorizing human needs or drives, motivation researchers today (e.g., Deci & Ryan, 1985), have focused on a small number of very generic needs, such as effectance motivation, with specificity (as in Bandura's work) applied mainly to situational variability within a single broad goal. This reflects: (1) the shift away from drives and towards an emphasis on intrinsic and self-motivating processes; (2) disillusionment over the questionable validity of need-based measures (such as need for achievement); and (3) greater interest currently in applying motivational constructs to problems of social institutions, such as schools and work places, rather than to problems of individual adaptation.

Reiss and Havercamp (1996) have attempted to revive interest in instinct salience by presenting a modern version, termed the "sensitivity theory." According to this theory, the maladaptive behaviors of people with MR are less a reflection of aberrant reinforcement history than it is a reflection of atypical "sensitivity" (enjoyment) of various goals or end-states. This could take the form either of having an unusually intense need for reinforcers (e.g., attention) that are typically experienced as pleasurable or for feeling states (e.g., anxiety) which in most people are experienced as unpleasant. Although Reiss and Havercamp (1996) pose a genetic explanation for this phenomenon, one could imagine non-genetic biological (e.g., brain injury) or experiential (e.g., social deprivation) causes for the possession of unusual reinforcement sensitivities. Nevertheless, the sensitivity theory does provide a much-needed emphasis on individual differences in goals as part of the explanation for maladaptive behavior in people with MR.

In addition to having aberrant goals, people with MR are less likely to have the meta-cognitive skills to be consciously aware of what their goals are. This puts them more at the mercy of external or affective pressures. Furthermore, as discussed earlier, people with MR lack the affective conservation skills to coordinate conflicting goals, especially where a less critical short-term goal (e.g., social relationship) may be more salient than a more critical (e.g., survival) long-term goal. The problem of goal coordination, however, which strikes me as quite important in understanding the behavior of people with MR, has been the subject of very little research.

Pinocchio's problems with goals are analogous to a Piagetian conservation experiment, in which a pre-operational child cannot keep in mind the most important fact about a phenomenon (e.g., that two clay balls started out identical) in the face of a perceptual transformation (e.g., rolling one into a cigar shape) that creates a salient illusion suggesting that one of the balls is now bigger than the other. In Pinocchio's case, he has difficulty in conserving the vital importance of keeping his original plan in the face of very salient temptations provided by various deluders. Among the arguments used to increase the salience of these temptations was the obviously phony claim that the goals were not really incompatible, in that the side trips would only take a short while and he could still make his rendezvous with Gepetto.

2. PERSONAL AGENCY BELIEFS

While the lack of salience of a particular goal may suggest a low sensitivity (preference) for that goal, it is also very likely to defensively reflect a belief that the goal is unattainable. This could be due to a poor evaluation of one's own competence (capability beliefs) or to a view that a specific environment is not likely to respond to one's efforts (context beliefs). In any complex social situation in which either form of poor PAB is activated, one is not likely to put in the effort needed to succeed. Ford's notion of PABs, especially capability beliefs, is derived largely from the work of Bandura (1997) on "self-efficacy." Although there has been little discussion of intelligence (and even less on people with MR) by Ford or

Bandura, their writings would appear to have considerable utility in explaining why people with MR would be likely to adapt poorly to high-pressure social situations. This is because: (1) there is much face validity in the idea that people with MR (who invariably have a long history of social incompetence) are likely to lack social self-efficacy; (2) this motivational model, unlike some others, explains behavior in interpersonal as well as in cognitive tasks; (3) the model is quite multi-faceted and takes into account a wide range of situational, biological, cognitive, and personality factors; and (4) the idea of interpersonal pressure (and interpersonal efficacy) has, in fact, been used by Bandura to discuss some forms of action.

In a recent book, Bandura (1997) illustrates the use of his model in explaining a category of behavior—unintended sexual behavior by adolescent females—that has some surface parallels to a topic of great current importance in the field of MR, namely the giving of police criminal confessions by people who are innocent (Clare & Gudjonsson, 1995; Perske, 1991). The basic outcome of competence required in Bandura's seduction scenario (saying "no, I won't do it") is similar to the one required in an interrogation scenario (saying "no, I didn't do it"), and both involve the ability to face interpersonal pressure and a variety of ploys (in the sexual realm, involving deceptive communications such as "everyone does it," and in the interrogation realm involving deceptive communications such as "your accomplice has already confessed").

While Bandura's model takes into account the multiplicity of contributors to any action, his most emphasized construct is self-efficacy, i.e., the degree to which one believes that one is capable of coping with a particular situation and of bringing about a desired intentional outcome in that situation. In the case of both scenarios used in the preceding text, this self-efficacy involves interpersonal efficacy, particularly around the belief that one can successfully assert their intentions in the face of interpersonal pressure. Bandura also illustrates the use of his model in explaining recovery or non-recovery from alcohol and drug abuse. Resistance to peer pressure is also quite relevant here, although less central (where efficacy around self-regulation of drug impulses is more paramount) than in sexual or confession behavior, where other pressures are a primary, rather than secondary, consideration.

The PABs are relevant to understanding Pinocchio's social vulnerability, as he repeatedly demonstrates little confidence in his ability to prevail in complex social situations. He refers to himself as "dumb" and tends to give up too easily, as was also true of his early school experiences. There is a general tendency for people to rely on others to define what is appropriate, and this tendency becomes even stronger when one feels as socially clueless as Pinocchio appears to feel.

3. AFFECT

Emotions play an important role in Ford's motivational theory: (1) as a clue to the goals that are important in a particular instance; (2) as a self-perpetuating influence on behavior even after goals are attained; and (3) as a force which works in tandem with PABs to affect decision-making and behavior. Ford (1992) sees a division of labor between PABs and emotion, in which the former has more impact on long-term goal-oriented behavior (such as staying the course in a program of study), while emotion has more impact on behavior in micro-situations (such as dealing with a humiliating encounter).

Anyone who has ever behaved foolishly while under the grips of a strong emotion (i.e., most readers of this paper) knows that one's affective state will often determine how capably one behaves in a given situation. Even one who habitually demonstrates skill and self-control in dealings with others is capable of over-reacting and behaving contrary to their goals or needs when under the influence of strong emotions. Goleman (1995) used the term "emotional hijacking" to refer to this phenomenon. An example of this is the interrogation scene in Orwell's (1949) *1984*. The mere threat to let rats nibble on his face activated the hero's deep fear of rats and caused him to lose any resolve or ability to resist.

While emotional self-regulation is obviously an important contributor to competent or incompetent social behavior, so too is one's ability to regulate and deploy attentional processes. People who are impulsive, i.e., who respond too quickly and without considering complexity, are less likely to perceive hidden dangers, even when they might otherwise possess the ability to spot those dangers. People with MR are more likely to have emotional or attentional problems, for a number of reasons, including backgrounds of rejection or isolation, underlying neurological abnormality, and concrete thinking (Schroeder et al., 1997). An interrogative ploy which might be an empty threat (such as to pursue the death penalty if one denies committing a murder) could trigger overwhelming anxiety in a person not able to detect deception cues, lacking understanding of the criminal justice system, or possessing a tendency to overreact to stress.

As a general rule, when strong affect enters the picture, reason and judgment are diminished, even in individuals who have an adequate understanding of what is taking place. In the case of the side trip to the Field of Wonders, Pinocchio appears to have been emotionally hijacked by greed. The idea of turning 5 (later only 4) gold coins into 2000 was too much for Pinocchio to resist. In that respect, he has a lot of company, ranging from the Dutch who were ruined by Tulipmania to modern-day Americans who lost their money investing in dot-com start-ups. If Pinocchio had possessed a better understanding of the risks and dubiousness of such an investment scheme, perhaps he could have been able to keep his emotions in check. In the case of the trip to Playtime Land, the idea of being on perpetual vacation, and never having to work or attend school, was also very affectively compelling. The skill of the manipulators lay, in part, in their ability to activate these affective schemas. Again, had Pinocchio been able to understand that it was a false sales tactic, perhaps the outcome would have been different.

4. MORALITY

Except when physical force is used, it is probably the case that someone cannot be made to do something that is absolutely anathema to him or her morally. Thus, for example, a saint-like person such as the Dalai Lama or Mother Theresa would probably choose death before agreeing to kill another human being. This has relevance for being duped, as exploiters often appeal to motives or promote actions that are somewhat immoral. (An example is conning someone into an investment scheme as a means of avoiding paying income tax.) Morality, in this sense, acts in a manner similar to the "super-ego" in Freud's topological personality model, in that it serves as a brake on any action that is outside the pale. Since few people are saints, and since other aspects of the model come into play—specifically, social intelligence (ego) and affect (id)—it is a mistake, however, to characterize all those who may give in to coercive pressures as "immoral."

An example of such a mistaken over-emphasis on conscience as the sole relevant criterion came from its use by defense attorneys in the infamous "Glen Ridge Rape" case (Lefkowitz, 1997). The case involved the notorious mistreatment of a female high school student with mild MR who was tricked into going to a basement setting in which she was violated vaginally with a pool cue and a toy baseball bat before a cheering crowd of high school wrestlers. Among the tricks used to overbear her stated wish to leave was an obviously phony, but affectively compelling, threat to tell the girl's parents.

Lawyers for the perpetrators argued that the girl would have fled had she possessed sufficient moral scruples, but this argument was appropriately rejected by the jury (although, outrageously, none of the convicted rapists spent a day in jail).

The MR field at the beginning of the 20th century grew out of eugenic notions in which people with MR were viewed as a criminal underclass lacking in conscience. This is reflected in Goddard (1914), who first used the term "moral imbecile" before eventually settling on the term "moron" to refer to people who today would be considered to have "cultural-familial" MR. This earlier view of people with MR as being amoral has been discredited. In fact, people with MR may be more morally upright than others, owing to their reliance on concrete moral judgments, reinforced by primitive ideas of immanent justice (e.g., God will punish you if you jaywalk).

The typical (i.e., Disney) take on Pinocchio is that his problems stem from an insufficiently developed conscience. This is probably an exaggeration. While Pinocchio is attracted to a life of ease and indolence (who isn't?), he is anything but a sociopath. For example, when the mastiff was drowning, Pinocchio used his superior buoyancy (an advantage of being made of wood) to save him, even though the dog had previously attacked him. It is true that Pinocchio was a little lacking in the area of moral development, which undoubtedly contributed to his susceptibility to bad influences. But conscience is only part of the picture, and Pinocchio's problems clearly stem more from being "dumb" than from being "bad."

D. Communicative Factors Contributing to Pinocchio's Difficulties

Communication, involving more than just language fluency, is important in a model of social adaptation, as one's possession of a repertoire of conventional communicative ploys (such as the "automated phone butler" who politely but firmly hangs up on all telephone solicitors) will increase one's likelihood of dealing successfully with challenging interpersonal situations. Conversely, the absence of a ready-bag of conversational tricks will increase feelings of helplessness and low interpersonal efficacy when facing confusing and conflictual situations.

Such communicative behaviors, typically referred to as "social skills," are relatively lacking in people with MR (Warren & Yoder, 1997) who, consequently, are frequently involved in behavioral interventions aimed at increasing the use of these skills (Matson & Fee, 1991). Social skills differ from social intelligence, in that social skills are isolated behaviors (e.g., eye contact, greeting behaviors) that are generally predictive of social acceptance, while social intelligence refers to the extent that one is "with it" or "out of it" in processing ambiguous social information. It is because so little attention is paid to social intelligence by social skills trainers that there is much bemoaning of the poor "generalization" effects of such training.

In Ford's model, one's social skill repertoire is referred to as the "behavior episode schemata" (relatively automatized behavior patterns) and are included under his "competence" rubric. I have chosen to depict communication as a separate element in the model, because such skills (as indicated in the preceding text) are not quite intellectual and communication is sufficiently important as to deserve separate treatment. Everyday intelligence comes into play as an activator of such relatively automatized communicative tactics (e.g., in labeling a situation as one in which an escape schema such as "see you" or "call my lawyer," rather than "schmoozing," is called for).

Pinocchio had adequate language skills and did not have apparent dysfluency or syntax problems. However, it took him some time to demonstrate adequate pragmatics, particularly in playing the "game" of social give-and-take with peers. This is not surprising, given that he had been hung on a wall previously, kind of like a wooden version of the "Wild Boy of Aveyron." Eventually, Pinocchio shows a flair for ritual insults, as when he realizes he had been duped into going to the shore to find the dogfish and he unleashes an impressive string of epithets. An ample repertoire of comebacks, put-downs, and diversionary techniques are useful for deflecting social manipulation, and Pinocchio is handicapped at the outset by not having a well-stocked supply of such social heuristics.

E. Role of Physical Incompetence in Pinocchio's Social Failures

In Ford's model of competence, there is a component termed "biology." In my proposed action model of social behavior, I have re-labeled it "physical competence." This reflects my view that biology is too broad a term, given that biological factors underlie limitations in many areas, including both everyday intelligence and affect. The broad role of biology is particularly evident in young children, where attentional and cognitive processes are highly dependent on such biological states as fatigue and hunger.

People with MR often have concomitant physical problems that affect endurance, strength, and coordination (Newell, 1997), and they are more likely to have neurological disorders or to use medications that affect concentration (Baumeister & MacLean, 1979; Tomporowski & Tinsley, 1997). Consequently, people with MR would appear to be at a disadvantage in dealing with interpersonal situations that are protracted and which cause unpleasant physical sensations such as fatigue, hunger, nicotine withdrawal, or the need to go the bathroom. Although physical competence is a less central contributor to social effectiveness than the other factors described earlier in this section, there are undoubtedly situations (e.g., the reported use of sleep deprivation in many police interrogations) where one's physical state can be the deciding factor in tipping the balance into what might be considered ineffective interpersonal behavior. This is because predatory exploiters intentionally take advantage of the disorganizing effect of fatigue and protracted sensory deprivation, as in the case of police interrogations that (typically) extend through the late-night hours. Individuals who have MR are doubly vulnerable in such situations, not only because they often have limited physical reserves, but also because they are more concrete in their goals and may, at such a time, value short-term comfort (such as the opportunity to get some sleep) over long-term survival. Other physical factors (e.g., inebriation, sensory impairment, lack of strength or coordination, and so on) undoubtedly contribute to social ineffectiveness as well.

Being made out of wood can be a handicap, as when Pinocchio falls asleep before a fireplace and his leg catches fire (Gepetto has to make him a replacement leg). Sometimes it can be an advantage, as when a predator tried to bite Pinocchio and he used his arm as a club to ward off the attacker. His other physical systems, such as hearing and vision, seemed to be intact. A very significant physical problem for a marionette, however, and one that undoubtedly explains many of Pinocchio's problems, is the absence of a brain.

There is growing evidence that social intelligence is localized in specific brain areas (Brothers, 1997). Some disorders, such as autism and Asperger disorder (an appropriate diagnosis for Pinocchio?) appear to be marked by specific social intelligence impairments and are most likely neurologically grounded, perhaps as a result of intrauterine infection. Given his absence of a brain, it is not surprising that Pinocchio had difficulties in processing social information. This is reflected not only in high-level social cognition (such as failure to categorize the Field of Wonders investment scheme as a scam) but also in more perceptual areas (such as seeing through disguises). (Pinocchio's difficulty in this area may be a sign of prosopagnosia, a difficulty in recognizing faces caused by brain damage.) In other physical areas, such as strength, endurance, and coordination, Pinocchio seems fairly normal, and motoric impairment does not appear to have played a role in his vulnerability to social pressure.

III. CAN SOCIAL INCOMPETENCE BE REMEDIATED?

Seeing Pinocchio finally achieve social competence provides hope for the rest of us. There are, however, structural limits to the extent of such remediation, and at times the best that can be done is to put protections (such as conservatorship arrangements) in place. Perhaps the best use for an action model of social effectiveness is that it can serve as a guide to particular interventions and protections that might be needed by a given individual.

Personally, I think the Fairy with Blue Hair had very little to do with Pinocchio's remarkable breakthrough, although all of us could benefit from someone watching over us and providing useful advice (even if, like Pinocchio, we ignore it at first). A contemporary equivalent of the Fairy With Blue Hair is Rosemary Crossley, the inventor of facilitated communication (FC), who claimed to make people with severe autism and MR socially normal by putting her hand over theirs, in a manner similar to the blessing which the fairy gives Pinocchio at the end of the book. Whatever the benefits of FC may be (and I think the stories of miraculous awakening are as much a fantasy as anything in *Pinocchio*), they likely stem more from encouragement and raised expectations than from anything it itself has to offer.

Pinocchio transformed himself into a *mensch*, and the fairy just put her stamp of approval on the result. How did it happen, and are there any lessons or cautions to be drawn from this story? First of all—lest anyone wonder whether I have lost touch with reality—*Pinocchio* is a fairy tale, and in the real world, and even sometimes in fairy tales (as in *AI*, Spielberg's sci-fi update of *Pinocchio*), endings are not always happy. Some people, including most of those with MR and related disorders, always remain relatively socially incompetent, and even a successful transformation project such as Pinocchio can unravel in a stressful or difficult moment. Still, the risk of disastrous social failure can be ameliorated somewhat, even in individuals who face significant handicaps, and Pinocchio's story, again examined in light of my heuristic model, may tell us about how that might happen.

In the book *By The Grace of Guile*, Rue (1994) observes that deceiving, being deceived, and avoiding being deceived, are at the core of what it means to be human. Almost anyone can be deceived occasionally, except for those who are paranoid, and they may be the most deceivable of all. The mark of a true incompetent is when he or she is deceived repeatedly, even by the same person, and even when the deception is clumsy and obvious. For most people, being deceived can be a learning experience, as was noted by Joseph Roux in *Meditations of a Parish Priest*, when he wrote: "That which deceives us and does us harm, also undeceives us and does us good." My point here is that being duped, despicable as is, can be of some benefit, especially if there is a helpful other person around who can sympathetically try to point out the lessons to be learned.

Pinocchio's eventual ability to resist trickery, as at the end when he encountered the fox and the cat, appears to have grown largely out of previous duping experiences, and the mediating efforts of the Fairy with Blue Hair and other teachers, including the (later revived) cricket. Social intelligence, particularly its crystallized component, is a likely aspect of intelligence that continues to develop throughout adulthood, as reflected in the common-folk belief that wisdom (experience-based insight, especially about social relationships) increases as one enters old age.

Motivational factors undoubtedly play a major role in helping people become less susceptible to being manipulated, and motivational methods can be as effective in the acquisition of social effectiveness as they can in the area of academic functioning. Pinocchio became more socially competent in large part because the goal of returning home became more salient, and the strong affect associated with becoming thwarted (especially the scare of becoming a donkey) became more negatively reinforcing. Gradually, with some success in resisting manipulators, Pinocchio began to develop interpersonal self-efficacy, so that he became more confident that he could prevail in social settings, just as he had already begun to do in academic settings. Then there is the little matter of a conscience. Pinocchio always had a kind heart, as the fairy pointed out at the end, but he needed to learn that "crime doesn't pay." Moral development for Pinocchio, as in the Kohlbergian sense, lay less in becoming a nice guy and more in learning that being nice needs to be balanced against the ability to say "no."

The final piece in the puzzle of becoming socially effective in challenging situations, at least for Pinocchio, was the acquisition of some verbal tricks, or heuristics, to call upon when being "fogged" by the tapestry of lies, inducements, and specious reasoning of con artists. Having friends probably helped Pinocchio, as he became quite adept at exchanging insults and "playing the dozens" (Pinocchio refrained from dissing the other kids' mothers, probably because that was a touchy subject for the motherless boy). Children's television shows, particularly those on cable channels, can be a useful source of modeling of ritual insults and social resistance techniques (it may be the only redeeming benefit of such shows), and Pinocchio's development as a player of such games may have been delayed because Gepetto did not have a television, let alone cable.

Where social incompetence has a neurological basis, as is likely the case with autistic people and with Pinocchio, there are more likely to be limits to how much social competence can be boosted, although even in such cases (as with Pinocchio) significant growth can occur. Pinocchio, as a youth, is still a social work in progress, and it is by no means certain at the end of the story that his hard-won competence is permanent or complete. Perhaps he prevailed over the cat and the fox because of their dispirited and bedraggled state, or because he recognized them for once. I imagine that it would not be too difficult to dupe Pinocchio again, as he was by the boys who talked him into playing hooky and going to the shore after he previously had appeared to turn over a new leaf. Pinocchio may always need a "supported living arrangement," where a caregiver such as the cricket or the fairy can keep a watchful eye over him. Still, there is reason to be cautiously optimistic about Pinocchio, as there is about every young person who shows signs of learning the rudiments of being an effective human. Unfortunately, being an effective human depends to a large extent, on one's ability to recognize and resist the tricks, traps, and deceptions of bad people.

This central reality has been recognized in numerous works of great literature, including the Bible (e.g., the serpent, Samson and Delilah), Shakespeare (Othello), Mark Twain (Tom Sawyer and his fence-painting scam), Melville (*The Confidence Man*), and current authors (e.g., most of the plays of David Mamet). Literature has much to tell us about gullibility and victimization in the face of lies. Social scientists need to address more attention to this topic, especially given its relevance to the social survival of at-risk populations such as the frail elderly and people with MR.

REFERENCES

Balla, D., & Zigler, E. (1979). Personality development in retarded persons. In N. R. Ellis (Ed.), *Handbook of mental deficiency: Psychological theory and research* (2nd ed., pp. 143–168). Hillsdale, NJ: Erlbaum.

Bandura, A. (1997). *Self-efficacy: The exercise of control.* New York: W. H. Freeman.

Baumeister, A. A., & MacLean, W. E. (1979). Brain damage and mental retardation. In N. R. Ellis (Ed.), *Handbook of mental deficiency: Psychological theory and research* (2nd ed., pp. 197–230). Hillsdale, N.J.: Erlbaum.

Brothers, L. (1997). *Friday's footprint: How society shapes the human mind.* New York: Oxford University Press.

Cantor, N., & Genero, N. (1986). Psychiatric diagnosis and natural categorization: A close analogy. In T. Millon & G. L. Klerman (Eds.), *Contempory directions in child psychopathology: Toward the DSM-IV* (pp. 233–256). New York: Guilford.

Cialdini, R. B. (1984). *Influence: How and why people agree to things.* New York: William Morrow.

Clare, I. C., & Gudjonsson, G. H. (1995). The vulnerability of suspects with intellectual disabilities during police interviews: A review and experimental study of decision-making. *Mental Handicap Research, 8,* 110–128.

Collodi, C. (1968/1881). *Pinocchio* (translated by J. Walker, illustrated by W. Dempster). Santa Rosa, CA: Classic Press, Inc.

Deci, E. L., & Ryan, R. M. (1985). *Intrinsic motivation and self-determination in human behavior.* New York: Plenum.

Doll, E. A. (1936). President's address: Current thoughts on mental deficiency. *Journal of Psycho-Asthenics, 18,* 40–41.

Feuerstein, R., Rand, Y., Hoffman, M. B., & Miller, R. (1980). *Instrumental enrichment: Intervention program for cognitive modifiability.* Baltimore: University Park Press.

Ford, D. H., & Lerner, R. M. (1992). *Developmental systems theory: An integrative approach.* Newbury Park, CA: Sage.

Ford, M. E. (1986). A living systems conceptualization of social intelligence: Processes, outcomes and developmental change. In R. J. Sternberg (Ed.), *Advances in the psychology of human intelligence* (Vol. 3, pp. 119–171). Hillsdale, NJ: Erlbaum.

Ford, M. E. (1992). *Motivating humans: Goals, emotions, and personal agency beliefs.* Newbury Park, CA: Sage.

Goddard, H. H. (1914). *Feeble-mindedness: Its causes and consequences.* New York: Macmillan.

Goleman, D. (1995). *Emotional intelligence.* New York: Bantam.

Greenspan, S. (1981). Defining childhood social competence: A proposed working model. In B. K. Keogh (Ed.), *Advances in special education* (Vol. 3, pp. 1–39). Greenwich, CT: JAI Press.

Greenspan, S. (1995). There is more to intelligence than IQ. In D. C. Connery (Ed.), *Convicting the innocent: The story of a murder, a false confession, and the struggle to free a "wrong man"* (pp. 136–151). Cambridge, MA: Brookline Books.

Greenspan, S. (1999). A contextualist perspective on adaptive behavior. In R. Schalock (Ed.), *Adaptive behavior: Conceptual basis, measurement and use* (pp. 61–80). Washington, DC: American Association on Mental Retardation.

Greenspan, S. (2003). Perceived risk status as a key to defining mental retardation: Social and everyday vulnerability in the natural prototype. In H. Switzky & S. Greenspan (Eds.), *What is mental retardation? Ideas for an evolving disability category*. Washington, DC: American Association on Mental Retardation (Published as an e-book, accessible at www.disabilitybooksonline.com).

Greenspan, S., & Driscoll, J. (1997). The role of intelligence in a broad model of personal competence. In D. P. Flanagan, J. L. Genshaft, & P. L. Harrison (Eds.), *Contemporary intellectual assessment: Theories, tests and issues* (pp. 131–150). New York: Guilford.

Greenspan, S., Loughlin, G., & Black, R. S. (2001). Credulity and gullibility in persons with mental retardation: A proposed framework for future research. In L. Masters-Glidden (Ed.), *International review of research in mental retardation* (Vol. 24, pp. 101–135). New York: Academic Press.

Greenspan, S., & Love, P. E. (1997). Social intelligence and developmental disorder: Mental retardation, learning disabilities, and autism. In W. E. MacLean (Ed.), *Ellis' handbook of mental deficiency, psychological theory, and research* (pp. 311–342). Mahwah, NJ: Lawrence Erlbaum Associates.

Greenspan, S., & Shoutlz, B. (1981). Why mentally retarded adults lose their jobs: Social competence as a factor in work adjustment. *Applied Research in Mental Retardation, 2,* 23–38.

Greenspan, S., Switzky, H., & Granfield, J. (1996). Everyday intelligence and adaptive behavior: A theoretical framework. In J. Jacobson & J. Mulick (Eds.), *Manual on diagnosis and professional practice in mental retardation* (pp. 127–135). Washington, DC: American Psychological Association.

Jones, K., & Day, J. D. (1997). Discrimination of two aspects of cognitive-social intelligence from academic intelligence. *Journal of Educational Psychology, 89,* 486–497.

Leffert, J. S., & Siperstein, G. N. (2002). Social cognition: A key to understanding adaptive behavior in individuals with mental retardation. *International Review of Research in Mental Retardation, 25,* 135–181.

Lefkowitz, B. (1997). *Our guys: The Glen Ridge rape and the secret life of the perfect suburb.* Berkeley: University of California Press.

Matson, J. L., & Fee, V. E. (1991). Social skill difficulties among persons with mental retardation. In J. L. Matson & J. A. Mulick (Eds.), *Handbook of mental retardation* (2nd ed., pp. 468–478). New York: Pergamon.

Newell, K. M. (1997). Motor skills and mental retardation. In W. F. MacLean, Jr. (Ed.), *Ellis' handbook of mental deficiency, psychological theory and research* (3rd ed., pp. 275–308). Mahwah, NJ: Erlbaum.

Orwell, G. (1949). *1984.* New York: Harcourt Brace.

Perske, R. (1991). *Unequal justice?: What can happen when persons with retardation or other developmental disabilities encounter the criminal justice system.* Nashville: Abingdon Press.

Reiss, S., & Havercamp, S. M. (1996). The sensivity theory of motivation: Implications for psychopathology. *Behavior Research and Therapy, 34,* 621–632.

Rue, L. (1994). *By the grace of guile: The role of deception in natural history and human affairs.* New York: Oxford University Press.

Schroeder, S. R., Tessel, R. E., Loupe, P. S., & Stodgell, C. J. (1997). Severe behavior problems among people with developmental disabilities. In W. F. MacLean, Jr. (Ed.), *Ellis' handbook of mental deficiency, psychological theory and research* (pp. 439–464). Mahwah, NJ: Erlbaum.

Siperstein, G. N., & Leffert, J. S. (1997). Comparison of socially accepted and rejected children with mental retardation. *American Journal on Mental Retardation, 101,* 339–351.

Spitz, H. (1988). Mental retardation as a thinking disorder: The rationalist alternative to empiricism. In N. Bay (Ed.), *International review of research in mental retardation* (Vol. 15, pp. 1–32). New York: Academic Press.

Sternberg, R. J. (1984). Macrocomponents and microcomponents of intelligence: Some proposed loci of mental retardation. In P. H. Brooks, R. Sperber, & C. McCauley (Eds.), *Learning and cognition in the mentally retarded* (pp. 89–114). Hillsdale, NJ: Lawrence Erlbaum Associates.

Switzky, H. N. (Ed.) (2001). *Personality and motivational differences in persons with mental retardation* Hillsdale, NJ: Lawrence Erlbaum Associates.

Switzky, H. N., Greenspan, S., Jacobson, J., & Glidden, L. (2002, August). *Symposium: The Tao of mental retardation for the 21st century?* Annual Meeting of the American Psychological Association, Division 33, Chicago, Illinois.

Switzky, H. N., Everington, C., Keyes, D., Baroff, G., Greenspan, S., & Fulero, S. (2003, August). *Symposium: Mental retardation and the law–Atkins v. Virginia.* Annual Meeting of the American Psychological Association, Divisions 33, 41, Toronto, Ontario, Canada.

Tomporowski, P. D., & Tinsley, V. (1997). Attention in mentally retarded people. In W. F. MacLean, Jr. (Ed.), *Ellis' handbook of mental deficiency, psychological theory and research* (3rd ed., pp. 219–244). Mahwah, NJ: Lawrence Erlbaum Associates.

Tredgold, A. F. (1922). *Mental deficiency.* New York: Wood.

Warren, S. F., & Yoder, P. J. (1997). Communication, language and mental retardation. In W. F. MacLean, Jr. (Ed.), *Ellis' handbook of mental deficiency, psychological theory and research* (3rd ed., pp. 379–404). Mahwah, NJ: Erlbaum.

Wilson, C., Seaman, L., & Nettelbeck, T. (1996). Vulnerability to criminal exploitation: Influence of interpersonal competence differences among people with mental retardation. *Journal of Intellectual Disability Research, 40,* 8–16.

Yalon-Chamovitz, S. (2000). *Everyday wisdom in people with mental retardation: Role of experience and practical intelligence.* Unpublished doctoral dissertation, University of Connecticut.

Zigler, E., & Yando, R. (1972). Outerdirectedness and imitative behavior of institutionalized and noninstitutionalized younger and older children. *Child development, 43,* 413–425.

Understanding the Development of Subnormal Performance in Children from a Motivational-Interactionist Perspective

JANNE LEPOLA, PEKKA SALONEN, MARJA VAURAS, AND
ELISA POSKIPARTA

UNIVERSITY OF TURKU, FINLAND

Recent theoretical formulations and empirical findings have challenged the simplistic deficit-explanations of subnormal cognitive performance. Subnormal cognitive performance in its varying forms (labeled, for instance, with terms like 'learning disability,' 'reading disability,' 'arithmetic disability,' or 'mental retardation'), seems to be a complex phenomenon that cannot be adequately explained on the basis of organic or psychological deficit models and linear-causal explanations dealing with hypothetical deficiencies in the constitution of the individual (Brooks & Baumeister, 1977; Cole & Bruner, 1971; Ginsburg, 1972; Harris, 1988; Kavale & Forness, 1985; Olkinuora & Salonen, 1992; Spear-Swerling & Sternberg, 1998; Stanovich, 1993; Switzky, 1997). It has been pointed out that more comprehensive, interactionist, dynamic, and systemic models are needed to detect the full complexity of subnormal performance (Charlesworth, 1978; Hargreaves, 1978; Sameroff, 1975; Schoggen, 1978). A comprehensive systemic view is capable of focusing on: (1) reciprocal, dynamic interplay between the person and his or her physical/social environment; (2) interactions between cognitive, motivational, and emotional functions; (3) the interplay of developmental processes at the microgenetic (i.e., moment-by-moment activity) level and the long-term developmental level; and (4) interactions between situational and instutional-cultural levels, to understand the sociocultural underpinnings of the interactive origins and maintenance of individual differences (Cicourel et al., 1974; Gutierrez et al., 1995; Howard-Rose & Rose, 1994; LCHC, 1982; Lehtinen et al., 1995; Mehan, 1988; Salonen et al., 1998a; Schultz, 1994).

Straightforward inferences from behavioral deficits (performance decrements) to an alleged trait of the individual (lack of competence based on an organic or phychological deficiency) have been questioned by interactionist, systemic, contextualist-functionalist, and socio-cultural views (Armour-Thomas, 1992; Charlesworth, 1976; Cole & Bruner, 1971; Endler & Magnusson, 1976; Pervin & Lewis, 1978), as well as by empirical research focusing on the variation of human activity under varying situational conditions (Ceci & Bronfenbrenner, 1985; Glutting & Youngstrom, 1996; Lave et al., 1984). Our conceptualization of the term 'subnormal performance' derives from the systemic-functionalist view that is best exemplified in the ethological approach (Charlesworth, 1978; Olkinuora & Salonen, 1992; Tinbergen & Tinbergen, 1983). An 'odd' behavior, in this case subnormal performance, is not defined in terms of 'lack' or 'deficiency' but in terms of functionality and adaptedness of behavior (Tinbergen & Tinbergen, 1983, p. 36). Similar to their 'normally' behaving counterparts, individuals showing symptomatic or deviant behaviors have undergone a history of adaptations, and have developed functional systems through which they have coped with adaptive demands in person-situation interaction. The strategic peculiarities and 'symptoms' associated with subnormal cognitive performance (e.g., mindless imitating, random guessing, passivity, inhibition, compulsive behavior, restlessness, stereotyped responses, acting-out behaviors), may thus indicate the adaptedness of behavior to certain (non-task) aspects of the environment (Salonen et al., 1998a).

There are empirical findings indicating that cognitive subnormality may indeed be a part of a more general (mal)adaptive condition. Recent research has shown that children with cognitive disorders usually manifest comorbid symptoms characteristic of several other symptom groups. Children with learning disorders and mental retardation (MR) often show severe motivational problems, emotional/behavioral disorders (EBD), serious emotional disturbance (SED), attention deficit/hyperactivity disorders (ADD/ADHD), and personality problems (August & Garfinkel, 1990; McConaughy et al., 1994; Rock et al., 1997; Switzky, 2001).

The tendency to form sharp-edged, narrow, and mutually exclusive diagnostic categories and definitions may (1) lead to theoretically and clinically arbitrary subdivisions of 'disabilities'; (2) prevent one from seeing possibly important common behaviors manifested by individuals despite their different diagnostic labels; (3) lead to a lack of consideration of the marked population with atypical symptom combinations; and (4) hinder the development of conceptual models focusing on cross-domain relationships, for instance, the concomitance of learning problems and emotional/behavioral/ motivational/personality problems (Rock et al., 1997). We are using a global and somewhat loose term 'subnormal cognitive performance' (referring to subaverage performance, irrespective of whether it is identified in classroom assessment situations, achievement tests, or standardized intelligence test settings) because we want to focus on the (mal)adaptive behavior that children, across the variety of allegedly cognitively 'deviant' groups, may have in common. If such commonalities are found, for instance, across the adaptive behavior of learning disability (LD), MR, and autistic children, this might contribute to a better understanding of the general maladaptive condition and the role of cognition within it.

We have questioned the trait-type conceptualizations and particularly the construct of IQ as the paramount distinctive factor among the subgroups of cognitive subnormality (Olkinuora & Salonen, 1992). An intelligence test performance, regularly used as an operational measure for the selection of the LD and MR samples, is assumed to reflect self-evidently and directly the individuals' innate potential, whereas an achievement test performance is seen to assess their current functioning (Siegel, 1999). We have argued that intelligence (or other 'aptitude') test scores, as well as school achievement test results, are only performances. From the point of view an individual's adaptation, his or her behavior in an intelligence test situation does not reflect a covert trait or capacity any more directly than other test scores (Olkinuora & Salonen, 1992). As Stanovich (1999) has pointed out, the poor reading of individuals with low or normal IQ cannot be explained by their IQ. What we need is a specific processing explanation for poor reading in both groups (Stanovich, 1999). A weak intelligence test performance needs a specific processing explanation as urgently as, for instance, a weak reading or math test performance (Olkinuora & Salonen, 1992). Consequently, we have to seek the explaining factors for both school achievement and aptitude test performances not among hypothesized cognitive competencies, but among more multifaceted and complex interactions that are occurring in the total process of adaptation within learning and performance situations. Thus, in addition to specific cognitive processes, emotional, motivational, and sociocultural aspects of adaptation gain importance (Armour-Thomas, 1992). Substantial empirical evidence for the relevance of such factors stems from the observational assessments of the children's behavior during aptitude test sessions: children with inappropriate motivational and socioemotional behaviors, such as avoidance, inattentiveness, and uncooperativeness, are likely to obtain markedly lower IQ scores than children with more suitable test-taking behaviors (Glutting & Youngstrom, 1996).

In the first part of the chapter, we focus on the motivational and emotional consequences of several less optimal adult-child teaching interactions. By using the scaffolding framework, traditionally applied to illustrate progressive developments, we aim to show its value in understanding the formation and development of non–task-oriented tendencies in early childhood.

In other words, the ideal instructional models typically do not alert us to the fact that the development of motivation and cognition, which are dependent on social interaction, may go awry (Harter, 1999, p. 167). In addition, we present our interactionist model for motivational orientations and coping strategies to describe how motivational tendencies are established and maintained (and reinforced) in a classroom context and how they interact with cognition. The second part of the chapter focuses on the interplay of the developmental patterns of motivation and cognition. The situational deterioration or progression of cognitive performance is embedded in long-term developmental processes in which the accumulation of situational interactions contribute to diverging learning careers. To illustrate the developmental dynamics of cognition and motivation, we will present results of three studies with children followed from preschool to the 8th grade. These studies relate motivational orientation and coping tendencies to cognitive prerequisites of reading and to reading skills such as decoding and text comprehension. Finally, we discuss the implications of the aforementioned theoretical perspective and empirical findings with respect to further research, remedial instruction, and classroom practices.

I. SCAFFOLDING AND THE SOCIALLY MEDIATED DEVELOPMENT OF COGNITION AND MOTIVATION

Most developmental theories presuppose that the growth of the child's adaptive capacity is based on the increasing organization and differentiation of mental and behavioral structures, progressively leading to growing self-regulation and independence of action from immediate external stimuli. The development of self-regulation is accompanied by a increasing sense of self-efficacy and motivation to initiate and maintain task-focused activities related to new environmental challenges.

According to Vygotsky's (1962, 1978) theoretical notion of the development of higher mental functions through social mediation, adults (and more skilled peers) initially take the major responsibility for organizing the developing child's action and articulating his/her cognitive processes. With time, this responsibility is ceded to the child who is expected to master the action independently and to take charge of his/her own thinking processes. The gradual increase of self-regulation becomes possible through systematically utilizing the child's *zone of proximal development* (ZPD) in the teaching-learning interaction. In a system of adult-child joint activity, the child's functions that are at the maturing stage are first segmented and organized by the adult. The adult aids and encourages the child from one level of competence to the next by structuring the task into subtasks, by modeling and prompting the execution of subskills and the integration of operations, and by introducing culturally prestructured heuristics and symbolic means for organizing the actions. During this process, the child is gradually given less assistance and encouraged to carry out larger units of action until he/she is capable of independently accomplishing the total task performance (Palincsar, 1986; Rogoff & Gardner, 1984).

Wood et al. (1976) originally used the '*scaffold*' *metaphor* to describe the ideal guiding role of the adult. In an optimal instructional interaction, the adult determines the child's 'region of sensitivity to instruction' and, through graduated intervention, 'adjusts the scaffolding to the child's developing capabilities' (Rogoff & Gardner, 1984, p. 101). Scaffolded instruction presupposes the growing of self-regulation through gradual internalization of a socially supported mediation process. In each phase of skill development, the learner is given appropriate supportive tools (e.g., directions, cueing) that provide a sufficient framework for reaching the next skill level and closing the gap between the actual developmental level and task requirements. Figure 1 illustrates, through a building construction analogy, the idea of a socially mediated process of development and, in particular, how a child is gradually able to accomplish more difficult tasks through successfully implemented scaffolding.

The optimal stimulating of the development of maturing competencies presupposes skilled *dosing* and *fading* of scaffolding support according to the growth of the child's independent functioning (Fig. 1; *Dosing*: constructing the minimal necessary scaffolding for the part of the building that is under

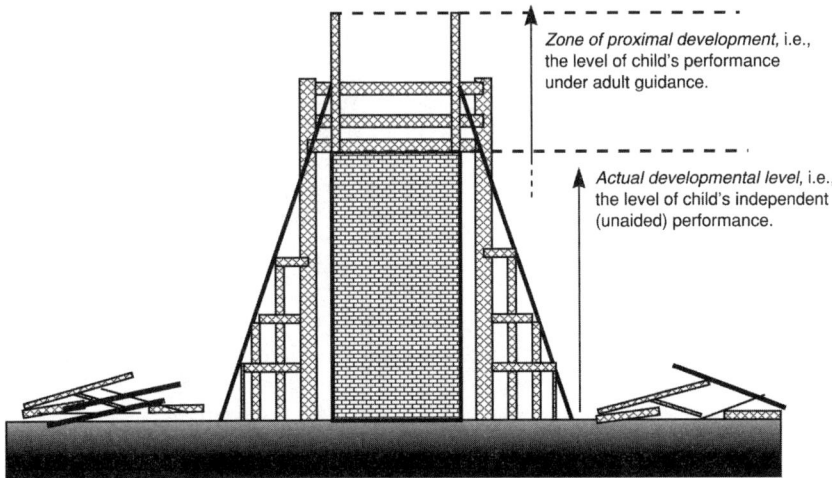

FIG. 1. A model of the zone of proximal development and the scaffolding process.

construction and cannot yet stand fast; *Fading*: tearing down the scaffolding from around the ready-made part of the building that is already capable to stand independently). In order to stimulate the child's optimal development, the teacher has to continuously adjust the subgoals to a slightly higher level than that represented by the child's momentary independent performance, as well as to appropriately provide a *minimal necessary support* for filling the gap between these two levels (Rogoff & Gardner, 1984). The notions of fading and minimal necessary support imply that the quality, amount, and phasing of the adult guidance should be dynamically adjusted to a particular child's momentary ZPD and to the actual microgenetic developmental processes occurring during a socially-mediated learning sequence. Thus, the reciprocal adjustments and regulations occurring during a scaffolding process are essentially based on continuous dynamic assessments.

The aforementioned characterization of the ideal scaffolding process implies the possibility of several less optimal alternatives based on the fact that the adults do not sufficiently pay attention to a particular child's changing needs during the scaffolding processes and cannot adjust their activities accordingly. Under such conditions, the child may begin to respond to environmental demands with growing externally-imposed regulation, or with emotional-behavioral dysregulation, accompanied by a decreasing sense of self-efficacy and strengthened non–task-focused motivation (Cherkes-Julkowski & Mitlina, 1999; Crittenden & DiLalla, 1988; Jacobsen et al., 1997; Marcus, 1975; Patterson & Bank, 1989; Sansbury & Wahler, 1992; Switzky, 2001). Theoretically, at least three types of interactional imbalance or dysfunctionality can be conceived.

1. Well-intentioned parents and teachers may utilize (over)controlling teaching strategies (Barrett & Boggiano, 1988; Boggiano & Katz, 1991; Flink et al., 1990; Wall & Dattilo, 1995). While delivering extrinsic incentives, many parents and teachers seem not to believe in the *minimal-sufficiency principle*, but think that, in accordance with the *maximal-operant principle*, it is better to provide the child with a 'maximal' dose of cues, rewards, and exhortations (Boggiano & Katz, 1991). Controlling parenting and teaching style comprises not only overdosing of extrinsic incentives, but also frequent acts of 'positive' intervening, as well as more directive and even coercive forms of control (for instance, just as the child is beginning to experiment with a newly acquired skill, the adult intrudes into the child's activity by saying: 'not that way, let *me* show!'). Even in the case where the child is willing and able to respond independently to the demands of the new task or skill level, he or she is bombarded with adult incentives appropriate to much lower skill levels. There is evidence that excessive or otherwise

inappropriate utilization of clues, external rewards, and control strategies will not only distort the child's independent functioning (self-regulation) within a skill domain, but will also undermine his or her intrinsic motivation and preference for challenge (Barrett & Boggiano, 1988; Deci & Ryan, 1987; Flink et al., 1990). Depending on the nature of controlling strategies, different kinds of adverse motivational, socio-cognitive, and emotional outcomes can be expected. If the child is overwhelmingly exposed to external clues, rewards, and frequent help, he or she is likely to show increased extrinsic motivational orientation and over-reliance on external cues and incentives. Since there is no gradual adjustment and fading of support, the responsibility of activity-control remains with the adult delivering directions and rewards, and the scaffolding process does not promote the child's task-related autonomy and sense of self-efficacy. Instead of the task dimension, the child will continue to build a sense of self-efficacy within the social dimension: instead of being directed toward the task, the child's approach motivation and coping efforts are increasingly directed toward the controlling social agent (authority) (Harter, 1978; Salonen et al., 1998a). The child not only learns to expect an adult's step-by-step guidance and rewards, but he or she also becomes accustomed to following and even eliciting supportive social cues from the guiding adult. As a function of excessive adult-guided interaction, the child may learn to respond to the environment rather than to initiate and participate in interactions (Busch-Rossnagel et al., 1995).

Controlling strategies sometimes include coercive or harsh forms of discipline and punishing evaluative elements that are often charged with negative affect (Barrett & Boggiano, 1988; Sansbury & Wahler, 1992). The more the teachers' or parents' over-controlling behavior takes directive, evaluative, and coercive forms, the more inhibited and negative emotion-charged compliant behavior can be expected. Children who have been exposed to the controllingness and harshness of an adult often show *'compulsive compliance'* or *'frozen watchfulness,'* i.e., they wait warily for demands, responding quickly and compliantly, and then return to the previous vigilant state (Crittenden & DiLalla, 1988). The approach motivation in both task and social dimensions is conflict-laden. Imposed (obedience-based) task-approach efforts will be inhibited by avoidance tendencies originating from earlier experiences of uncontrollable failure feedback and its emotional consequences. In a similar vein, socially-directed approach motivation enters into conflict with avoidance tendencies originating from aversive social experiences (Elliott, 1999). It is apparent that interactions leading to such a distortion of approach motivation and emotion-charged inhibition (wariness) in both important dimensions of socially-mediated learning, do not represent an optimal scaffolding process.

2. Parents and teachers may permanently provide a child with too few clues or withdraw their support prematurely (e.g., 'you're already so old that you should do it yourself'). Ambitious and hurried parents or teachers, who are stressing on the mastery of the whole curriculum, may set pretentious demands for the child's development and too hastily aspire to the child's autonomous functioning during the formation of a complex skill. Cumulative experiences of insufficient support and/or too rapid fading of support distort the formation of independent functioning. Since the gap between the child's actual developmental level and task requirements remains repeatedly unfulfilled during many successive scaffolding episodes, the child will be exposed to chronic failure experiences with the sense of uncontrollability and stress. On one hand, the child has not yet developed sufficient skills to autonomously master the new task requirements and, on the other hand, he or she does not succeed in getting appropriate support from the withdrawn adult. The child, being chronically over-demanded, is likely to develop a poor sense of self-efficacy in both task and social dimensions. The child will probably show avoidance motivation tendencies directed towards both the task and the guiding adult. The motivational processes and mechanisms related to over-demanding and insufficient support-giving are, so far, theory-based hypotheses. Although there is rather ample empirical evidence concerning cognitive-developmental outcomes of imbalanced communication patterns in adult-child dyads (Lyytinen et al., 1994; Tiegermann & Siperstein, 1984), studies concerning the motivational and socio-emotional effects of insufficient or improperly phased support-giving in instructional and scaffolding settings are almost non-existent (Nelson-LeGall, 1981; Nelson-LeGall & Glor-Scheib, 1985).

3. Due to their own life situation and socio-emotional problems, parents and teachers may respond to the child's momentary needs in instructional and scaffolding settings in a roughly inconsistent, indeterminate, or asynchronous manner. Such responses include parental over-compliance (i.e., extreme compliance in the face of the child's momentary demands and refusals) and asynchronous feedback (i.e., responses lacking reciprocity and coordination in relation to the joint task or the child's activity), randomly given aversive and positive responses (e.g., punishing and rewarding based on the adult's current mood), as well as occasional and chronic unresponsiveness (Tiegerman & Siperstein, 1984; Wentzel, 1994). The inconsistency of parents or teachers is likely to bring extensive threatening elements into the whole process of socially-mediated construction of learning tasks. Although avoidance motivation is established particularly due to the lack of contingency between the child's efforts and their social consequences, his or her sense of self-efficacy will be distorted also in the task dimension; the lack of systematic autonomy-supporting social regulation (or mediation) inhibits the child's

adequate progressing within the ZPD and blocks the feeling of growing task-related competence.

The attachment literature has also pointed out how parental unresponsiveness (i.e., caregivers' insensitivity to child's signals) is related to children's insecure attachment, because parental under-attunement does not provide the necessary tools for the child to attend to and label his or her emotional states. Furthermore, the opposite of unresponsiveness, parental over-attunement or intrusiveness, according to Stern (as cited in Harter, 1999, p. 173), represents a form of 'emotional theft' in which the parent determines how the infant should feel rather than how the infant actually does feel. According to Harter (1999), this kind of pattern in turn may lead to emotional imbalance.

The scaffolding process is essentially reciprocal. Just as parents and teachers influence the course of socialization during childhood, the child participating in the transaction can be viewed as a source of influence over his or her own development (Marcus, 1975). Self-reinforcing transactional cycles seem to be essential in the early development of not only cognitive but also motivational and socio-emotional dispositions. Parents and teachers tend to reinforce the particular child behavior dominant at the time and shift their interactional styles according to the type of child behavior (Marcus, 1975). For instance, dependent behavior in children has been found to elicit greater encouragement of dependence and directiveness from parents, whereas independent conduct elicits greater encouragement of dependence and directiveness from parents (Marcus, 1975; Osofsky, 1971; Osofsky & O'Connell, 1972; Yarrow et al., 1971). Thus, the origins of early motivational and socio-emotional adaptations leading to diverging developmental pathways characterized by increasing vulnerability versus resilience can be traced to the mutuality and reciprocity of social transactions (Sameroff, 1975).

A. Three-Part Model for Motivational Orientations

Our analysis of the situational and developmental transactions between a child's adaptive efforts and the instructor's controlling and reward styles led us to construct a three-part model comprising basic motivational orientation dimensions and corresponding sets of coping strategies and emotional behaviors (Lehtinen et al., 1995; Olkinuora & Salonen, 1992; Salonen, 2000; Salonen et al., 1998a). According to this model, a generalized orientation tendency manifests itself as certain sets of situation-specific coping strategies and emotional responses. A typical set of coping strategies and/or emotional responses tends to be launched when a certain orientation tendency interacts with appropriate situational cues. The three motivational orientations are: (1) task orientation; (2) ego-defensive orientation; and (3) social dependence orientation (Olkinuora & Salonen, 1992; Salonen et al., 1998a). Each orientation dimension can be characterized by its adaptive focus (task, self, instructor), its activated functional system (approach, avoidance), and its constellation of self-efficacy beliefs or perceived competence (for a summary, see Table I) (Elliott, 1999; Tinbergen & Tinbergen, 1983). On the basis of earlier empirical findings concerning children's coping strategies and achievement-related emotional responses (Heckhausen & Roelofsen, 1962; Heckhausen & Wagner, 1965; Moriarty, 1961; Murphy & Moriarty, 1976), we created a taxonomy for coping strategies and emotional behaviors for each of the three motivational orientations (Salonen, 1988, 2000). Emotional responses manifesting positive, negative, or conflict-type responding to the task or social aspects (Wentzel, 1996) of the learning environment were added because certain achievement-related emotional responses are highly indicative of motivational tendencies (Heckhausen & Roelofsen, 1962; Moriarty, 1961).

1. TASK ORIENTATION

Task orientation is indicated by the child's intrinsically motivated tendency to approach, explore, and master the challenging or otherwise problematic aspects of the environment (Harter, 1981; White, 1959). When confronted with a learning task, the task content and the challenges (e.g., novelties and ambiguities) provided by the materials to be learned predominate over other situational demands (i.e., the task at hand comprises the main adaptive focus for the child).

The child's task-related exploratory activity is directed by the major functional system of *approach* (Tinbergen & Tinbergen, 1983, p. 31–32; for the construct of approach motivation, also see Elliott, 1999). In the case of task-oriented activity, this functional system coordinates behavioral subsystems that contribute to moving toward the task and attending to the task, as well as exploring and manipulating the task elements (Tinbergen & Tinbergen, 1983). The task-oriented child shows a strong sense of self-efficacy (or competence) with regard to the task. This is indicated by the child's high-grade personal involvement and persistence in his/her efforts to overcome obstacles, to make sense of the materials, and to attain mastery (Harter, 1981; Diener & Dweck, 1978). Any inconsistencies, obstacles, or even the instructor's task-related prompts and criticism, are interpreted as challenges to be responded to with growing persistence and more elaborated task-related strategies and not, for instance, with avoidance, inhibition, or immediate help-seeking (Salonen et al., 1998a).

The task-oriented child's main adaptive focus does not lie on the instructor, but this does not mean that he/she shows avoidance motivation (or inhibitory) tendencies as regards the guiding adult. Since the child's social

TABLE I
THE QUALITATIVE FEATURES AND SOCIO-COGNITIVE ORIGINS OF MOTIVATIONAL ORIENTATIONS

Qualities of orientations	Motivational Orientations			
	Task Orientation	Ego-Defensive Orientation	Social Dependence Orientation	
Adaptive focus	Mastery of the task	Self: Reducing emotional distress	Instructor: Approval-seeking, fulfilling expectations, and pleasing	
Activated functional system	Approach: Task (instructor)	Avoidance/inhibition: Avoidance-approach conflict with regard to task, instructor	Approach: Instructor (task)	
Self-efficacy beliefs	Strong: Task (instructor)	Weak: Task and instructor	Strong: Instructor (task)	
Coping strategies and emotions	Problem-focused: Positive, optimistic	Emotion-focused: Negative, depressive, irritated	Socially-focused: Positive, optimistic	
Cognitive performance	Deep-level processing: Integrity of action	Superficial level of processing: Disorganized, associative, random trials	Superficial level of processing: Mindless imitating, associative responses	
Scaffolding history	Optimal dosing and fading of support; task-focused positively charged or neutral feedback	Insufficient and inconsistent support; overdemanding; asynchronous or disoriented control; negatively charged feedback	Overresponsive/overwhelming dosing of support; overdirective control; socially focused positively charged feedback	

efforts are subordinated to task-related mastery goals, his/her approach motivation is directed toward the instructor only occasionally (i.e., when the child needs a minimal necessary amount of instrumental help) (Salonen et al., 1998a).

Several studies indicate that students with task-focused motivational or goal orientation tend to use deeper-level cognitive and self-regulatory strategies, such as linking new information to prior knowledge, identifying main ideas, monitoring their comprehension, and finding new or alternative learning strategies when difficulties arise (Entwistle & Ramsden, 1982; Graham & Golan, 1991; Meece et al., 1988; Nolen, 1988; Pintrich & DeGroot, 1990; Pintrich & Schrauben, 1992; Pintrich et al., 1994). It is plausible that task-focused orientation and the quality of cognitive performance are interrelated primarily because the task-oriented child is able to ignore incidental, distracting stimuli and maintain the integrity of action (Järvelä et al., 2001; Salonen et al., 1998a).

Task orientation bears a close resemblance to problem-focused coping, a construct that has been introduced in recent research on coping with stressful situations (Carver et al., 1989; Endler & Parker, 1990; Lazarus & Folkman, 1984). Problem-focused coping strategies, aimed at attacking a problem and altering the conditions causing the difficulty, imply principally task-oriented goal setting and belief in task-related personal control or self-efficacy (Endler & Parker, 1990, p. 846).

Our taxonomy of coping strategies and emotional behaviors (Salonen, 2000) presents the following behaviors to exemplify task-oriented coping:

1. Concentrated on-task activity (e.g., attentiveness with regard to task instructions, intensive working on the task, perseverance).
2. Verbalizations expressing positive emotions (e.g., verbalizations anticipating success, positive verbalizations related to the learning situation/product of activity).
3. Non-verbal expressions of positive emotions (e.g., signs of enthusiasm while approaching the task, signs of enthusiasm/joy in the face of difficulties or after finding the solution).

We assume that task-oriented coping strategies cumulatively reinforce the child's resilience in the face of new learning tasks and developmental challenges because of the self-reinforcing transactional cycles occurring in scaffolding processes (Lehtinen et al., 1995). It has been found that the independent and autonomous conduct of children elicits greater encouragement of independence and non-directiveness from parents, whereas children's dependence tends to elicit greater encouragement of dependence and directiveness (Marcus, 1975; Osofsky, 1971; Osofsky & O'Connell, 1972; Yarrow et al.,

1971). The same reciprocal pattern to foster dependency among the elderly people by dependency-supportive behavior of the staff has been demonstrated by Baltes (1996). There is evidence that task-oriented coping strategies are also substantiated in the scaffolding interactions occurring in the classrooms. High-achieving, task-oriented children, because of their more self-regulated and less disruptive behavior, fit better the autonomy-expectancies of the teachers and are likely to receive more autonomy-inducing or informational feedback (Deci & Ryan, 1996). During scaffolding interactions, the child's sense of self-efficacy is reinforced in the task dimension because his or her intrinsically motivated mastery efforts are responded to by minimal necessary instrumental support and by providing well-synchronized fading of support. Due to the fact that the responsibility is progressively shifted to the child, the child probably learns to attribute his or her progress to his or her own efforts and gradually growing capacity. They tend to become increasingly sensitized to task-intrinsic incentives, experience growing task-related personal control, enjoy the feelings of mastery, and seek new self-imposed challenges (Boggiano & Katz, 1991; Schultz & Switzky, 1990; Switzky, 2001). Under such conditions, it is unlikely that the instructor will become the primary focus of the child's further adaptive efforts. Yet the child's sense of self-efficacy will be reinforced also within the social dimension: the child learns that in the case that his or her own resources do not momentarily suffice, he or she will receive the necessary instrumental help that is needed for renewed task-related efforts (Nelson-LeGall & Glor-Scheib, 1985; Salonen et al., 1998a).

2. EGO-DEFENSIVE ORIENTATION

The main adaptive focus of ego-defensive orientation is the child's own self. The child, experiencing his/her self as an object-like entity rather than as an active agent, is sensitized to situational factors suggesting ego-related threat or risk (e.g., task-difficulty cues, signs expressing instructor's negative responses). The child's self-focused alarm or emergency system recognizes threats through the emotional signs of not-well-being (emotional tension, negative affects). This system tends to alleviate emotional tension or restore well-being either through eliciting inhibition of activity (e.g., freezing) and withdrawal behavior (e.g., avoidance, flight) or through more manipulative and active-aggressive forms of behavior (e.g., acting-out, fighting) (Elliott, 1999; Rotenberg & Boucsein, 1993; Tinbergen & Tinbergen, 1983).

If the child's belief in his/her personal control or self-efficacy is particularly low both in task and social dimensions, it is plausible that the learner's goals will be directed toward altering his or her self-system rather than transforming the task or social environment. Instead of a deliberate task approach or social problem-solving effort, the learner is likely to alleviate distress through emotion-focused coping strategies, such as self-preoccupation, behavioral and mental disengagement, avoidance, and denial (Boekaerts, 1993; Carver et al., 1989; Endler & Parker, 1990; Nicholls, 1984).

The following behaviors extracted from our taxonomy exemplify ego-defensive coping and emotional responses:

1. Verbalizations expressing negative emotion (e.g., anticipation of failure or blame, negative emotional verbalizations directed at one's own ego, instructor, or situation, or product of activity).
2. Non-verbal expressions of negative emotion (depressive-inhibited behavioral signs of anxiety or tension, such as blocked staring, sighing, and swallowing; active-aggressive, 'acting-out' emotional behaviors indicating agitation and reactance, such as outbursts, banging the desk, daubing or tearing the task materials).
3. Avoidance behavior (e.g., physical or imaginary flight, withdrawal gestures, inhibition of action, inhibited intention movements, verbal refusal, manipulation of the situation with the purpose of avoiding).
4. Substitute and subsidiary activities (e.g., simple routines performed instead of the task, such as drawing and playing with materials; gesture substitutes).
5. Social manipulation of the situation with the purpose to avoid (e.g., physical aggression and threatening, intentional or 'tactical' tantrums, giving orders to the guiding adult, social threatening, emotional appealing or fawning, distracting the guiding adult from the task, changing roles, persuasion).
6. Defensive regulation of the level of aspiration (e.g., choosing the easiest tasks, choosing the most difficult tasks).
7. Justifying an anticipated failure (e.g., lowering one's readiness to act and publicly expressing it, i.e., 'self-handicapping,' lowering one's own effort before or during the performance, and conveying the impression of effortlessness to others).
8. Defensive coping with the emotional consequences of failure (e.g., denying the failure, covering or passing the failure, denying the relevance of failure, insisting that the failure was insignificant or unimportant, attributing the cause of failure to an external factor outside one's control, explaining failure as intentional, using humor to cover negative feelings or to relieve inner conflict, compensating for the effects of failure) (Salonen, 2000).

Subnormally performing children with ego-defensive coping and emotional response sets are particularly vulnerable in inclusive classrooms but also in sophisticated small-group remedial instruction settings in which the training is much more accommodated to the special needs of the child (Vauras et al.,

1999a,b). Ego-defensively coping children frequently confront inadequate and ill-synchronized amounts of support and control. Their stubborn passive-avoidant or active-aggressive coping behavior, perceived as more or less 'deviant', is likely to lead either to excessive teacher control efforts or, ultimately, to giving up (Salonen et al., 1998a). Several studies show that children at risk are given more help and incentives, but also more direction, criticism, reprimands, and rejection (Barker & Graham, 1987; Boggiano & Katz, 1991; Jordan et al., 1997; McNaughton, 1981). Teachers seemingly experience pressures to normalize the 'deviant' behavior of ego-defensively oriented subnormally performing children through increasing the dose of social incentives and control (Olkinuora & Salonen, 1992; Salonen et al., 1998a). Although children at risk receive more attention and feedback than their 'normal' task-oriented counterparts, the 'controlling' nature of the feedback may make them more sensitized to task-extrinsic incentives, external control, and social threats (Boggiano & Katz, 1991; Deci & Ryan, 1996).

In addition, particularly in inclusive classrooms, subnormally performing children tend to fall chronically behind their normally achieving classmates (Crijnen et al., 1998), and the teachers in such vastly heterogeneous groups rarely have resources for sufficiently individually-adjusted and adequately-timed scaffolded instruction (Salonen et al., 1998a; Vauras et al., 2001, p. 297–298). Because children with ego-defensive coping strategies rarely receive adequate support and evaluative feedback that would enable the gradual growth of independent functioning, continuous feelings of being over-demanded and over-controlled undermine the child's sense of self-efficacy in the task and social dimensions. As these children confront the rapid introduction of new skills and the progress of their accelerating peers, they are likely to experience a loss of self-efficacy, feelings of inferiority, and to fall into deepening passivity, task-avoidance, or acting-out behavior (Boggiano & Katz, 1991; Boggiano et al., 1987; Crijnen et al., 1998; Schultz & Switzky, 1990).

3. SOCIAL DEPENDENCE ORIENTATION

In this case, the child's paramount adaptive focus in learning and performance situations is not the task or the self, but the instructor (Table I). Social dependence orientation is indicated by the child's extreme sensitivity to social cues and feedback, as well as the child's attempts to seek approval, to please the instructor and comply with her or him. One could say that the agency (or intellectual responsibility) has been shifted from the child to the guiding adult. Several, partly overlapping, constructs, such as outer-directedness, over-compliance, over- or cue-dependence, approval motivation, and conformity, have been applied in various theoretical approaches to describe analogous extrinsically motivated tendencies (Crittenden & DiLalla, 1988; Crombie & Gold, 1989; Crombie et al., 1991; Crutchfield, 1962; for reviews, see Switzky, 2001; Zigler & Balla, 1981; Zigler & Hodapp, 1991).

As in the case of task orientation, the child's activity is directed by the major functional system of *approach*, but instead of trying to directly attack the task or problem at hand, the child is engaged in efforts to approach the instructor. The child is primarily prepared to fulfill the instructor's momentary expectations and wishes, and to receive a maximal amount of help comprising detailed, stepwise advice, and feedback (e.g., rewards), following every minor step of performance (Salonen et al., 1998a). The socially dependent child shows a strong sense of self-efficacy within the social dimension (i.e., with regard to the instructor). This is indicated by the child's persistent social efforts as he or she strives to receive teacher help and approval. The child continues to respond to the instructor's task-related prompts and criticism by tracking the instructor's behavioral cues and responding in a trial-and-error manner until the instructor accepts his or her response (Holt, 1964; Lehtinen et al., 1995; Salonen et al., 1998a). The motivational tension-maintaining dependence-type efforts (e.g., blind guessing, imitating) last until the instructor responds with approval or signalizes that he or she does not expect a further answer. The child's sense of self-efficacy within the task dimension is in itself weak or instrumental. As the child's task-related efforts are subordinated to social goals, he or she is not prepared to approach the task autonomously or with the minimal amount of instrumental help. However, no inhibiting emotions or social avoidance tendencies arise even in the case of successive failure feedback because of the child's belief that sooner or later he or she will be piloted toward the acceptable solution and reward (Salonen et al., 1998a).

What is characteristic of social dependence orientation is the superficial processing of the learning tasks. With regard to task requirements, the child's responses remain random and inconsistent. The child's motivation is not focused on exploring, transforming, or reorganizing the task elements, but instead, he or she follows arbitrary associative links between his or her earlier trials and the teacher's support/rewards (Crombie & Gold, 1989; Crombie et al., 1991; Holt, 1964; Lehtinen et al., 1995; Salonen et al., 1998a).

Recent coping literature, having expanded the traditional two-dimensional coping constructs (e.g., problem-focused vs. emotion-focused) into multidimensional models, has suggested additional dimensions, such as 'seeking social support' (either for instrumental or emotional reasons) (Carver et al., 1989; Endler & Parker, 1990; Lazarus & Folkman, 1984). Our conceptualization of social dependence coping strategies is derived not from these coping dimensions but from the motivational analyses of unsuccessful social regulatory (scaffolding) processes that may counteract the growth of intrinsic orientation as well as the formation of a self-reward system and a system of internal standards or mastery goals (Barrett & Boggiano, 1988; Boggiano et al., 1987; Harter, 1978, 1981). On the basis of theoretical analyses and extensive observational data, we designed the following coping categories representing social dependence orientation (Olkinuora & Salonen, 1992; Salonen, 2000; Salonen et al., 1998a):

1. Following of social cues (e.g., attending to the instructor with the purpose of getting cues, utilizing the instructor's or peer's gestures, signs, verbal cues, or feedback to 'pilot' one's activity, complying with an external model for performance, mindless imitating).

2. Active efforts to elicit supportive cueing or help from the instructor. Active efforts can be manifested by two main variants of coping strategies: (1) babyish (regressive) emotional appealing behaviors (e.g., helpless gaze, appealing smile, baby talk), and (2) more advanced social tactics for eliciting supportive cueing from the adult (e.g., 'gift of the gab,' enticement, persuasion). Examples of active efforts are, e.g., tactical waiting and pausing when giving an answer with the purpose of inducing the instructor to give a verbal or non-verbal hint for the direction of the acceptable solution, help-seeking gestures directed toward the instructor or peer, verbal help requests focused on the instructor or peer in order to seek the direct 'answer' to the problem).

Children with an excessive tendency to seek help and social feedback particularly appeal to the teacher's professional role as a help-giving, supporting, and rewarding agent. As a reflection of the social balancing acts typical of school (and home, as well), both helplessly smiling babyish children and socially active, 'nice' children who guess uninhibitedly and give fluent but inconsistent answers tend to be far more over-helped and rewarded than called to account (Holt, 1964; Salonen et al., 1998a). Socially-dependent children, who are extremely sensitive to teachers' wishes, fulfill most of the expectations with regard to social management. Social balance will be established through the complementary functions of the child's dependent coping and the teacher's reciprocal role as a possibly over-helping and over-protecting emotional caregiver (McLaughlin, 1991; Salonen et al., 1998a). Thus, the social balancing mechanisms may disturb the optimal dosing and fading of support that is required in a successful scaffolding process.

II. COGNITIVE AND MOTIVATIONAL FACTORS IN THE DEVELOPMENT OF SUBNORMAL READING ACHIEVEMENT

The socially mediated formation of a complex skill, such as reading, is the most appropriate domain to study the interplay of cognitive, motivational, and emotional processes contributing to the quality of cognitive performance. For many children, early reading experiences in school involve intensive coping efforts. The child may be continuously over-taxed due to deficits or difficulties in some of the cognitive prerequisites or subskills of reading. The formation of cognitive prerequisites and subskills of reading is not always adequately scaffolded, and it is likely that beginning readers will be over-demanded (or over-controlled) as they try to meet the growing demands of early reading situations. Additionally, they may encounter negative adult prejudices, social comparisons, and evaluative pressures that are often characteristic of public classroom reading performances. It is plausible, especially if the child already shows non–task-oriented coping tendencies originating from pre-school learning situations, that such difficulties increase his or her non–task-orientation and weaken subsequent learning opportunities (Salonen et al., 1998b).

The acquisition of reading skills has been considered mainly in isolation from social mediation, i.e., the scaffolding process, even though reading as a skill is not learned naturally, such as speech through participation, but is a culturally formed act that presupposes at least minimal explicit teaching by parents, teachers, or peers. In fact, there is a growing body of cognitive-oriented research on how children learn to read. To become a competent reader involves, for instance, linguistic awareness, gradually automating multilevel decoding processes, hierarchically organized strategies for text comprehension, and comprehension monitoring skills (Adams, 1991; Gough et al., 1996; Kinnunen & Vauras, 1995). Ideally, a child becomes aware of words in speech, syllables in words, and finally the sounds of the words through optimal adult guidance, all of which facilitate learning to read and write.

One of the most powerful cognitive predictors of reading acquisition is linguistic sensitivity, particularly *phonemic awareness*, i.e., the skill to perceive a spoken word as composed of a sequence of individual sounds (Bradley & Bryant, 1983; Lundberg et al., 1980; Vellutino & Scanlon, 1987). Another strong predictor is knowledge of the alphabet (Adams, 1991), which probably reflects the beginning reader's print awareness. In relation to early reading difficulties, recent research has shown that the phonological view is incomplete without reference to *naming speed*. The studies examining the relationship between phonological awareness, rapid naming (of a series of visually presented stimuli) and reading progress have found that 'the double deficit' group (i.e., those children with deficits in both naming speed and phonological skills), especially have more severe reading problems than children with either deficit alone (Bowers et al., 1999; Wolf & Bowers, 1999). These critical sub-skills of reading explain the lion's share of individual differences in word reading achievement. In fact, children who show weak phonological awareness when they begin school have been found to be almost certainly poor readers in the 4th grade, if no remedial instruction had been given (Juel, 1988). The (poor) development of these phonological processes has proved to be one important source of the Matthew effects in early reading, illustrating the well-known educational polarization process in which the rich-get-richer and the poor-get-poorer (Stanovich, 1986, 2000).

In addition, research on text comprehension skills in regular classrooms has provided evidence for diverging learning careers. Vauras et al. (1994) analyzed, through a longitudinal design, the development of elementary students' text-processing skills from grades 3 to 5. Students were allocated into the three groups on the basis of teacher interview: high, average, and low achievers in grade 3. The students' reading comprehension of expository text was analyzed at micro (sentence), local (paragraph), and global (whole text) level processing skills (van Dijk & Kintsch, 1983). The results revealed a clear progression in the construction of coherent meaning units among the high and average achievers. The most rapid progression of text-processing skills was observed among students who were initially skilled. In contrast, low achievers showed no progression to the higher-level (local and global) text-processing skills during the two school years. Since the emphasis in upper grades is increasingly on self-regulated learning from text, it is likely that the gap between low- and high-achievers increases with age and school practice.

In summary, skilled reading requires competence in both word recognition and comprehension. The reader needs to identify letters, form a representation of a word in a text, and integrate the meaning of these words and sentences, in order to construct a valid interpretation of what is being read. This view is based on the Hoover and Gough model (1990) of reading ability, which postulates that reading comprehension is determined by decoding and language comprehension skills. It is emphasized that both components are necessary for skilled reading (Gough et al., 1996).

In addition to the skill *acquisition* process, the application of those skills in and out of school is even more central to understanding why school alone cannot succeed in eliminating the initial differences between children. Schools try to provide equal opportunities for learning to read; however, differences in learning reading skills exist as well as individual differences that manifest themselves in the use of these skills outside the school and classroom contexts (Stanovich, 2000, p. 151). Hayes and Grether (1983) documented interesting evidence of the role of self-teaching and out-of-school learning in terms of polarization in reading. They analyzed the gains in reading comprehension and vocabulary both during the school year and during the summer period, and found that the summer period explained more of the developmental gap between the high-achieving and the low-achieving students than the period when the children were in school. Furthermore, it has been observed that voluntary reading in and out of school diverges drastically as a function of skill and grade. In fact, the average good reader in grade 4 reads at home almost four nights per week, whereas the average poor reader reads at home only once a week. Thus, poor readers tend to fulfill their prophecy by not reading much, whereas good readers tend to self-reinforce their reading and motivation by reading more (Juel, 1988). Allington (1977) has pointed out, "if they don't read much, how they ever gonna get good?" This indicates that optimally developing children are likely to produce a facilitative learning environment for themselves. Ryan (1980) has described the interactive nature of language acquisition among subnormally and 'normally' performing children, and the way in which the difference in self-produced learning environments is also related to human interaction (Rueda & Mehan, 1986).

The aforementioned findings concerning the origins of the cognitive prerequisites of reading and the role of self-teaching activity may lead to straightforward linear-causal inferences on the development of subnormal reading skills. However, longitudinal studies have shown that linguistically disadvantaged children may display developmental trajectories, which are non-linear, for example, slow starters with curvlinear acceleration patterns (Cox, 1987; McGee et al., 1988). Also, children with unpredictable success in early reading have been identified (Lepola et al., 2000).

As a response to the preceding discussion about the cognitive determinants of subnormal reading achievement, we next present findings from our longitudinal studies on motivation and reading. In fact, there have been insufficient longitudinal data to allow the determination of whether the pervasive developmental effects of linguistic awareness and letter knowledge represent a direct reflection of (socio-)cognitive disadvantage, or whether this is also mediated by motivational factors. Therefore, we have considered that the development of a socially mediated complex skill, such as reading, depends not only on cognitive prerequisites but also on the child's motivational tendencies and coping strategies.

A. Longitudinal Studies on the Formation of Motivational and Reading Competencies

The follow-up data for these studies include children's development from preschool to grade 8. The presented studies are a part of the DECOM research and intervention program on decoding, comprehension, and motivation, which was started in the early 1990s. Besides the extensive analyses of motivational-cognitive development, intervention programs for remediation of learning difficulties were systematically put in practice in the early school years (e.g., linguistic awareness training in grade 1, computer-assisted reading intervention in grade 2, and integrated strategy intervention in grade 3) (Niemi et al., 1998; Poskiparta et al., 1999; Vauras et al., 1999b). However, the overview of the promising findings of each intervention is beyond the scope of this chapter.

The first study focuses on how children's motivational tendencies in preschool are related to motivational-emotional vulnerability differences, to the quality of prospective cognitive performance, and to the gradual yet different reading trajectories during the first school year. In the second study, we examine the development of motivational vulnerability from preschool to grade 2 as a function of prospective good, average, and poor readers. The question of developmental concomitance of difficulties in learning to read and write and maladaptive coping behavior is analyzed. The third example presents results from a recent study on the long-term development of motivation and learning, focusing on the parallel development of children's motivational orientations in a classroom context and reading skills from preschool to grade 8.

1. DEVELOPMENTAL INTERACTION OF MOTIVATION AND READING SKILL DURING THE FIRST SCHOOL YEAR

The aim of the study by Salonen et al. (1998b) was to predict the reading skill at the end of the first school year on the basis of preschool motivational orientations, situational coping strategies, knowledge of the alphabet, and phonemic awareness. In addition, we explored how children's motivational vulnerability differences are related, on the one hand, to early motivational tendencies, and, on the other hand, to the gradual yet different individual reading careers during the first school year.

We assumed that progression in reading would be associated with high preschool phonemic awareness and high task orientation, whereas regression in reading skill would be linked to low preschool phonemic awareness and low task orientation, particularly with increased non–task-orientation. Moreover, we assumed that children with high preschool ego-defensiveness or multiple non–task-orientation (i.e., ego-defensive plus social dependence) were, independent of their initial reading readiness, likely to cope with the difficulties or obstacles with dysfunctional coping strategies that tend to increase their emotional vulnerability and undermine their progress in reading.

Thirty-two six-year-old preschool non-readers participated in this study (Salonen et al., 1998a). The participants were selected from 151 preschool children on the basis of the teacher's (n = 12) and experimenter's motivational orientation ratings. The three *motivational orientations* were rated on three to four Likert-type scales. *Task orientation* items addressed concentration on task, verbal behavior indicating task involvement, and willingness to think and experiment in play and problem-solving situations. *Social dependence orientation* items related to verbal help-seeking, imitative behavior, and compliance-type task-approaching behavior. *Ego-defensive orientation* items addressed avoidance behavior, inhibition of action, and negative utterances referring to the self or one's own performance. On the basis of the orientation ratings, the participants were assigned according to their dominating motivational disposition to one of the four motivational orientation extreme groups: (1) task orientation (n = 8); (2) social dependence orientation (n = 8); (3) ego-defensive orientation (n = 8); and (4) social dependence plus ego defensive orientation, i.e., "multiple non–task-orientation" (n = 8).

The participants' phonemic awareness was assessed and knowledge of the alphabet was tested at the preschool level. Children's *coping behavior* was observed in preschool and in school in *play-like LEGO construction* tasks involving three induced pressure situations, one competition, and two obstacle tasks. The entire play-like construction process with intermittent pressure episodes, i.e., the obstacle and competition sub-tasks, was videotaped. Children's non-verbal and verbal behaviors were transcribed from the videotapes (Järvelä, Salonen, & Lepola, 2001). The smallest unit used in the time analysis was a three second episode of the same kind of behavior. Task-oriented, ego-defensive, and social dependence type coping strategies were classified according to a coping taxonomy system (Salonen, 2000). The duration of the different coping behavior episodes was computed across the whole situation and across free-play episodes, as well as across the pressure episodes only. Then, at the end of grade 1 the children's word reading skills were assessed and motivational orientations were rated by the classroom teacher.

The results concerning the acquisition of reading skills were in accordance with previous findings showing that progression versus regression in early reading was strongly associated with phonemic awareness and letter knowledge. Moreover, task orientation rated at preschool level by the teacher significantly improved the prediction of reading achievement beyond phonemic awareness. In fact, group comparisons for reading in the end of grade 1 revealed that task-oriented (TO) preschoolers progressed much further in their reading skills than those who were ego-defensive oriented (EDO) or multiple non–task-oriented (SEO). Actually, children rated as ego-defensive showed the poorest performance on a word reading test (Fig. 2, left panel). We also found that children rated as task-oriented (TO) and ego-defensive (EDO) differed with regard to preschool phonemic awareness (Fig. 2, right panel). This underscores the interrelatedness of early motivational dispositions and reading

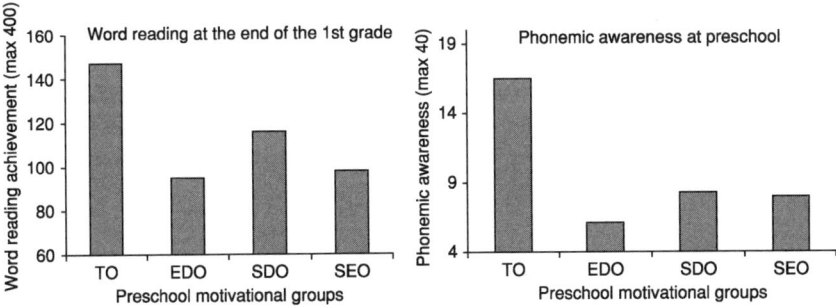

FIG. 2. Word reading skill (left panel) and phonemic awareness (right panel) as a function of the preschool motivational group. TO = task-oriented; EDO = ego-defensive oriented; SDO = social-dependence oriented; SEO = ego-defensive plus social-dependence oriented group.

prerequisites, and suggests that reading careers have their starting points in both linguistic and motivational factors that have been formed interactively before the start of grade 1.

Together, these motivational-developmental findings suggested that children high in ego-defensiveness may be motivationally more vulnerable to the new demands of learning to read than task-oriented children, and this vulnerability in turn influences their cognitive development. Firstly, to test this vulnerability hypothesis, we analyzed the dynamics of children's coping behavior at preschool in consecutive LEGO construction tasks involving both free-play and pressure episodes (Salonen et al., 1998b).

As shown in Table II, task-oriented (TO) children displayed significantly less ego-defensive coping behavior both in the total play situation and in pressure situations than children with high ego-defensive orientation (EDO) or multiple non-task orientation (SEO). It was also found that children's ego-defensive coping increased when shifting from free-play to pressure tasks. From the motivational vulnerability point of view, we found a striking difference between task and ego-defensive children in their tendency to shift to ego-defensive coping in the face of growing task demands: task-oriented children did not respond to pressures by shifting to non–task-oriented coping, whereas ego-defensively oriented children's ego-defensive coping behavior doubled in the pressure situations. This underlines not only the validity of preschool teacher orientation ratings, but also the difference in vulnerability between task-oriented and ego-defensive children.

In the study by Salonen and Lepola (1993), we analyzed how the interaction of situational pressure factors and children's motivational tendencies contributes to the quality of cognitive performance. This was done by

TABLE II
PERCENTAGE OF EGO-DEFENSIVE COPING BEHAVIOR IN
TOTAL SITUATION VS PRESSURE EPISODES

Setting	Motivational Groups at Preschool			ANOVA	Post Hoc Test
	TO M (SD)	EDO M (SD)	SDO M (SD)	SEO M (SD)		
Total situation	4.5 (4)	16.8 (11)	8.2 (6)	13 (8)	Group, F(3, 27) = 5.07, p < 0.01	TO < EDO = SEO
Pressure tasks	9 (7)	35 (25)	10.6 (5)	19.8 (12)	Setting, F(1, 27) = 24.51, p < 0.01	TO < EDO = SEO
					Group × Setting, F (3, 27) = 4.92, p < 0.01	

TO = task-oriented; EDO = ego-defensive-oriented; SDO = social dependence; SEO = ego-defensive plus social-dependence oriented group; ANOVA = analysis of variance; > = refers to significant difference at p < 0.01 tested by the LSD procedure; Pressure tasks = the mean percentage of time spent on ego-defensive coping in two obstacle and one competition tasks. M = mean; SD = standard deviation.

examining children's spelling achievement as a function of preschool motivational tendency and performance context. The role of motivation in spelling skills was investigated at the end of grade 1 by two parallel sentence writing tests, one given in a more familiar individual setting and the other in a more formal classroom setting. The classroom test was supposed to comprise more social comparison and competition elements and evaluative features than the individual test setting. The individually administered and classroom tests were matched. Both tests consisted of 10 orally presented two-to-five word sentences. The individual test was given one month before the classroom test. One point was given for each correctly written sentence. The maximum score was 10.

4 (motivation group) × 2 (context) ANOVA revealed a significant main effect for motivation group, $F(3, 25) = 4.09$, $p < 0.05$, and for performance context, $F(1, 25) = 7.47$, $p < 0.01$. In addition, a significant interaction effect was found, $F(3, 25) = 3.11$, $p < 0.05$. On the one hand, these results show that students' writing achievement was poorer in the classroom setting compared to the individual setting, even though the individual test was given earlier. On the other hand, task-oriented children performed significantly better than multiple non–task-oriented (i.e., SEO group) children across the settings. However, a more interesting finding was that task-oriented students performed equally well or even better in the more formal and more evaluative-laden classroom setting (Fig. 3). An opposite pattern was observed among the non–task-oriented groups. The spelling achievement of ego-defensive children dropped the most drastically from individual to classroom setting of all orientation groups. In fact, two students, both from the EDO group, refused to write in the classroom evaluation, which itself indicates an extreme avoidance behavior and the validity of motivational orientation assessment.

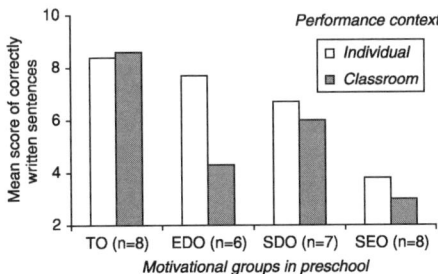

FIG. 3. Sentence spelling achievement as a function of motivational orientation and performance context. TO = task oriented; EDO = ego-defensive-oriented; SDO = social dependence; SEO = ego-defensive plus social-dependence oriented group.

The aforementioned findings are in line with recent research indicating that students who have an extrinsic motivational (EM) orientation are more susceptible to helplessness than pupils with an intrinsic motivational (IM) orientation under evaluative and controlling cues (Boggiano et al., 1992). In addition, it has been found that EM children tend to show motivational impairment in tasks involving negative evaluative feedback, whereas IM children tend to show increased motivation in an evaluative setting (Boggiano et al., 1992). In summary, these findings suggest that the initial motivational tendencies predispose children either to regressive or progressive motivational-cognitive cycles. Progression is reflected as increased tuning to learning and mastering the tasks, whereas regression is characterized by increased tuning to task-extrinsic factors.

2. DEVELOPMENT OF MOTIVATIONAL VULNERABILITY AND READING AND WRITING DIFFICULTIES

Poskiparta et al. (2003) examined the development of motivational-emotional profiles from preschool to grade 2 among three groups classified as *poor readers, good decoders* (hereinafter referred to as *average readers*), and *good readers* in grade 2. The aim was to explore to what extent differences in motivational-emotional vulnerability exist before school, or whether vulnerability is a by-product of early school experience and occurs concomitantly with the emergence of cognitive differences. The use of maladaptive coping strategies, i.e., ego-defensive and social dependence orientations, in stress situations indicated motivational-emotional vulnerability, while the use of task orientation suggested motivational-emotional resilience (Olkinuora et al., 1984).

One hundred and twenty-seven children participated in the study from preschool up to grade 2. Two different methods were used to assess motivational-emotional vulnerability. First, researchers at preschool and classroom teachers (n = 12) in grades 1 and 2 rated children's task, ego-defensive, and social dependence orientations. Secondly, an experimental situation was arranged each year where children's play behavior with LEGO bricks was observed in induced pressure situations, and their coping strategies scored.

The results indicated that, on the basis of researchers' perceptions, at preschool age, no differences in vulnerability between the prospective reading level groups were found. Prospective good readers were more task-oriented than prospective poor readers, but the latter group and prospective average readers were equally task-oriented. On the contrary, in grades 1 and 2, classroom teachers rated poor readers as less task-oriented and more ego-defensive and socially dependent compared to average and good readers (Fig. 4). An interesting finding was a high correspondence between classroom

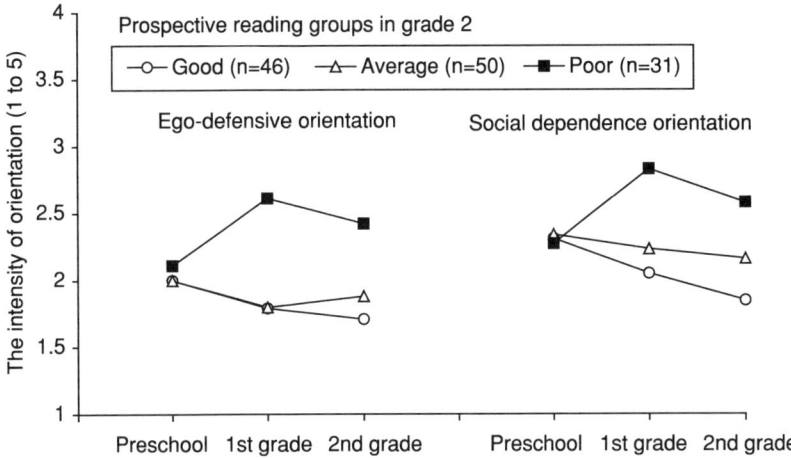

FIG. 4. Development of non-task orientations from preschool to grade 2 of prospective reading groups.

teachers' orientation ratings and children's basic skills in reading and writing. In grades 1 and 2, average readers' decoding and spelling, as well as their motivational tendencies, were more like those of good readers. In contrast, poor readers were cognitively, as well as motivationally, inferior compared to the other two groups.

Researchers' and teachers' ratings and observational data based on representative samples of prospective poor, average, and good readers' task-oriented and ego-defensive type of coping behavior yielded rather similar results. At preschool age, no differences were found in motivational-emotional vulnerability between the reading groups. Generally, children's task-oriented coping behavior decreased and their ego-defensive coping behavior increased when under pressure, this effect being similar for each of the three reading groups at preschool age (Fig. 5). However, in grade 1, prospective poor readers showed clear tendencies towards increased emotional vulnerability in situations where competition and obstacles were present. Interestingly, in the freeplay situation, no differences in coping behaviour were found among the three prospective reading groups whereas the differences were marked in the pressure situation. Poor readers were significantly less task-oriented and more ego-defensive oriented compared to average and good readers. Among good readers, there was neither a decrease in task-oriented behavior nor an increase in ego-defensive coping behavior in pressure situations. In contrast, poor readers' ego-defensive coping behavior increased many-fold when they

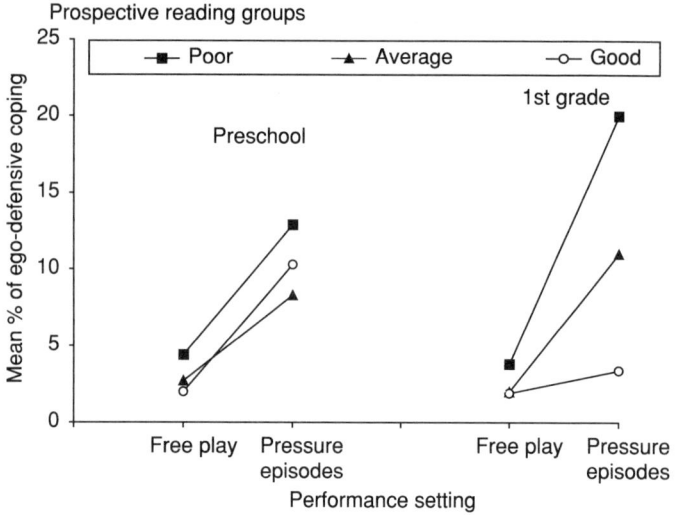

FIG. 5. Ego-defensive coping behavior as a function of reading group and performance context.

encountered pressure and, consequently, they spent less time on task-oriented behavior (Fig. 5). The average readers' ego-defensive behavior also increased in pressure situations but the total amount of it was only one-half that of poor readers. It is worth noting that all of this took place although vulnerability was measured in LEGO construction play situations which had nothing to do with reading or writing.

The results of Poskiparta et al. (2003) suggest that early problems in learning to read and write have immediate consequences for school motivation. Moreover, the results led to the conclusion that there was something less favorable in the classroom context for children with problems in learning to read and write. Skinner and Belmont's (1993) study with 3rd to 5th graders revealed reciprocal effects of children's motivation on teacher behavior (Lehtinen et al., 1995). In other words, teachers modified their behavior toward individual children on the basis of their perception of the child's behavioral and emotional engagement. According to teachers' self-reports they tended to respond to children who were passive and showed negative emotion by being less involved, less structured, or less autonomy-supporting than with children with positive initial engagement. Because the maladaptive motivational tendencies of children in Skinner and Belmont's study (1993) resemble those of poor readers in the study by Poskiparta et al. (2003), it is possible that, in our study too, many teachers responded to poor readers' performance in a way that enhanced the initial maladaptive motivational pattern. Teacher anger after academic failure is not an effective way to enhance subsequent effort in younger children. Butler (1994) found that teacher anger after failure was directly and negatively correlated with younger (grade 3) children's predictions of subsequent effort, but enhanced the effort of older (grade 6) children. Future efforts were most positive at both ages in a situation where the teacher offered an opportunity for a guided second attempt. Furthermore, the Turner (1995) findings on the effects of instructional contexts on children's motivation for literacy in grade 1 revealed that so-called open tasks in which children had opportunities for challenge, for pupil control, for satisfying interests, and for collaboration, were the strongest predictors of favorable motivation. However, Turner (1995) stressed that the applicability of her results should be studied in other populations, especially among low-achieving readers.

The results of the Poskiparta et al. (2003) study can also be explained by the late school entrance of Finnish children (at age seven) compared to many other countries. Could it be that Finnish children begin school at an age when they are more susceptible to social comparison because of a developed normative conception of ability compared to younger children who have a more undifferentiated conception of ability (Butler, 1999)? Moreover, a longitudinal study by Chapman and Tunmer (1997) showed that at the age of seven and a half (although after two years of schooling), but not before, reading performance started to contribute to children's reading self-concept.

3. TRACING THE TRAJECTORIES OF LEARNING AND MOTIVATION FROM PRESCHOOL TO GRADE 8

In our recent study (Lepola et al., 2002), we have traced the long-term development of students' reading and motivation trajectories from preschool to secondary school (comprising grades 7 to 9). The objectives of this study were first to examine motivational-linguistic origins of diverging reading careers, and second to analyze the developmental changes in motivational tendencies of prospective poor, average, and good readers in grade 8.

To analyze the formation of motivation and reading skill, we applied a prospective design similar to that used in the study above by Poskiparta et al. (2003). First, we grouped the participants (N = 76) at the end of grade 8, on the basis of their reading comprehension achievement, into groups of good, average, and poor readers. The reading group classification was based on achievement on the Comprehensive School Reading Test (Lindeman, 1998). The criterion for being assigned to the prospective poor reading group was scoring one standard deviation below the mean in the reading rest and to the prospective good reading group, one standard deviation above the mean score, based on the achievement of 301 students. Actually, the poor readers' reading comprehension was on the same level as an average grade 6 student's performance. This procedure yielded the following reading groups in grade 8: (1) prospective good readers (n = 13, 17%), average readers (n = 45, 59%), and poor readers (n = 18, 24%).

To chart motivational and cognitive-linguistic developments of prospective reading groups, children's reading prerequisites were evaluated in preschool, decoding in grades 1 and 2, listening comprehension from grades 1 to 3, and reading comprehension from grades 2 to 8 (for the detailed test, see Poskiparta et al., 2003). Children's motivation was assessed at five time-points. Classroom teachers in the primary grades (1 to 6) and subject teachers in grade 8 assessed the participants motivational orientations (i.e., task orientation, ego-defensive, and social dependence orientation) on the basis of the student's behavior in the classroom (Vauras et al., 2001).

The priority of reading competence as a target of our studies was also motivated by the fact that it has been cherished in the Finnish culture since the end of the 1600s after reading became a compulsory prerequisite for a marriage license in Finland and Sweden (Lundberg & Nilsson, 1986). Thus, reading is still viewed as the main goal of primary education. In fact, one of the main challenges during the first two primary school years (in Finland) is learning fluent decoding and spelling skills. In grade 3, a student has to cope with new demands related, on the one hand, to higher order skills in math and language (i.e., verbal problem-solving skills), and on the other hand, to new school subjects, such as environmental science and the first foreign language. Mastering the contents of new subjects and simultaneously moving upward in a more hierarchically organized knowledge structure presuppose that the basic skills are not only well-automated but are also applied as tools for learning. At the same time, the teacher's role is changing from a help-giver to a knowledge facilitator and learning coach. These changes in the learning environment as a whole presuppose increasing responsibility, self-regulated learning, and task-focused motivation from the student's point of view.

In terms of diverging reading careers, we assumed that the differences in reading comprehension between prospective poor, average, and good readers start to emerge in grade 3, since from then onwards emphasis is put more on learning from texts. Furthermore, we hypothesized that motivational factors are related to (relative) progression or regression in the reading career. Thus, we assumed that prospective good readers will respond to the increasing demands in grade 3 by task-focused motivation, whereas prospective poor readers are assumed to respond to the new demands of learning by non–task-focused motivation.

Results concerning the cognitive-linguistic origins of diverging reading comprehension careers showed that prospective reading groups did not differ either in pre-reading skills or cognitive prerequisites at preschool level (Table III). There were no differences between the high, average, and poor reading groups in the acquisition of word reading skill in grades 1 and 2. However, prospective poor readers displayed inferior listening comprehension compared with prospective good readers, already in grade 1. In addition, the prospective good readers showed progression in listening comprehension from grades 1 to 3, unlike the prospective poor readers, whose gains were weaker (Table III).

Concerning the development of reading comprehension, the polarization phenomenon between the reading groups was observed across the school years (Fig. 6). This was portrayed as a growing achievement gap between prospective good and poor readers. In fact, poor, average, and good reading careers started to diverge from grade 3 and onwards, underlining our assumption about the critical role of grade 3 in learning to understand what is read. The above findings concerning the positive slope of reading comprehension of the good readers and the negative slope of the poor readers cannot be straightforwardly interpreted as illustrating Mathew effects in reading. Stanovich (2000, p. 154) clearly stated that "no fan-spread could be demonstrated with percentiles or any type of standard score ... and by definition, the standardization wipes out the possibility of increasing variability with age." Consequently, it should be stated that our results on the developmental differences in reading comprehension did not reveal failure or success in reading achievement at an individual level, but rather showed the emergence and stabilization of the difference between the good and the poor readers across the school years.

Results concerning the relatedness of motivational tendencies to the reading achievement of prospective reading groups revealed that the poor readers had a significantly weaker task orientation already in grade 1 than the prospective good readers. From the developmental point of view, prospective poor readers were less task-oriented and more non–task-oriented than prospective average or good readers from primary to secondary school (Fig. 7A and B). Again, grade 3 appeared to be critical, since motivational differences were very marked at the end of the grade. In grade 3, the difficulties in reading comprehension of the prospective poor readers were all the more clearly reflected as increasing non–task-orientation. On the contrary, prospective good and average readers were more self-regulated in the classroom context.

In summary, it seems that the prospective good and average readers' dominating task orientation led them to respond in a task-oriented way to increasing demands of learning. On the contrary, the prospective poor readers' comprehension difficulties and weaker task orientation led them to use non–task-oriented coping in the face of new learning demands. These opposite motivational patterns interacting with reading comprehension

TABLE III
Reading Prerequisites, Decoding, and Listening Comprehension Skills From Preschool to Grade 3 of Prospective Good, Average and Poor Readers

Tests	Grade	Prospective Reading Groups			ANOVA	Tukey HSD Test
		Poor n = 18 M (SD)	Average n = 45 M (SD)	Good n = 13 M (SD)		
Phonemic awareness (max. 40)	Preschool	5.6 (6.1)	8.7 (7.3)	8.6 (10.2)	$F(2, 56) = 0.87, p = ns$	
WISC-R (verbal)	Preschool	88 (11.7)	88 (9.3)	92 (8.9)	$F(2, 68) = 0.72, p = ns$	
WISC-R (performance)	Preschool	92 (10.6)	95 (11.6)	98 (9.9)	$F(2, 66) = 1.13, p = ns$	
Word recognition skill (max 400)	1st Grade	125 (38)	149 (58)	161 (40)	$F(2, 72) = 2.08, p = ns$	
Reading speed*	2nd Grade	1.60 (0.65)	1.59 (0.84)	1.21 (0.43)	$F(2, 73) = 1.43, p = ns$	
Listening comprehension†	1st Grade	31 (18)%	34 (14)%	43 (14)%	Group $F(2, 72) = 7.4, p < 0.001$	$P < G$
	2nd Grade	40 (10)%	46 (15)%	53 (12)%	Time $F(2, 144) = 22.6, p < 0.001$	$P < G$
	3rd Grade	39 (10)%	45 (11)%	58 (10)%	Group × Time §$F(4, 144) = 0.9, p = ns$	$P = A < G$

*The reading time of the 95-word story was divided by the number of correctly read words to achieve the average reading time per word. †Listening comprehension = the mean percentage of understanding main ideas of narrative and expository texts; ‡Tukey (HSD) test to compare between-groups differences at each grade level; P = prospective poor, A = average, G = good readers. §3 (reading groups) × 3 (grade/time) within-subject ANOVA for listening comprehension. WISC-R = Wechsler Intelligence Scale for Children-Revised (1984).

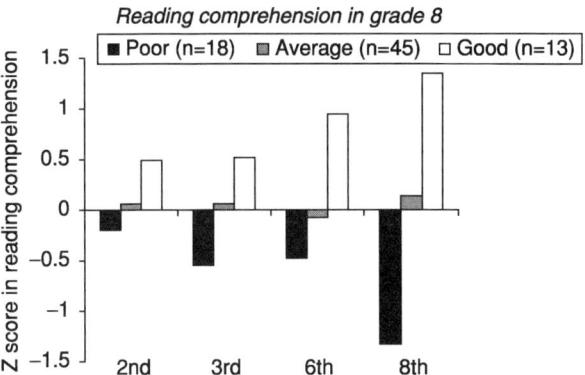

FIG. 6. Development of reading comprehension from grade 2 to grade 8 among prospective good, average, and poor readers.

differences seemed to co-determine favorable and unfavorable learning trajectories (Schneider et al., 1997; Schultz & Switzky, 1993).

III. SUMMARY AND CONCLUSIONS

In this chapter we outlined the systemic and functionalist view to capture the complexity of situational and developmental interactions related to the formation of subnormal cognitive performance. The rationale for our interactionist approach to subnormal achievement was based on the analysis of the limitations of decontextualized approaches founded on the assumption of static differences in the individual's motivational or cognitive traits (e.g., IQ). We proposed that in order to understand the origins and manifestations of subnormal cognitive performance or otherwise distorted behavior (MR, ADHD, LD, reading disability), the explaining factors should be sought from the situational and developmental interactions between cognitive, motivational, and emotional processes occurring in the individual's adaptation to different contexts, rather than from cognitive factors alone.

The starting point of our analysis was Vygotsky's (1978) theoretical view of the development of higher mental functions through an optimal instructional interaction. We used the Vygotsky-based scaffolding metaphor to illustrate both the *favorable* and *less favorable* development of cognition and motivation under the adult's regulation (i.e., the giving and fading of support). The adult's regulative skills in determining the child's region of sensitivity to instruction and, simultaneously, in adjusting the scaffolding support to the

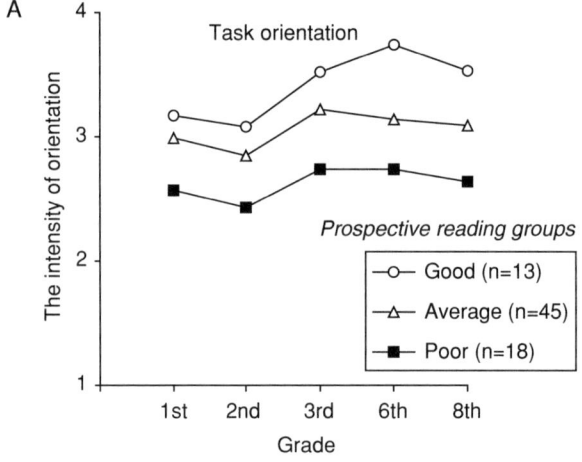
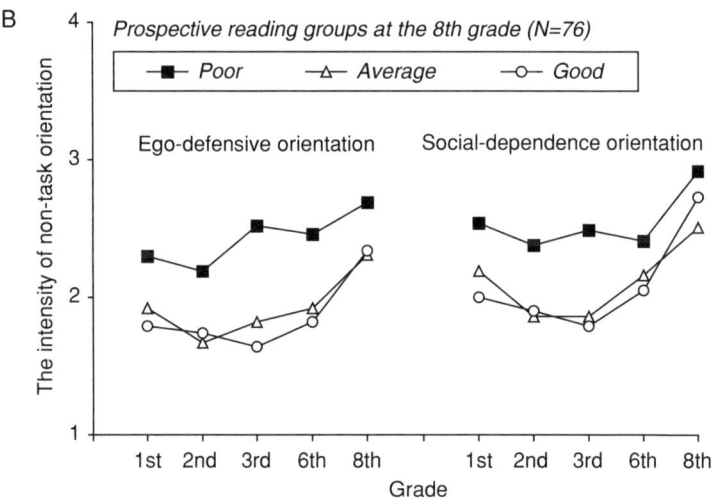

FIG. 7. Development of motivational orientations of prospective good, average, and poor readers in grade 8.

child's developing competencies are crucial in promoting the child's independent functioning in the ZPD. The analysis of interpersonal processes, and especially biased or unbalanced scaffolding processes, provided us with a model to outline the interactive formation of non–task-oriented coping strategies in early childhood years. Three less optimal scaffolding patterns that seem to have an influence on the development of children's motivational and emotional vulnerability, and later learning and behavioral problems, were identified: (1) over-supporting or over-controlling instructional strategies; (2) insufficiently supporting (and over-demanding) instructional strategies; and (3) inconsistent, asynchronous, or unresponsive interaction patterns.

On the basis of the developmental analysis of optimal and less optimal forms of instructional interactions, we introduced a typology of task-directed, ego-defensive, and social dependence type of motivational orientations, and a taxonomy of corresponding coping strategies and emotional responses. We hypothesized that task-oriented coping efforts are associated with a deep level of cognitive processing, promote the integrity of cognitive activity, and lead to the progressive organization of cognitive structures. In contrast, ego-defensive and social dependence-type coping strategies are associated with a superficial level of cognitive processing and the disorganization of cognitive activity.

The cognitive-motivational interactions connected with task- and non–task-oriented coping were illustrated through three follow-up studies focusing on the development of motivation and reading and writing skills. Together, the findings of our three longitudinal studies (Lepola et al., 2002; Poskiparta et al., 2003; Salonen et al., 1998b) indicated, first, that motivational tendencies in the early school years are related to emotional vulnerability differences, which in turn seem to influence the quality of cognitive performance, especially under pressure and social comparison feedback conditions. Second, early problems in learning to read and write were concomitantly reflected as children's increased motivational-emotional vulnerability and non-task orientation, underscoring the reciprocal development of cognition and motivation, as well as the interactive formation of learning difficulties in the classroom context. Third, the development of children's learning disabilities can be traced during early childhood years, and their origins are related both to cognitive-linguistic and motivational tendencies that have been formed interactively in family and day-care contexts. Furthermore, the predictions of cognitive development became more accurate if not precise, when using both the pre-reading measures focusing on linguistic awareness and the typology of motivational orientation. Through our theoretical model of motivational orientation and corresponding situation-specific coping behaviors, we were better able to understand the formation and long-term development of subnormal learning trajectories. In conclusion, individual reading careers seem to bifurcate not only due to differences in the ease of learning to read (Stanovich, 2000, p. 293) but also due to early interactions of cognitive prerequisites and coping tendencies as well as (less) optimal adjustment of teaching (scaffolding support) to the child's developing competencies.

A. Implications for Further Research

Our findings indicate that children's regressive and progressive learning careers had their starting points in both cognitive prerequisites and skills, as well as in motivational-emotional tendencies manifesting in instructional situations. Furthermore, our results suggested that these competencies and dispositions have been formed during early childhood years in day-care and family contexts. The teachers' and parents' orientation to guiding and scaffolding the progress of children's skills has been found to exert an effect on the child's further opportunities and motivation to learn (Heckhausen, 1987; Hokoda & Fincham, 1995). The difference in the quality of guidance can be assumed to be related to the development of the child's motivational and emotional dispositions. To understand individual differences in motivational vulnerability and resilience, further research is needed to explore the relationship between early parenting and scaffolding practices and the child's non–task-oriented versus task-oriented coping tendencies.

Teacher-child interaction in day-care and in the classroom are contexts in which the motivational, social, and cognitive differentiation may also occur. We have illustrated elsewhere (Salonen et al., 1998a) how teachers who interact with a student of excessive social dependence themselves tend to increase the reciprocal attachment characterized by their weakening self-governed orientation toward the task and subject matter. In students with extreme avoidance and acting out behaviors, teachers tend to normalize and control the situation either by reducing the students' demands for self-regulated learning or withdrawing themselves from the dialogue. This kind of social balancing or distancing, based on reciprocal avoidance, may produce from a student point of view a short-term sense of control but, in the long-run, may lead to total resistance to education and non-commitment to learning. A similar multiplier effect in which the consequences of a particular child's coping strategy is amplified by the teacher's strategy is reported in studies by Skinner and Belmont (1993) and Pollard (1986). However, until now there have been extremely few studies relating children's intellectual efforts, motivational orientations, and coping strategies to instructors' reciprocal tendencies and regulation strategies.

Although there are studies examining the role of classroom participatory structures on learning (Gutierrez et al., 1995), more socioculturally-oriented research is needed to reveal how instructional frame factors constrain and regulate teachers' motivation-relevant interaction with children differing in their cognitive, motivational, and emotional characteristics (Howard-Rose & Rose, 1994; Meadows, 1996).

On the one hand, our findings indicated that the first graders' spelling achievement was clearly associated with the performance context and motivational tendencies. Moreover, the results suggested that motivational vulnerability plays a central role in learning and performing in the classroom context. Further studies are needed to analyze, from a motivational and cognitive point of view, how children with subnormal achievement in reading and/or math perform in academic tasks in everyday life situations which they may interpret as more meaningful than the formal test-like setting. The performance variation as a function of context could provide important diagnostic information about a student's learning potential for the implementation of remedial and classroom teaching. In addition, it would be interesting to investigate whether poor readers' greater vulnerability also manifests itself in situations outside school, and with a reference group other than their classmates, or whether classroom as a learning environment handicaps their performance potential.

One of our major methodological conclusions is that narrow diagnostic categories developed for accurate clinical identification of deviant individuals have created artificial boundaries between symptom groups (e.g., cognitive disabilities, emotional-behavioral disorders, personality and motivational problems, and so on) and have ruled out relevant approaches and hypothetical constructs originating from alternative research paradigms. Particularly sharp-edged, mutually exclusive definitions of clinical groups have prevented researchers from seeking possibly important common behaviors manifested by individuals despite their different diagnostic labels. It would be fruitful, at least provisionally, to abandon the sharp-edged definitions with implicit causal presuppositions (e.g., IQ-based, brain-based, genetically determined) connected with subnormally performing clinical groups. The focus could be shifted from comparing the performance of a deviant group and 'normals' on certain measures, to comparing the adaptive and cognitive behavior across various cognitively, motivationally, and behaviorally 'deviant' groups (e.g., LD, MR, ADHD, autistic).

In summary, we propose that is it fruitless to locate the unfavorable motivation and poor achievement only in the individual's dispositions or the knowledge acquisition process. To understand the origins and developmental nature of these tendencies and skills, we have to analyze the situations in which they are interactively formed. This is in line with the current theories of learning, proposing that the knowledge acquisition perspective should be supplemented by learning as a participation perspective. One key to promoting self-regulated learning and progressive achievement is to understand the social and interactive nature of development. This provides teachers and adults an important role in providing an emotionally and intellectually stimulating context for children, in adjusting the scaffolding to the child's developing competence, and in challenging his or her developmental potential.

ACKNOWLEDGMENTS

The preparation of this chapter was made possible by Grant No. 52039 from the Academy of Finland to the first author, and the research reported in this chapter was supported by Grants No. 1071265 and No. 4131 from the Council for Social Sciences Research, Academy of Finland, to the third author and to Pekka Niemi (University of Turku).

REFERENCES

Adams, M. J. (1991). *Beginning to read. Thinking and learning about print* (2nd ed.). Cambridge, MA: The MIT Press.

Allington, R. L. (1977). If they don't read much, how they ever gonna get good? *Journal of Reading, 21,* 57–61.

Armour-Thomas, E. (1992). Intellectual assessment of children from culturally diverse backgrounds. *School Psychology Review, 21,* 552–565.

August, G. J., & Garfinkel, B. D. (1990). Comorbidity of ADHD and reading disability among clinic-referred children. *Journal of Abnormal Child Psychology, 18,* 29–45.

Baltes, M. M. (1996). *The many faces of dependency in old age.* New York: Cambridge University Press.

Barker, G. P., & Graham, S. (1987). A developmental study of praise and blame as attributional cues. *Journal of Educational Psychology, 79,* 62–66.

Barrett, M., & Boggiano, A. K. (1988). Fostering extrinsic orientations: Use of reward strategies to motivate children. *Journal of Social and Clinical Psychology, 6,* 293–309.

Boekaerts, M. (1993). Being concerned with well-being and with learning. *Educational Psychologist, 28,* 149–167.

Boggiano, A. K., Barrett, M., Weiner, A. W., McClelland, G. H., & Lusk, C. M. (1987). Use of maximal-operant principle to motivate children's intrinsic interest. *Journal of Personality and Social Psychology, 53,* 866–879.

Boggiano, A. K., & Katz, P. (1991). Maladaptive achievement patterns in students: The role of teachers' controlling strategies. *Journal of Social Issues, 47,* 35–51.

Boggiano, A. K., Shields, A., Barrett, M., Kellam, T., Thompson, E., Simons, J., & Katz, P. (1992). Helplessness deficit in students: The role of motivational orientation. *Motivation and Emotion, 16,* 271–294.

Bowers, P. G., Sunseth, K., & Golden, J. (1999). The route between rapid naming and reading progress. *Scientific Studies of Reading, 3,* 31–53.

Bradley, L., & Bryant, P. E. (1983). Categorizing sounds and learning to read—a causal connection. *Nature, 301,* 419–421.

Brooks, P. H., & Baumeister, A. A. (1977). A plea for consideration of ecological validity in the experimental psychology of mental retardation: A guest editorial. *American Journal of Mental Deficiency, 81,* 407–416.

Busch-Rossnagel, N. A., Knauf-Jensen, D. E., & DesRosiers, F. S. (1995). Mothers and others: The role of the socializing environment in the development of mastery motivation. In R. H. MacTurk & G. A. Morgan (Eds.), *Mastery motivation: Origins, conceptualizations, and applications: Vol. 12. Advances in applied developmental psychology* (pp. 117–145). Norwood, NJ: Ablex.

Bulter, R. (1994). Teacher communications and student interpretations: Effects of teacher responses to failing students on attributional inferences in two age groups. *British Journal of Educational Psychology, 64,* 277–294.

Butler, R. (1999). Information seeking and achievement motivation in middle childhood and adolescence: The role of conceptions of ability. *Developmental Psychology, 35,* 146–163.

Carver, C. S., Scheier, M. F., & Weintraub, J. K. (1989). Assessing coping strategies: A theoretically based approach. *Journal of Personality and Social Psychology, 56,* 267–283.

Ceci, S. J., & Bronfenbrenner, U. (1985). Don't forget to take the cupcakes out of the oven: Strategic time-monitoring, prospective memory, and context. In M. M. Gruneberg, P. Morris, & P. Syke (Eds.), *Practical aspects of memory* (Vol. 2, pp. 243–256). London: Wiley.

Chapman, J. W., & Tunmer, W. E. (1997). A longitudinal study of beginning reading achievement and reading self-concept. *British Journal of Educational Psychology, 76,* 279–291.

Charlesworth, W. (1976). Human intelligence as adaptation. In L. Resnick (Ed.), *The nature of intelligence* (pp. 147–168). Hillsdale, NJ: Erlbaum.

Charlesworth, W. (1978). Ethology: Its relevance for observational studies of human adaptation. In G. Sackett (Ed.), *Observing behavior: Theory and applications in mental retardation* (Vol. 1, pp. 7–32). Baltimore, MD: University Park Press.

Cherkes-Julkowski, M., & Mitlina, N. (1999). Self-organization of mother-child instructional dyads and later attention disorder. *Journal of Learning Disabilities, 32,* 6–21.

Cicourel, A. V., Jennings, K., Jennings, S., Leiter, K., Mackay, R., Mehan, H., & Roth, D. (1974). *Language use and school performance.* New York: Academic Press.

Cole, M., & Bruner, J. S. (1971). Cultural differences and inferences about psychological processes. *American Psychologist, 26,* 867–876.

Cox, T. (1987). Slow starters versus long term backward readers. *British Journal of Educational Psychology, 57,* 73–86.

Crijnen, A. M., Feehan, M., & Kellam, S. G. (1998). The course and malleability of reading achievement in elementary school: The application of growth curve modeling in the evaluation of a mastery learning intervention. *Learning & Individual Differences, 10,* 137–157.

Crittenden, P. M., & Di Lalla, D. L. (1988). Compulsive compliance: The development of an inhibitory coping strategy in infancy. *Journal of Abnormal Child Psychology, 16,* 585–599.

Crombie, G., & Gold, D. (1989). Compliance and problem-solving competence in girls and boys. *Journal of Genetic Psychology, 150,* 281–291.

Crombie, G., Pilon, D., & Xinaris, S. (1991). Children's problem-solving performance: The effects of compliance and cognitive factors. *Journal of Genetic Psychology, 152,* 359–369.

Crutchfield, R. (1962). Conformity and creative thinking. In H. Gruber, G. Terrell, & M. Wertheimer (Eds.), *Contemporary approaches to creative thinking* (pp. 120–140). New York: Prentice-Hall.

Deci, E. L., & Ryan, R. M. (1987). The support of autonomy and the control of behavior. *Journal of Personality and Social Psychology, 53,* 1024–1037.

Deci, E. L., & Ryan, R. M. (1996). Need satisfaction and the self-regulation of learning. *Learning & Individual Differences, 8,* 165–183.

Diener, C. I., & Dweck, C. S. (1978). An analysis of learned helplessness: Continuous changes in performance, strategy, and achievement cognitions following failure. *Journal of Personality and Social Psychology, 36,* 451–462.

Elliott, A. J. (1999). Approach and avoidance motivation and achievement goals. *Educational Psychologist, 34,* 169–189.

Endler, N. S., & Magnusson, D. (1976). Towards an interactional psychology of personality. *Psychological Bulletin, 83,* 956–974.

Endler, N. S., & Parker, J. D. (1990). Multidimensional assessment of coping: A critical evaluation. *Journal of Personality and Social Psychology, 58,* 844–854.

Entwistle, N. J., & Ramsden, P. (1982). *Understanding student learning.* London: Croom Helm.

Flink, C., Boggiano, A. K., & Barrett, M. (1990). Controlling teaching stategies: Undermining children's self-determination and performance. *Journal of Personality and Social psychology, 59*, 916–924.

Ginsburg, H. (1972). *The myth of the deprived child.* Englewood Cliffs, NJ: Prentice-Hall.

Glutting, J. J., & Youngstrom, E. A. (1996). Situational specificity and generality of test behaviors for samples of normal and referred children. *School Psychology Review, 25*, 94–107.

Gough, P. B., Hoover, W. A., & Peterson, C. L. (1996). Some observations on a simple view of reading. In C. Cornoldi & J. Oakhill (Eds.), *Reading comprehension difficulties: Processes and Intervention* (pp. 1–13). New Jersey: Lawrence Erlbaum.

Graham, S., & Golan, S. (1991). Motivational influences on cognition: Task involvement, ego involvement, and depth of information processing. *Journal of Educational Psychology, 83*, 187–194.

Gutierrez, K. D., Larson, J., & Kreuter, B. (1995). Cultural tensions in the scripted classroom: The value of subjugated perspective. *Urban Education, 29*, 410–442.

Hargreaves, D. (1978). Deviance: The interactionist approach. In B. Gillham (Ed.), *Reconstructing educational psychology* (pp. 67–83). London: Croom Helm.

Harris, K. R. (1988). Learning disabilities research: The need, the integrity, and the challenge. *Journal of Learning Disabilities, 21*, 267–270.

Harter, S. (1978). Effectance motivation reconsidered: Toward a developmental model. *Human Development, 1*, 34–64.

Harter, S. (1981). A new self-report scale of intrinsic versus extrinsic orientation in the classroom: Motivational and informational components. *Developmental Psychology, 17*, 300–312.

Harter, S. (1999). *The construction of the self: A developmental perspective.* New York: The Guilford Press.

Hayes, D. P., & Grether, J. (1983). The school year and vacations: When do students learn? *Cornell Journal of Social Relations, 17*, 56–71.

Heckhausen, H., & Roelofsen, I. (1962). Anfänge and Entwicklung der Leistungsmotivation: (I.) im Wetteifer des Kleinkindes [The origin and development of achievement motivation: (I.) in the competition tendency of the child]. *Psychologische Forschung, 26*, 313–397.

Heckhausen, H., & Wagner, I. (1965). Anfänge und Entwicklung der Leistungsmotivation: (II.) in der Zielsetzung des Kleinkindes. Zur Genese des Anspruchsniveaus [The origin and development of achievement motivation: (II.) in the goal-setting of the child. The origin of the level of aspiration]. *Psychologische Forschung, 28*, 179–245.

Heckhausen, J. (1987). Balancing for weaknesses an challenging developmental potential: A longitudinal study of mother-child dyads in apprenticeship interactions. *Developmental Psychology, 23*, 762–770.

Hokoda, A., & Fincham, F. D. (1995). Origins of children's helpless and mastery achievement patterns in the family. *Journal of Educational Psychology, 87*, 375–385.

Holt, J. (1964). *How children fail.* New York: Pitman.

Hoover, W. A., & Gough, P. B. (1990). The simple view of reading. *Reading and Writing, 2*, 127–160.

Howard-Rose, D., & Rose, C. (1994). Students' adaptation to task environments in resource room and regular class settings. *Journal of Special Education, 28*, 3–26.

Jacobsen, T., Huss, M., Fendrich, M., Kruesi, M., & Ziegenhain, U. (1997). Children's ability to delay gratification: Longitudinal relations to mother-child attachment. *Journal of Genetic Psychology, 158*, 411–426.

Jordan, A., Lindsay, L., & Stanovich, P. (1997). Classroom teachers' instructional interactions with students who are exceptional, at risk, and typically achieving. *Remedial & Special Education, 18,* 82–93.

Juel, C. (1988). Learning to read and write: A longitudinal study of 54 children from first through fourth grades. *Journal of Educational Psychology, 80,* 437–447.

Järvelä, S., Salonen, P., & Lepola, J. (2001). Dynamic assessment as a key to understanding student motivation in a classroom context. In P. Pintrich & M. Maehr (Eds.), *Advances in motivation and achievement: Methodology in motivation research: New directions in measures and methods* (Vol. 12, pp. 217–240). Greenwich, CT: JAI Press.

Kavale, K. A., & Forness, S. R. (1985). *The science of learning disabilities.* San Diego: College-Hill Press.

Kinnunen, R., & Vauras, M. (1995). Comprehension monitoring and the level of comprehension in high- and low-achieving primary school children's reading. *Learning and Instruction, 5,* 143–165.

Lave, J., Murtaugh, M. M., & de la Roche, O. (1984). The dialectic of grocery shopping. In B. Rogoff & J. Lave (Eds.), *Everyday cognition: Its development in social context* (pp. 67–94). Cambridge, MA: Harvard University Press.

Lazarus, R., & Folkman, S. (1984). *Stress, appraisal, and coping.* New York: Springer-Verlag.

LCHC (Laboratory of Comparative Human Cognition) (1982). Culture and intelligence. In R. J. Sternberg (Ed.), Handbook of human intelligence (pp. 642–719). New York: Cambridge University Press.

Lehtinen, E., Vauras, M., Salonen, P., Olkinuora, E., & Kinnunen, R. (1995). Long-term development of learning activity: Motivational, cognitive, and social interaction. *Educational Psychologist, 30,* 21–35.

Lepola, J., Salonen, P., & Vauras, M. (2000). The development of motivational orientations as a function of divergent reading careers from pre-school to the second grade. *Learning and Instruction, 10,* 153–177.

Lepola, J., Vauras, M., & Poskiparta, E. (2002). Pitkittäistutkimus lukutaidon ja motivaation kehityksestä esikoulusta kahdeksannelle luokalle [A longitudinal study of reading and motivation from preschool to the eight grade]. *Psykologia, Journal of the Finnish Psychological Society, 37*(1), 33–44.

Lindeman, J. (1998). *Ala-asteen Lukutesti (ALLU)* [Standardized, comprehensive school reading test]. Jyväskylä, Finland: Gummerus.

Lundberg, I., & Nilsson, L-G. (1986). What church examination records can tell us about the inheritance of reading disability? *Annals of Dyslexia, 36,* 217–236.

Lundberg, I., Olofsson, Å., & Wall, S. (1980). Reading and spelling skills in the first school years predicted from phonemic awareness skills in kindergarten. *Scandinavian Journal of Psychology, 21,* 159–173.

Lyytinen, P., Rasku-Puttonen, H., Poikkeus, A-M., Laakso, M-L., & Ahonen, T. (1994). Mother-child teaching strategies and learning disabilities. *Journal of Learning Disabilities, 27,* 186–192.

Marcus, R. F. (1975). The child as elicitor of parental sanctions for independent and dependent behavior: A simulation of parent-child interaction. *Developmental Psychology, 11,* 443–452.

McConaughy, S. H., Mattison, R. E., & Peterson, R. L. (1994). Behavioral/emotional problems of children with serious emotional disturbances and learning disabilities. *School Psychology Review, 23,* 81–98.

McGee, R., Williams, S., & Silva, P. A. (1988). Slow starters and long-term backward readers. A replication and extension. *British Journal of Educational Psychology, 58,* 330–337.

McLaughlin, H. J. (1991). Reconciling care and control: Authority in classroom relationships. *Journal of Teacher Education, 42,* 182–195.

McNaughton, S. (1981). Low progress readers and teacher instructional behavior during oral reading: The risk of maintaining instructional dependence. *Exceptional Child, 28,* 167–176.

Meadows, S. (1996). *Parenting behaviour and children's cognitive development: Essays in developmental psychology.* Hove: Erlbaum.

Meece, J. L., Blumenfeld, P. C., & Hoyle, R. H. (1988). Students' goal orientations and cognitive engagement in classroom activities. *Journal of Educational Psychology, 80,* 514–523.

Mehan, H. (1988). Educational handicap as a cultural meaning system. *Ethos, 16,* 73–91.

Moriarty, A. (1961). Coping patterns of pre-school children in response to intelligence test demands. *Genetic Psychology Monographs, 64,* 3–127.

Murphy, L. B., & Moriarty, A. E. (1976). *Vulnerability, coping, & growth: From infancy to adolescence.* London: Yale University Press.

Nelson-LeGall, S. (1981). Help-seeking: An understudied problem-solving skill in children. *Developmental Review, 1,* 224–246.

Nelson-Le Gall, S., & Glor-Scheib, S. (1985). Help-seeking in elementary classroom: An observational study. *Contemporary Educational Psychology, 10,* 58–71.

Nicholls, J. G. (1984). Achievement motivation: Conceptions of ability, subjective experience, task choice, and performance. *Psychological Review, 91,* 328–346.

Niemi, P., Poskiparta, E., Vauras, M., & Mäki, H. (1998). Reading and writing difficulties do not always occur as the researcher expects. *Scandinavian Journal of Psychology, 39,* 159–161.

Nolen, S. B. (1988). Reasons for studying: Motivational orientations and study strategies. *Cognition and Instruction, 5,* 269–287.

Olkinuora, E., & Salonen, P. (1992). Adaptation, motivational orientation, and cognition in a subnormally-performing child: A systemic perspective for training. In B. Wong (Ed.), *Intervention research in learning disabilities: An international perspective* (pp. 190–213). New York: Springer-Verlag.

Olkinuora, E., Salonen, P., & Lehtinen, E. (1984). *Toward an interactionist theory of cognitive dysfunctions.* Research Monographs of the Faculty of Education, University of Turku, B10.

Osofsky, J. D. (1971). Children's influences upon parental behavior: An attempt to define the relationship with the use of laboratory tasks. *Genetic Psychology Monographs, 83,* 147–169.

Osofsky, J. D., & O'Connell, E. (1972). Parent-child interaction: Daughters' effects upon mothers' and fathers behaviors. *Developmental Psychology, 7,* 157–168.

Palincsar, A. S. (1986). The role of dialogue in providing scaffolded instruction. *Educational Psychologist, 21,* 73–98.

Patterson, G. R., & Bank, L. (1989). Some amplifying mechanisms for pathologic processes in families. In M. R. Gunnar & E. Thelen (Eds.), *Systems and development: Minnesota symposia on child psychology* (Vol. 22, pp. 167–209). Hillsdale, NJ: Erlbaum.

Pervin, L., & Lewis, M. (1978). *Perspectives in interactional psychology.* New York: Plenum.

Pintrich, P. R., & DeGroot, A. M. (1990). Motivational and self-regulated learning components of classroom academic performance. *Journal of Educational Psychology, 82,* 33–40.

Pintrich, P. R., Roeser, R. W., & DeGroot, A. M. (1994). Classroom and individual differences in early adolescents' motivation and self-regulated learning. *Journal of Early Adolescence, 14,* 139–161.

Pintrich, P. R., & Schrauben, B. (1992). Students' motivational beliefs and their cognitive engagement on classroom tasks. In D. H. Schunk & J. Meece (Eds.), *Students perceptions in the classroom: Causes and consequences* (pp. 149–183). Hillsdale, NJ: Lawrence Erlbaum Associates.

Pollard, A. (1986). Coping strategies and the multiplication of differentiation in infant classrooms. In M. Hammersley (Ed.), *Case studies in classroom research* (pp. 30–48). Milton Keynes: Open University Press.

Poskiparta, E., Niemi, P., Lepola, J., Ahtola, A., & Laine, P. (2003). Motivational-emotional vulnerability and difficulties in learning to read and spell. *British Journal of Educational Psychology, 73*, 187–206.

Poskiparta, E., Niemi, P., & Vauras, M. (1999). Who benefits from training linguistic awareness in the first grade and what components of it show training effects? *Journal of Learning Disabilities, 32*(5), 437–446, 456.

Rock, E. E., Fessler, M. A., & Church, R. P. (1997). The concomitance of learning disabilities and emotional/behavioral disorders: A conceptual model. *Journal of Learning Disabilities, 30*, 245–263.

Rogoff, B., & Gardner, W. (1984). Adult guidance and cognitive development. In B. Rogoff & J. Lave (Eds.), *Everyday cognition: Its development in social context* (pp. 95–116). Cambridge, MA: Harvard University Press.

Rotenberg, V. S., & Boucsein, W. (1993). Adaptive versus maladaptive emotional tension. *Genetic, Social & General Psychology Monographs, 119*, 207–232.

Rueda, R., & Mehan, H. (1986). Metacognition and passing: Strategic interactions in the lives of student with learning disabilities. *Anthropology & Education Quarterly, 17*, 145–165.

Ryan, J. (1980). The silence of stupidity. In J. Morton & J. C. Marshall (Eds.), *Psycholinguistic: Developmental and Pathological* (pp. 101–124). New York: Cornell University Press.

Salonen, P. (1988). Learning disabled children's situational orientations and coping strategies. *Nordisk Pedagogik, 8*, 70–75.

Salonen, P. (2000). *Subnormally performing children's coping strategies in situational context: Field-theoretical foundations, taxonomy, and case analysis.* Center for Learning Research, University of Turku (Unpublished manuscript).

Salonen, P., & Lepola, J. (1993). *The development of children's coping strategies and reading skills during the first school-year.* Paper presented in M. Vauras (Chair) Motivation and classroom interaction. Symposium conducted at the 5th European Conference for Research on Learning and Instruction, Aix-en-Provence, France.

Salonen, P., Lehtinen, E., & Olkinuora, E. (1998a). Expectations and beyond: The development of motivation and learning in a classroom context. In J. Brophy (Ed.), *Advances in research on teaching* (Vol. 7, pp. 111–150). Greenwich, CT: JAI Press.

Salonen, P., Lepola, J., & Niemi, P. (1998b). The development of first graders' reading skill as a function of pre-school motivational orientation and phonemic awareness. *European Journal of Psychology of Education, 13*, 155–174.

Sameroff, A. J. (1975). Early influences on development: Fact or fancy. *Merrill-Palmer Quarterly, 21*, 267–294.

Sansbury, L. L., & Wahler, R. G. (1992). Pathways to maladaptive parenting with mothers and their conduct disordered children. *Behavior Modification, 16*, 574–592.

Schneider, W., Stefanek, J., & Dotzler, H. (1997). Erwerb des Lesens und des Rechtschreibens: Ergebnisse aus dem SCHOLASTIC-Projekt [Achievement in Reading and Spelling: Results from SCHOLASTIC Project]. In F. E. Weinert und & A. Helmke (Hrsg.) (Eds.), *Entwicklung im Grundschulalter.* Beltz: Psychologie VerlagsUnion.

Schoggen, P. (1978). Ecological psychology and mental retardation. In G. Sackett (Ed.), *Observing behavior: Theory and applications in mental retardation* (Vol. 1, pp. 33–62). Baltimore, MD: University Park Press.

Schultz, G. F., & Switzky, H. N. (1990). The development intrinsic motivation in students with learning problems. *Preventing School Failure, 34*, 14–20.

Schultz, K. (1994). "I want to be good; I just don't get it." A fourth-grader's entrance into a literacy community. *Written Communication, 11*, 381–413.

Schultz, G. F., & Switzky, H. N. (1993). The academic achievement of elementary and junior high school students with behavior disorders and their nonhandicapped peers as a function of motivational orientation. *Learning and Individual Differences, 5*, 31–42.

Siegel, L. S. (1999). Issues in the definition and diagnosis of learning disabilities: A perspective on Guckenberger v. Boston University. *Journal of Learning Disabilities, 32*, 304–319.

Skinner, E. A., & Belmont, M. J. (1993). Motivation in the classroom: Reciprocal effects of teacher behaviour and student engagement across the school year. *Journal of Educational Psychology, 85*, 571–581.

Spear-Swerling, L., & Sternberg, R. J. (1998). Curing our 'epidemic' of learning disabilities. *Phi Delta Kappan, 79*, 397–401.

Stanovich, K. E. (1986). Matthew effects in reading: Some consequences of individual differences in the acquisition of literacy. *Reading Research Quarterly, 21*, 361–406.

Stanovich, K. E. (1993). Dysrationalia: A new specific learning disability. *Journal of Learning Disabilities, 26*, 501–515.

Stanovich, K. E. (1999). The sociopsychometrics of learning disabilities. *Journal of Learning Disabilities, 32*, 350–361.

Stanovich, K. E. (2000). *Progress in understanding reading: Scientific foundations and new frontiers*. New York: The Guilford Press.

Switzky, H. N. (1997). Mental retardation and the neglected construct of motivation. *Education and Training in Mental Retardation and Developmental Disabilities, 32*, 194–196.

Switzky, H. N. (2001). Personality and motivational self-system processes in persons with mental retardation: Old memories and new perspectives. In H. N. Switzky (Ed.), *Personality and motivational differences in persons with mental retardation* (pp. 57–143). Mahwah, NJ: Erlbaum.

Tiegerman, E., & Siperstein, M. (1984). Individual patterns of interaction in the mother-child dyad: Implications for parent intervention. *Topics in Language Disorders, 4*, 50–61.

Tinbergen, N., & Tinbergen, E. (1983). *'Autistic' children: new hope for cure*. London: Allen & Unwin.

Turner, J. C. (1995). The influence of classroom contexts on young children's motivation for literacy. *Reading Research Quarterly, 30*, 410–441.

van Dijk, T. A., & Kintsch, W. (1983). *Strategies in discource comprehension* (p.163). London: Academic Press.

Vauras, M., Kinnunen, R., & Kuusela, L. (1994). Development of text-processing skills in high-, average- and low-achieving primary school children. *Journal of Reading Behaviour, 26*, 361–389.

Vauras, M., Kinnunen, R., & Rauhanummi, T. (1999a). The role of metacognition in the context of integrated strategy intervention. *European Journal of Psychology of Education, 14*, 555–569.

Vauras, M., Rauhanummi, T., Kinnunen, R., & Lepola, J. (1999b). Motivational vulnerability as a challenge for educational interventions. *International Journal of Educational Research, 31*, 515–531.

Vauras, M., Salonen, P., Lehtinen, E., & Lepola, J. (2001). Long-term development of motivation and cognition in family and school contexts. In S. Volet & S. Jarvela (Eds.), *Motivation in learning context: Theoretical and methodological implications* (pp. 295–315). Pergamon Press: Amsterdam.

Vellutino, F., & Scanlon, D. (1987). Phonological coding, phonological awareness, and reading ability: Evidence from a longitudinal and experimental study. *Merrill-Palmer Quarterly, 33*, 321–363.

Vygotsky, L. S. (1962). *Thought and language.* New York, NY: Wiley.
Vygotsky, L. S. (1978). *Mind in society.* Cambridge, MA: Harvard University Press.
Wall, M. E., & Dattilo, J. (1995). Creating option-rich learning environments: Facilitating self-determination. *Journal of Special Education, 29,* 276–294.
Wentzel, K. R. (1996). Social and academic motivation in middle school: Concurrent and long-term relations to academic effort. *Journal of Early Adolescence, 16,* 390–416.
Wentzel, K. R. (1994). Family functioning and academic achievement in middle school. *Journal of Early Adolescence, 14,* 268–291.
White, R. W. (1959). Motivation reconsidered: The concept of competence. *Psychological Review, 66,* 297–333.
Wolf, M., & Bowers, P. G. (1999). The double-deficit hypothesis for the developmental dyslexia. *Journal of Educational Psychology, 91,* 1–24.
Wood, P., Bruner, J., & Ross, G. (1976). The role of tutoring in problem solving. *Journal of Child Psychology and Psychiatry, 17,* 89–100.
Yarrow, M., Waxler, C., & Scott, P. (1971). Child effects on adult behavior. *Developmental Psychology, 5,* 300–311.
Zigler, E., & Balla, D. (1981). Issues in personality and motivation in mentally retarded persons. In M. Begab, H. Haywood, & H. Garber (Eds.), *Psychosocial influences in retarded performance* (Vol. 1, pp. 197–218). Baltimore: University Park Press.
Zigler, E., & Hodapp, R. M. (1991). Behavioral functioning in individuals with mental retardation. *Annual Review of Psychology, 42,* 29–50.

Toward Inclusion Across Disciplines: Understanding Motivation of Exceptional Students

HELEN PATRICK

PURDUE UNIVERSITY

ALLISON M. RYAN

UNIVERSITY OF ILLINOIS, URBANA-CHAMPAIGN

ERIC M. ANDERMAN

UNIVERSITY OF KENTUCKY

JOHN KOVACH

NORTHERN ILLINOIS UNIVERSITY

Why do some students enjoy learning new things and value schoolwork while others do not? Why do some students exert effort to accomplish academic tasks while others expend as little effort as possible or find ways to avoid engaging at all? Motivational questions such as these are vital to address because they have significant implications for students' learning, adjustment and, ultimately, success beyond school. In addition to students without disabilities, they are relevant to students with cognitive disabilities, such as those with mental retardation or learning disabilities. Because motivation energizes and directs behavior, it plays a different role from ability. Regardless of ability level or the presence of learning-related disabilities, motivation to learn can maximize all students' chances to realize their full academic potential.

The study of achievement motivation is currently one of the most central and prolific areas of research in the field of educational psychology (Smith et al., 2003). Current theories that guide motivational research are social-cognitive—that is, they involve individuals' perceptions of themselves, their abilities and intentions, and the perceived supports and demands of others and of the environment (Pintrich & Schunk, 2002). Although they were developed for students without disabilities, researchers (e.g., Switzky, 1999) have suggested that these motivation theories are also appropriate for use with exceptional students. Therefore, is somewhat disquieting to observe that the recent productivity within the motivation field, with its significant theoretical developments and empirical findings, has not extended far into the field of special education. Motivation researchers have tended to exclude exceptional students from their research. Furthermore, special education researchers do not typically use the theoretical perspectives that are used predominantly by motivation researchers. Consequently, there seems to be a less than desirable interchange between both fields of research, despite the considerable overlap in concern with students' motivation and learning. Nevertheless, there have been some calls to integrate theories and research within both these fields (e.g., Deci & Chandler, 1986; Switzky, 1999). This present volume, with its contributors representing both fields of motivation and special education, is an excellent example of efforts to stimulate more research that integrates state-of-the-art approaches from both fields.

In that spirit, we focus in this chapter on the integration of motivation research and the field of special education. We begin by suggesting some of the reasons why research in motivation and special education has not been integrated as much as it might have. Identifying barriers may make it easier for researchers to overcome them. We focus next on a few of the dominant theoretical approaches within both fields of research. These include intrinsic motivation, goal theory, expectancy-value theory, and social motivation. After reviewing the theories and associated findings from research with non-exceptional students, we examine studies that have been conducted with exceptional students. We also discuss some preliminary results from a recent study of sixth graders' motivation that included students in self-contained special education classes. We compare the patterns of their responses with those of students in regular classes who were not identified as having special needs. We conclude the chapter by discussing directions for future research that would continue the integration of theory and research between special education and educational psychology.

I. BARRIERS TO INTEGRATING RESEARCH WITHIN FIELDS OF MOTIVATION AND SPECIAL EDUCATION

We suspect that there are a number of reasons why interdisciplinary research encompassing motivation and special education has not been as plentiful as it might have, and conjecture on what some of those might be. They include the specialized nature of knowledge and terminology, concern with construct validity, and measurement issues.

A. Specialization

Both the motivation and special education fields involve a high degree of specialized knowledge, and researchers do not usually have sufficient appreciation of both. However, sound research, particularly that which will expand the understanding of exceptional students' achievement motivation past the simple or trivial, requires specialized knowledge of motivation and special education. The complexities inherent in each field mean that efforts to investigate the motivation of exceptional students are fraught with unknown perils for the ill-prepared researcher.

There is a seeming plethora of terminology within motivation and special education. The associated inherent complexity can deter informed research outside one's own specialty. For example, the meanings of terms and labels have changed over time, similar terms exist for the same construct, and terminology sometimes has a different meaning from that in everyday use. Therefore, there are minefields of potential misconceptions on both fronts.

1. MOTIVATION

Motivation research has myriad terms for constructs that are actually very similar—a state of affairs that is not without some concern within the field (Murphy & Alexander, 2000). For example, perceptions of self-competence, self-efficacy, and expectancies are all similar constructs in that they involve evaluations or appraisals of how good one is or will be in a task or domain. These perceptions (self-competence, self-efficacy, expectancy) are all believed to be associated positively with students choosing tasks that are optimally challenging, persisting despite setbacks, using effortful but effective learning strategies, and ultimately associated with learning and achievement (Pintrich & Schunk, 2002). Although they are not used interchangably, because each is from a different theoretical approach or tradition and can be differentiated at a fine level (e.g., Bong & Clark, 1999), they are thought of in very similar terms. However, they are all very different from another "self" construct—self-esteem, which involves an affective sense of worth and, therefore, differs from the very cognitive appraisals inherent in the previous constructs (Beane & Lipka, 1980).

As if that is not sufficiently complex, motivation theories include terminology that is used in everyday language, but that has a different or more specific meaning. One example involves the construct of performance goals within goal theory. A performance goal does not refer to wanting to perform well, but instead to engaging in achievement-related behavior with the purpose of demonstrating, rather than developing, competence (Ames, 1992). The difference between everyday and specialized meanings of terminology can render motivation research perplexing to those in other fields. For example, the negative correlates and outcomes associated typically with performance goals may not make sense if performance goals are (mis)construed as wanting to perform or do well.

As with all fields of active research, there is ongoing refinement and evolution within the array of motivation theories. For example, the view of motivation as being either intrinsic or extrinsic has been refined by Deci and Ryan to include four different classifications of extrinsic motivation, one of which is similar to an intrinsic orientation. They also situated the classifications within their theory of self-determination (Deci & Ryan, 1985; Ryan & Deci, 2000). Other approaches, such as goal theory, conceptualize different motivational orientations toward achievement tasks as being orthogonal, or unrelated to each other. This allows for students to be oriented to multiple goals, or have multiple purposes for engaging in tasks, at the same time (e.g., Pintrich, 2000b). Another development that has influenced goal theory in particular involves a distinction between individuals' tendency to either approach or avoid a situation. Therefore, goal theorists now distinguish between performance-approach goals (i.e., a desire to look more competent than others) and performance-avoid goals (i.e., a desire to avoid looking less competent than others) (Elliot & Harackiewicz, 1996; Middleton & Midgley, 1997).

2. SPECIAL EDUCATION

There is a similar degree of complexity within special education. As with motivation, there is a plethora of different terms for the same exceptionality. For example, in the study of learning disabilities, terms such as "learning disabled," "minimal brain injury," and "slow learner" are often used interchangeably. On a national level, there are a number of accepted definitions of learning disabilities, including the federal definition and the National Joint Committee for Learning Disabilities' definition. The complexity of this issue is noted (Hallahan & Kauffman, 1997). In addition, even general terms such as "exceptionality," "handicap," and "disability" are often used quite freely by researchers, teachers, and practitioners.

Similarly, labels or sub-categories have changed over time. For example, within the domain of mental retardation, there are a variety of terms that have been used to describe the severity of retardation. For example, classification systems based on IQ cut-off scores used categorizations such as "mild retardation" and "moderate retardation," whereas newer categorizations are based on the levels of support needed by individuals, and use terms such as "intermittent" and "limited" mental retardation (AAMR Ad Hoc Committee on Terminology and Classification, 1992).

In addition to changes in the definitions and labels for different disabilities, there have been marked shifts over time in how terms have been used, and for whom terms have referred to. For example, prior to the 1990s, students with attention-deficit-hyperactivity disorder (ADHD) were often considered to be learning disabled. However, research now clearly indicates that students with ADHD are not necessarily always learning disabled (e.g., Reid et al., 1994). Additionally, students who would have been classified with educable mental retardation (EMR) tend now to be labeled as learning disabled. Consequently, the population of students with learning disabilities has become more like those who used to be labeled as having EMR or mild mental retardation, and the mild mental retardation population has become more like those who used to be classified as having moderate mental retardation. (Hallahan et al., 1996).

B. Construct Validity Issues

A reason that motivation researchers have typically excluded exceptional students from their research may involve the social-cognitive nature of motivation theories. That is, the theories focus on individuals' cognitive appraisals of themselves and their situation, and these beliefs and perceptions are seen as contributing to different kinds of motivated behavior. Motivational theories involve addressing questions such as: "Can I succeed at this task?", "Do I want to succeed?", "Why do I want to succeed?", "What will count as success?", "What would it cost me to succeed?", and "What would it cost me not to succeed?" Perhaps there is uncertainty about the extent to which students with cognitive disabilities think about and conceptualize these questions, or even whether these questions have the same meaning or relevancy for these students. Such caution has also to be seen in the context of most motivation researchers' limited knowledge about special education.

C. Measurement Issues

Issues related to the measurement of motivation may also contribute to the typical practice of motivation researchers not including exceptional students in their research. Because motivation theories emphasize students' beliefs and perceptions, measurement has focused principally on students' self-reports in response to survey items and likert-scales. Surveys are typically administered in groups, such as whole classes. Although it is typical for surveys to be administered by at least two researchers—one to read items aloud and at least one to monitor students and be available to answer questions—this format raises significant concerns for exceptional students. The reliability may be questionable when used with students who have difficulties with reading, comprehension, cognitive processing, or maintaining attention. It may be necessary to ask fewer questions of these students, resulting in scales with fewer items; this no doubt will tend to lessen the internal reliability of the scales. Furthermore, the likert scales (typically with 5 or 7 points) may not be appropriate for students with mental retardation. Scales may need to be adjusted in line with those used for young students, such as having much fewer (e.g., 3) responses to choose from (e.g., Gottfried, 1990) or responses represented pictorially (e.g., Harter & Pike, 1984). Also, because there tend to be so fewer exceptional students, compared to the number of regular students, the decision to exclude the former group from data collection, and so avoid these concerns, is understandable.

In short, the potential benefits of including a relatively small number of students to the pool of participants may often not seem to outweigh the immediate concerns with reliability, validity, pragmatics, and inconsistency regarding student classification. Over the long term, however, this leads to the situation of motivation and special education research developing separately and thus not informing each other.

II. IMPORTANCE OF INTEGRATING MOTIVATION AND SPECIAL EDUCATION RESEARCH

There are strong reasons why research in motivation and special education should inform each other. Motivation is crucial to exceptional students (Robinson et al., 2000), just as it is to regular students; school success at all ability levels requires intentional, motivated behavior. There are theoretical questions of importance to be addressed. For example, to what extent and in what ways are the motivational beliefs of students who are mentally disabled or learning disabled similar to, or different from, those of non-exceptional students? To what degree do the motivational beliefs of exceptional students relate similarly to achievement behaviors compared to those of students without special needs or who represent the middle of the normal curve? The promise of benefits for educators is enormous as well. The processes of understanding student motivation and facilitating adaptive motivational patterns is complex. Within the diversity of students who require special education, it may be even more so. Teachers and other educators need the expertise that both fields can contribute.

III. EXAMINING MOTIVATION OF EXCEPTIONAL AND NON-EXCEPTIONAL STUDENTS

One step toward integration of motivation and special education is cross-fertilization of ideas and theoretical approaches, where researchers address the same topic from their different specializations. Our objective is to contribute to this cross-fertilization process. We begin by reviewing a selection of theories of motivation (intrinsic motivation, goal orientations, expectancy-value theory, and social motivation approaches). We briefly review current and representative research with regular students as well as review the little research within those theoretical frameworks that have included exceptional students.

A. Intrinsic Motivation

Intrinsic motivation theories conceptualize motivation as being either *intrinsic* (engaging in tasks for their own purpose) or *extrinsic* (engaging in tasks to either receive some type of reward or to avoid some type of punishment) (e.g., Harter, 1981). That is, individuals' predominant disposition is portrayed as one "versus" the other. This theory is intuitively appealing and understandable. Furthermore, considerable research has indicated that holding an intrinsic orientation is more adaptive for a range of learning-related outcomes than holding an extrinsic orientation. For example, intrinsic motivation is related positively to interest, perceptions of competence and internal control, higher-quality learning and achievement, and psychological well-being (Deci et al., 1999; Gottfried, 1985, 1990; Ryan & Deci, 2000). Intrinsic motivation is also related negatively to anxiety (Gottfried, 1985, 1990).

The research regarding exceptional students' motivation has been predominantly within an intrinsic motivation framework (Switzky, 2001). There have typically been two kinds of studies: (1) those that have investigated associations between students' motivational orientation (intrinsic or extrinsic) and achievement, and (2) those that have compared mean levels of intrinsic motivation between groups of regular and exceptional students.

1. ASSOCIATIONS BETWEEN EXCEPTIONAL STUDENTS' INTRINSIC MOTIVATION AND ACHIEVEMENT

As has been found with non-exceptional students, there appear to be clear benefits for students with mental retardation in being intrinsically motivated. That is, in general, an intrinsic orientation is associated with adaptive patterns of engagement and achievement. A review of studies of students with mental retardation indicated that intrinsic motivation is associated positively with achievement (Switzky, 1999). Furthermore, Switzky found that the intrinsic orientation of these students was related even more strongly to achievement than it was for students of average intelligence; "the effects of motivational orientation intensified as the intellectual ability levels of the students decreased" (Switzky, 1999, p. 78). Perhaps partly accounting for the association between intrinsic motivation and achievement, intrinsic motivation is related positively to effort for people with mental retardation (Zewdie, 1995, in Switzky, 1999). Specifically, those individuals who were more intrinsically motivated completed more tasks and worked longer than those who were less intrinsically motivated.

Similar to the research of students with mental retardation, a review of studies that investigated the motivation of students with learning disabilities concluded that intrinsic motivation is related strongly to their academic achievement (Dev, 1998). Some researchers (e.g., Adelman & Chaney, 1982) have suggested that the underachievement of children with learning disabilities is caused in part by them having an extrinsic motivational orientation. However, not all research has supported that view; Reeve and Loper (1983) found no significant correlation between the motivational orientation and academic achievement of children with learning disabilities.

There have been fewer studies examining the intrinsic motivation of students with behavior disorders. Schultz and Switzky (1993) found that for students with behavior disorders being intrinsically, rather than extrinsically, oriented was related significantly to both their reading comprehension and math achievement. However, there was no significant effect of motivational orientation for the students without disabilities. The researchers suggested that having an intrinsic focus may help to compensate for emotional problems, whereas an extrinsic focus may further intensify their negative effects on achievement.

2. COMPARISONS BETWEEN EXCEPTIONAL AND NON-EXCEPTIONAL STUDENTS' INTRINSIC MOTIVATION

In contrast to the rather consistent findings that an intrinsic orientation to school work is related positively to achievement for exceptional students, there is considerable discrepancy in the research about whether or not these students tend to have lower levels of intrinsic motivation than non-exceptional students.

A few studies have compared the intrinsic motivation of students with learning disabilities with that of students without disabilities. The results have been somewhat mixed. For example, Wilson and David (1994) compared the mean intrinsic motivation score for a sample of learning-disabled students with the scale's mean, taken from the published norms calculated for students without disabilities. They found that, on average, students with learning disabilities were significantly less intrinsically motivated than the students without disabilities. However, Fulk, Brigham, and Lohman (1998) found no difference in mean level intrinsic motivation among groups of students with learning disabilities, behavior disorders, and students without disabilities.

3. EFFECTS OF REWARDS ON INTRINSIC MOTIVATION

In addition to the evidence of positive perceptions and behaviors associated with intrinsic motivation, there is considerable research indicating that the use of extrinsic rewards often undermines intrinsic motivation (e.g., Deci et al., 1999; Lepper et al., 1973). According to Deci and Ryan, tangible extrinsic incentives or rewards (e.g., gold stars, grades, money) are perceived by individuals as controlling, and consequently decrease students' sense of autonomy and intrinsic motivation (Deci et al., 2001).

Nevertheless, despite the known effects of extrinsic incentives on intrinsic motivation, special educators often use extrinsic rewards to motivate exceptional children to engage in targeted behaviors. For example, token economies and response-cost programs often are used to modify behaviors of mentally retarded individuals (e.g., Chen, 1990; Sisson & Dixon, 1986), learning-disabled individuals (e.g., Salend & Henry, 1981; Salend & Lamb, 1986), and even individuals with behavior disorders (e.g., Comaty et al., 2001). Interestingly, special education research, for the most part, has not focused on potential detrimental effects of extrinsic motivators. Whereas a host of studies suggest that extrinsic rewards can effectively be used to modify behaviors in exceptional populations, research to date has not examined or considered the potential detrimental effects of such practices.

An intrinsic motivation approach to conceptualizing students' motivation appears to be most popular within special education. However, there are many other theoretical approaches used currently by researchers in educational psychology that are expanding and enriching the understanding of regular students' motivation. In the following sections, we will highlight some of those theories.

B. Goal Theory

Goal theory addresses the purpose and meaning that individuals ascribe to their achievement behavior. This includes considering students' *goal orientations*, or reasons for involvement in academic tasks and their conceptions of success (Ames, 1992). People may simultaneously have multiple reasons for their achievement-related behavior; thus, goal orientations are independent of each other.

Research has identified two goal orientations that capture meaningful distinctions in how individuals orient themselves to achieving competence in the academic setting (Elliot & Harackiewicz, 1996; Middleton & Midgley, 1997; Pintrich, 2000a; Skaalvik, 1997). A *mastery goal orientation* concerns a focus on developing competence and gaining understanding or mastery. In contrast, a performance goal orientation concerns a focus on demonstrating competence. A *performance-approach goal orientation* concerns a focus on gaining favorable judgments of one's ability and a *performance-avoid goal orientation* concerns a focus on avoiding negative judgments of one's ability. With a performance-approach goal orientation, the focus is performing better than others and with a performance-avoid goal orientation the focus is not performing worse than others.

These achievement goal orientations represent disparate purposes for involvement regarding academic tasks and have been linked to different achievement-related processes. Goal orientations are conceptualized as a precursor to achievement-related processes (i.e., why students do something precedes whether, if, and how they actually do it) and thus are viewed as setting in motion cognitive, affective, and behavioral processes on any given task.

A mastery goal orientation sets in motion adaptive achievement-related processes for learning and achievement. With a focus on developing competence, students are more likely to engage in tasks in a manner that maximizes their opportunities to learn. Research has found that a mastery goal orientation is associated with preference for challenging tasks, persistence, adaptive learning strategies, asking for help when it is needed, and positive affect (see Anderman et al., 2002; Pintrich & Schunk, 2002; Urdan, 1997, for recent reviews).

A performance-avoid goal orientation sets in motion maladaptive achievement-related processes for learning and achievement. A focus on demonstrating that one does not have less ability relative to others has been linked to self-handicapping, a disorganized approach to studying, use of more surface and less deep processing strategies, lack of persistence, avoidance of help seeking, anxiety, and lower exam performance (Elliot et al., 1999; Middleton & Midgley, 1997; Urdan et al., 2002).

Research on a performance-approach goal orientation does not provide a clear picture regarding achievement-related processes as the mastery or performance-avoid goal orientations. There seems to be both the potential for adaptive and maladaptive achievement-related processes. On the one hand, a performance-approach goal orientation has been linked with increased effort and persistence while studying for an exam (Elliot et al., 1999), efficacy (Bong, 2001; Pajares, Britner, and Valiante 2000; Skaalvik, 1997; Wolters et al., 1996, study 1; and Middleton & Midgley, 1997 and Pajares et al., 2000, study 2) and high exam performance (Harackiewicz et al., 2002; although this is less consistent with younger students). On the other hand, a performance-approach goal orientation has been associated with a disorganized approach to studying, surface level processing strategies (Elliot et al., 1999), and avoidance of help seeking (Middleton & Midgley, 1997; Ryan & Pintrich, 1997; Ryan et al., 1997).

1. COMPARISONS BETWEEN EXCEPTIONAL AND NON-EXCEPTIONAL STUDENTS' GOAL ORIENTATIONS

There has been very little research within goal theory with exceptional students. However, the few studies that have compared the goal orientations of students with learning disabilities with those of regular students found no difference in the average level of mastery orientation (Anderman & Young, 1994; Pintrich et al., 1994).

After comparing the means of students with and without learning disabilities on different measures, Pintrich and his colleagues (1994) investigated how a range of motivation constructs, including mastery goals, tended to cluster with metacognition and comprehension across all students. They found three different profiles: (1) high motivation, metacognition, and comprehension; (2) high motivation but low metacognition and comprehension; and (3) low motivation and moderate metacognition and comprehension. The second cluster—high motivation but low metacognition and comprehension—was comprised only of students with learning disabilities. However, interestingly, there were learning-disabled students in all three clusters. That is, some students had profiles that resembled students without disabilities, whereas others' profiles were significantly different and somewhat less adaptive. This finding suggests that motivational issues are not necessarily equivalent for all students who fit a specific special education profile. Indeed, just as individual differences in motivation are evident in non-exceptional populations, they also are evident among exceptional students.

C. Expectancy-Value Theory

Another theory of achievement motivation is expectancy-value theory (Eccles, 1983; Wigfield, 1994). This theory posits that students' motivation is influenced by both their expectancy of success in a task or subject and by their valuing of the task or subject.

Expectancy involves perceptions of one's competence or ability and also confidence regarding future success, or self-efficacy (Eccles & Wigfield, 2002). Students' current self-perceptions of ability and their self-efficacy are related positively to indicators of motivation (e.g., effort, persistence, choosing challenging tasks), learning-related behaviors (e.g., problem-solving, use of cognitive and self-regulatory learning strategies), adaptive beliefs (e.g., increased value for academics), and achievement (Anderman et al., 2001; Bandura, 1993; Pintrich & De Groot, 1990; Zimmerman, 2000). Self-efficacy is also related negatively to anxiety (Bandura, 1993).

Eccles and Wigfield (2002; Wigfield & Eccles, 1992) refer to four different types of value. *Importance* refers to the attainment value or personal significance of the task or activity; *intrinsic value* is the enjoyment and interest the individual experiences when doing the task or activity; *utility value* concerns the usefulness of the task or activity for the individual in light of future goals; and *cost* refers to perceptions of negative aspects of involvement with the task. There has been considerable research that has shown that students' valuing of academic subjects is related to the choices they make (Wigfield & Eccles, 1992) and to other motivational beliefs (Anderman et al., 2001). When students report valuing learning about a subject, they tend to also report use of cognitive and self-regulatory learning strategies (Krapp et al., 1992; Pintrich & De Groot, 1990). Value is also associated with achievement, no doubt due to the mediating role of deep processing strategies (Schiefele et al., 1992).

One of the most important findings in the research on expectancies and values concerns the predictive nature of these constructs. Specifically, in longitudinal studies, research demonstrates that expectancy beliefs are predictive of achievement, whereas values are predictive of choice (e.g., enrollment in specific courses in the future) (Eccles, 1983; Wigfield & Eccles, 1992).

1. COMPARISONS BETWEEN EXCEPTIONAL AND NON-EXCEPTIONAL STUDENTS' EXPECTANCIES AND VALUES

Perhaps not surprisingly, some studies have indicated that students with learning disabilities tend to perceive their academic competence as lower than students without learning disabilities (e.g., Anderman & Young, 1994;

Bear, Minke, & Manning, 2002; Frederickson & Jacobs, 2001; Grolnick & Ryan, 1990). However, this is not unequivocal; Pintrich and colleagues (1994) found similar mean levels of self-efficacy for students with and without learning disabilities.

There has been very little research about exceptional students' value beliefs regarding academics. Anderman and Young (1994) found no significant difference between students with and without learning disabilities in their beliefs about the value of learning science. Although Wilson and David (1994) did not refer to a value framework, the Motivation for Schooling scale they used involves values in that it is concerned with students' views of the importance of school and their willingness to participate in school. They found that the scores of the students with learning disabilities were not significantly different from the published norms of the measure, created from samples of students with average achievement. On the basis of the limited evidence, therefore, it appears that exceptional students tend to value schoolwork as much as non-exceptional students do. In an interesting view of value, however, Fulk et al. (1998) asked students about the degree to which they agreed that the purpose of school is to prepare them for jobs that result in wealth and luxuries. They found that students with learning disabilities endorsed this view to a greater extent than either students with behavior disorders or non-exceptional students.

D. Social Motivation

There has been growing interest among motivation researchers in the association between the academic and social domains of students' lives. School success does not only involve academics; schools and classrooms are inherently social places, and students approach their work in the presence of many peers. There has been increasing attention, therefore, to understanding how relationships with others at school are associated with students' achievement motivation. Rather than being a separate theory of motivation, however, there have been different approaches to considering social motivation. Some approaches have involved elaborating on existing motivation theories, incorporating the social domain into them. Other approaches have focused on constructs that are used more commonly in psychology to understand adjustment, such as perceptions of support or belonging. In general, however, research addressing social motivation has indicated that students' perceptions about their relationships with both peers and teachers have significant implications for adaptive patterns of motivation and engagement (e.g., Juvonen & Wentzel, 1996; Patrick et al., 2002).

1. SOCIAL GOALS

Some researchers (e.g., Anderman, 1999b; Wentzel, 1989) have examined different social goals that students may pursue in relation to learning-related outcomes. Wanting to be socially responsible and meet the formal social demands of the classroom (social responsibility goal) is related to positive learning-related beliefs, including academic efficacy (Patrick et al., 1997), increased mastery goal orientation (Anderman & Anderman, 1999), positive affect at school (Anderman, 1999a), and to grades (Wentzel, 1989). Wanting to form close relationships with peers (social relationship goal) is associated with positive affect at school (Anderman, 1999a) and also with increased performance-approach goal orientation (Anderman & Anderman, 1999). A goal of wanting visibility and high social status is related to more negative beliefs and behaviors, including increased performance-approach goal orientation (Anderman & Anderman, 1999) and reports of not asking for help with schoolwork when help is needed (Ryan et al., 1997).

More recently researchers have examined achievement goal orientations in the social domain (Ryan et al., 2004). A social mastery goal orientation concerns a focus on developing positive, supportive relationships. A social performance-approach goal orientation concerns a focus on demonstrating social desirability and gaining positive judgments from others. A social performance-avoid goal orientation concerns a focus on demonstrating that one is not socially undesirable and not doing anything to incur negative judgments from others. These social goal orientations relate to students' social adjustment in a similar manner to how academic goal orientations relate to academic adjustment. A social mastery goal orientation is positively associated, whereas a social performance-avoid orientation is negatively associated, with social adjustment (i.e., self-esteem, social satisfaction). In the social domain, the effect of performance-approach goals seems to depend on the level of social mastery goals. Ryan et al. (2004) found no effect of performance-approach goals on students' self-esteem and social satisfaction if social mastery goals were high. However, if social mastery goals were low, performance-approach goals had a positive effect. Thus, a social performance-approach goal orientation does not have any additional benefits beyond a mastery goal orientation, but it can compensate for the lack of a mastery goal orientation.

2. SOCIAL EFFICACY

Students' confidence in their ability to interact effectively with others, or social self-efficacy, is related to their beliefs about school and academics. Relationships with peers and with teachers are different in nature (Hartup, 1989) and, therefore, students need different knowledge and behaviors (e.g., knowing and following different social norms and rules) for each type of relationship. Accordingly, self-efficacy with peers and with teachers are associated independently with academic outcomes.

Perceived efficacy for relating positively and satisfactorily with peers is associated with self-efficacy for school work (Patrick et al., 1997). This is believed to be, in part, because peers serve as potential sources of instrumental help with schoolwork, and a belief that one can ask for clarification of instructions, help with specific tasks, or general reassurance that what one is doing is correct bolsters confidence in learning. Students who feel confident relating to their teachers also report feeling efficacious about their ability to learn and succeed academically (Patrick et al., 1997). The association between academic efficacy and a positive teacher-student relationship is arguably because communicating effectively with the teacher inspires confidence that students will receive maximum support and assistance when necessary, and thus lessens anxiety and facilitates learning and achievement. Feeling confident relating to the teacher is associated also with students' self-regulated learning, and associated negatively with disruptive behavior in that teacher's class (Ryan & Patrick, 2001).

3. PERCEPTIONS OF SUPPORT

Perceptions of support may come from either teachers or peers. Both are uniquely associated with student motivation. Teacher support refers to students' beliefs that their teachers care about them, and value and establish personal relationships with them (Fraser & Fisher, 1982; Trickett & Moos, 1973). There are positive associations between perceptions of teacher support and students' adaptive motivational beliefs and engagement behaviors. For example, when students view their teachers as supportive they report higher levels of interest, valuing, effort, and enjoyment in their schoolwork (Fraser & Fisher, 1982; Midgley et al., 1989; Trickett & Moos, 1974), a more positive academic self-concept (Felner et al., 1985), and greater expectancies for success (Goodenow, 1993). Further, support from teachers is related to how students feel about themselves, including their general self esteem (Felner et al., 1985). Perceiving teachers as supportive is also related positively to asking for help with school work when needed (Newman & Schwager, 1993), use of self-regulated learning strategies (Ryan & Patrick, 2001), and a desire to comply with classroom rules (Wentzel, 1994); it is related negatively to absenteeism (Moos & Moos, 1978) and disruptiveness in the classroom (Ryan & Patrick, 2001).

Students may also perceive support from classmates, believing that other students care about them and will help them, whether instrumentally, socially, or emotionally. Because peer relationships involve reciprocity and similar levels of power (Hartup, 1989), support from classmates comprises a different type of support than that from teachers. However, both types of support are important for students. Peer support is related to students' desire to behave responsibly in the classroom (Cauce et al., 1982; Wentzel, 1994). Arguably similar to peer support, students' perception of cohesion or affiliation within the classroom is related positively to their liking and interest of academics, satisfaction with school, and achievement (Goh et al., 1995; Trickett & Moos, 1974). Conversely, a perception of friction or unfriendliness among students is related negatively to those outcomes (Goh et al., 1995; Haertel et al., 1981).

The research reviewed here has been conducted with non-exceptional students. However we believe that relationships in the classroom are also vital to the motivation and learning of exceptional students. Furthermore, there are additional socialization and relationship factors associated with students who have mental retardation or learning disabilities, and these are likely to affect their achievement motivation as well.

4. SOCIAL RELATIONSHIPS OF EXCEPTIONAL STUDENTS

Research has yet to address the social motivation of exceptional students, including associations with motivation for learning and achievement-related outcomes. However, this is likely to be a very fruitful area of investigation, as it continues to be for regular students. There are additional factors related to the social perceptions and experiences of exceptional students that may need to be taken into consideration. Students with learning disabilities tend to have lower perceptions of their social competence compared to students without disabilities (Bear et al., 2002). They, in addition to students with mental retardation, tend also to have poor social skills, including perceiving others' intentions, social problem-solving, and responding appropriately non-verbally or verbally (Vaughn et al., 2001). Consequently, they are more likely to experience social difficulties with peers at school, including rejection and low peer acceptance, compared to non-exceptional students (Gresham & MacMillan, 1997; Haager & Vaughn, 1995; La Greca, 1987). Relatedly, some research suggests that exceptional students who are included at times in regular classrooms are disliked by the regular status students (Sale & Carey, 1995). Extending this finding, however, Haager and Vaughn (1995) compared the social status of students with learning disabilities in regular classes to students with either low achievement or average to high achievement. They found no significant differences between the learning disabled and low achievement students, although both groups of students were less known and less liked than the average to high achieving students. The researchers suggested that students' reactions may have been in part because of their poor achievement, rather than their social skills.

Nevertheless, the attitudes of non-exceptional students in the regular classrooms toward exceptional students can be improved if those students are prepared for the inclusion of exceptional peers (e.g., York et al., 1992). Of interest is the finding in one study that learning-disabled students in self-contained classes had better social and emotional adjustment than similar students in regular classes (Schmidt, 2000). In line with these findings, Vaughn and her colleagues (2001) have suggested that educational placement decisions for students with learning disabilities should consider factors involving the social domain.

The higher incidence of peer relationship difficulties for exceptional students may mean that the teacher-student relationship plays a particularly vital role in supporting motivation. There is considerable evidence that students with mental retardation or learning disabilities tend to be more reliant on teacher direction and feedback than non-disabled students (Silon & Harter, 1985). However, there are factors that may make it difficult for students with disabilities to maintain positive relationships with their teachers. A review of studies addressing the social relationships of children with learning disabilities found that these students tend to receive more negative attention from teachers, and also be ignored by teachers more often, relative to students without learning disabilities (La Greca, 1987). However, some research contradicts those summaries. For example, Moore and Simpson (1983) conducted an observational study of self-contained special education classes and regular classes in which they compared teacher and peer classroom interactions of students with and without disabilities. They found that students with learning disabilities and those with behavior disorders engaged in a significantly greater proportion of disruptive, negative statements with their teacher, compared to students without disabilities. Interestingly, there were no differences in the proportion of negative comments between students with learning disabilities and those with behavior disorders. Despite the greater occurrence of negative verbalizations made by students, the study found no differences between teachers of special education and of regular classes in the proportions of positive verbalizations they made. This finding was supported by another observational study that found that teachers' instructional interactions did not differ for students with and without learning disabilities in their class (Parker et al., 1989).

E. Summary

In summary, researchers in educational psychology currently use a number of theories to investigate and explain students' motivation for academics. Although these theories are in many ways quite similar, each deals with specific and somewhat unique aspects of the motivation equation. For example, intrinsic motivation theories deal with the types of incentives used to motivate students, goal theory examines the reasons why students engage in various academic tasks, and expectancy-value theory is concerned with the effects of self-perceptions of ability and achievement values on both choices and achievement. Although all of these theories have been incorporated into some research with exceptional students, the work is nascent, and most studies involving these populations has been limited in that it has only utilized one motivational perspective at a time. Thus, being mindful of the value of investigating exceptional students' motivation in terms of current and dominant motivational theories, we sought to include students in self-contained special education classes in a recent research project; ordinarily we would have collected data only from students in regular classes. We discuss our efforts and findings in the following section.

IV. MOTIVATION OF EARLY ADOLESCENTS IN SPECIAL EDUCATION CLASSES

The larger research project addressed sixth grade students' perceptions and beliefs about a range of motivation constructs, and associations with measures of engagement. Therefore, in addition to administering surveys to students in regular classes, we created slightly shorter versions of the survey for use with the students in the self-contained special classes. We chose a smaller number of constructs to ask the exceptional students; these included mastery and performance goal orientations, value for school work, and perceptions of teacher support. We also included a measure of positive engagement (effort for school work) and a measure of negative engagement (disruptive classroom behavior).

One objective was to investigate whether the constructs and measures that we had used in other studies with early adolescents in regular classrooms could also be used with students at the same grade level who had been diagnosed with significant learning-related disabilities. That is, given the barriers that we discussed at the beginning of this chapter, could these exceptional students respond to our measures reliably and in a manner that indicated understanding and validity? Our second objective was to examine the descriptive information regarding the exceptional students' reported motivation and engagement and, in the tradition of previous research, to compare the means with those of the non-exceptional students. This allowed us to compare the findings with similar previous research, in part to address validity of the measures. However, we also sought to move beyond addressing mean level differences, to consider associations among motivation and engagement. More specifically, we were interested in investigating whether the motivation measures were associated with engagement in the same way for the exceptional students as they are for the students in regular classes (Pintrich & Schunk, 2002).

We collected data from 50 students (14 girls, 36 boys) in seven self-contained special education classes within three elementary schools. According to school records, all students were classified as learning disabled. In addition to their learning-disabled classification, 16 of those students were identified as behaviorally disordered, 4 also had emotional impairments, and 2 also had physical disabilities.

We could not administer the survey to students as whole classes, as we did with the regular classes. Instead we were faced with many of the challenges we referred to in the opening section of this chapter, including concerns that students understood the questions and also maintained attention throughout the process. Therefore, the students in the special education classrooms were given a shorter version of the survey than the regular students received; some measures were omitted and others were shortened by one or two items. Both groups of students responded to the items on a 5-point scale. Additionally, the students in special education classes took the survey either individually or in small groups of between two and five students, depending on the teachers' recommendations. Perhaps due in part to these efforts, the data we collected from the students in special education classes mostly formed scales with acceptable internal consistency. Thus, we found that despite requiring greater time and more individualized attention to administer the items, early adolescent exceptional students can respond reliably to the same measures of motivation that are used frequently with regular students.

Because we were interested in comparing the responses of the exceptional students with those of students in regular classes, we created a similarly-sized comparison group by randomly selecting 52 students from those who were not receiving special education services. We present here some of our preliminary findings about student motivation and engagement behavior.

We sought to first examine the mean levels of the various measures for students in special education classes and for students in regular classes. These are shown in Table I. We found that students in the two groups did not differ in measures of performance goal orientation, value of school work, perceived teacher support, effort, or disruptive behavior. However, students in special education classes reported being more mastery goal oriented (M = 4.32) than students in regular classes (M = 3.93, $p < 0.05$).

These findings are similar to those from others studies, in that we found few mean level differences in measures of motivation and disruptive behavior between the exceptional and non-exceptional students. It was

TABLE I
MEANS AND GROUP DIFFERENCES FOR MEASURES OF MOTIVATION, TEACHER RELATIONSHIP, AND ENGAGEMENT

	Non-Exceptional Students ($n = 52$)	Exceptional Students ($n = 50$)	t Statistic
Mastery goal orientation	3.93	4.32	2.29*
Performance goal orientation	3.81	3.77	0.13
Value	3.83	3.80	0.20
Teacher support	3.79	3.99	0.96
Effort in academics	4.12	4.17	0.27
Disruptive behavior	2.76	3.02	−1.21

Note: Items scored on a 1–5 scale. *$p < 0.05$.

interesting to note that, in contrast to concern that students receiving special education are less intrinsically motivated, the exceptional students in our sample reported on average a greater mastery orientation than non-exceptional students in regular classes.

We next investigated whether patterns of associations among the measures of motivation, teacher relationship, and disruptiveness differed between the two groups of students. To do this we examined the correlations separately for both groups; these are presented in Table II.

Many of the relations were similar for both groups. Mastery and performance goal orientations were not correlated with each other, consistent with theory and other research (Midgley et al., 1998). Students' mastery goal orientation was correlated positively with value beliefs, perceptions of teacher support, and effort for academics. Thus, students who were focused on doing their work for improving their skills and intrinsic reasons were more likely to report valuing school, positive teacher relationships, and putting effort into their school work. Students' performance goal orientation was not related significantly to any of the other measures.

Value for one's schoolwork was associated positively with teacher support and effort for both groups of students. Thus, good relationships with one's teachers and trying hard in school tend to be associated with a belief that the work in school is both useful and interesting. Teacher support was related positively to effort for both groups of students, indicating that when students perceive that their teacher cares about them they are more likely to try hard in school.

Because we were interested in investigating whether the pattern of correlations among variables differed significantly for the two groups of students, we conducted Fisher's Z-score transformations. There were several

TABLE II
Correlations Among Measures of Motivation, Teacher Relationship, and Engagement

	1	2	3	4	5	6
1. Mastery goal orientation	—	0.20	0.83†	0.50†	0.60†	−0.37†
2. Performance goal orientation	0.26	—	0.07	0.19	0.12	0.07
3. Value	0.55†	0.08	—	0.41†	0.54†	−0.41†
4. Teacher support	0.42†	0.28	0.41†	—	0.15	−0.36*
5. Effort in academics	0.35*	0.29	0.46†	0.33*	—	−0.62†
6. Disruptive behavior	0.03	−0.22	−0.02	0.17	−0.29*	—

Note: Correlations for exceptional students are shown below the diagonal and correlations for non-exceptional education students are shown above the diagonal. $*p < 0.05$; $^{\dagger}p < 0.01$.

significant differences between the two groups. First, whereas the direction of the relationship regarding a mastery goal orientation and value for school work was similar for both groups, the magnitude was significantly different ($Z = 2.87$, $p < 0.01$). Mastery goal orientation and value were associated more strongly for students in regular classes ($r = 0.83$, $p < 0.01$) than for students in special education classes ($r = 0.55$, $p < 0.01$).

There were interesting differences between the two student groups in terms of the pattern of relations regarding disruptive behavior and the motivation, social relationship, and effort measures. Specifically, correlations between disruptive behavior and mastery goal orientation, value for schoolwork, teacher support, and effort were significantly different for students in special education classes and students in regular classes ($Zs = -2.05, -2.69,$ and -2.09, respectively). In general, students in regular classes who reported being disruptive showed a maladaptive profile, whereas those in special education classes did not. Students in regular classes who reported getting into trouble for their conduct tended to be the students with a low mastery goal orientation ($r = -0.37$, $p < 0.01$), low value for school work ($r = -0.41$, $p < 0.01$), and who perceived their teacher as less supportive ($r = -0.36$, $p < 0.05$), compared to less disruptive students. In contrast, disruptive behavior was not associated with a mastery goal orientation ($r = 0.03$, $p > 0.05$), value ($r = -0.02$, $p > 0.05$), or teacher support ($r = 0.17$, $p > 0.05$) for students in special education classes. Thus, students in special education classes who reported getting into trouble for their conduct in class were neither more or less likely to report maladaptive motivational beliefs and teacher relationships than those who did not. The direction of the relation between disruptive behavior and effort for school work was similar for both groups. The correlation, however, was stronger for students in regular ($r = -0.62$, $p < 0.01$), compared to special education ($r = -0.29$, $p < 0.05$; $Z = 2.09$, $p < 0.05$), classes. Thus, all students who reported being disruptive in class were less likely to report high effort, but the association was much stronger for students in regular education classes.

A. Summary

In summary, we found that researchers can reliably measure important motivational constructs with exceptional students in self-contained classes, albeit with some accommodations during survey administration. This is an important finding that may encourage further, and much-needed, research that combines a focus on exceptional students and current approaches to conceptualizing motivation. In examining the descriptive data, we found that the exceptional students in self-contained classes and the non-exceptional students in regular classes reported mostly very similar levels, on average, of motivation and engagement. The only difference was that the exceptional students reported greater mastery orientation. Of greatest interest, however, was the finding that the pattern of correlations among motivation and engagement measures differed significantly for both groups of students. Specifically, being disruptive in class was associated with maladaptive motivational beliefs and perceiving lower levels of teacher support for non-exceptional students. This was not the case, however, for the exceptional students, many of whom were classified as having behavior disorders. For example, their disruptiveness was not accompanied by low value for school work or a low focus on learning and understanding. This finding illustrates the usefulness of going beyond comparing mean levels of motivation for different groups of students, and suggests the necessity of considering the process—how motivation is related to other important outcomes, and what factors may be associated with that process.

The finding that the exceptional students in our study were more mastery-oriented than the non-exceptional students in regular classes is intriguing, particularly given the general concern that exceptional students tend to have low intrinsic motivation. This finding suggests the need to examine the educational context, including instructional practices of special education teachers. The motivation theories that we have presented thus far involve an individual differences perspective. That is, they assume that motivation is 'within the individual.' There is growing evidence, however, that the classroom context contributes powerfully to students' motivation beliefs and engagement behaviors. We review this research in the following section.

V. THE CLASSROOM ENVIRONMENT AND STUDENT MOTIVATION

A focus of motivational research within educational psychology that is currently and especially active involves investigating the role of the educational context with respect to student motivation (e.g., Anderman & Anderman, 2000). An increasing body of research indicates that teachers' practices and how they are perceived by students are related strongly to students' adaptive (or maladaptive) achievement-related perceptions, beliefs, and behaviors (e.g., Patrick et al., 2003; Ryan et al., 1998; Turner et al., 1998, 2002). Furthermore, there is considerable evidence that how students perceive their classroom in terms of the social interactions and relationships afforded is also associated with their adaptive motivation and engagement in school work (e.g., Ryan & Patrick, 2001). To understand students' motivation, therefore, we must attend to different messages that are conveyed in the classroom about schoolwork and social relationships.

A. Classroom Goal Structures

An integral aspect of goal theory is the assumption that students' motivation is influenced not only by their individual personal dispositions and beliefs but by their environment, including classroom practices (Ames, 1992; Maehr & Anderman, 1993). Classroom practices are believed to contribute to creating motivational environments that emphasize different goal orientations. Thus, classroom environments are considered with respect to the purposes and meanings that are communicated to, and perceived by, students for engaging in academic tasks (i.e., the classroom goal structures).

A classroom *mastery goal structure* conveys a perception that students' learning and understanding, in contrast to mere memorization, are valued and that success is accompanied by effort and indicated by personal improvement. Classrooms that are perceived as being mastery-focused are most adaptive. Students' perceptions that their teacher emphasizes a mastery orientation have been related significantly to a personal mastery goal orientation (Midgley et al., 1995). These students also tend to use more effective learning strategies (Ames & Archer, 1988), use more positive coping strategies after experiencing failure (Kaplan & Midgley, 1999), and report more positive affect in school (Anderman, 1999a). Additionally, classrooms that are perceived as being mastery-focused have the lowest rates of maladaptive student behavior, such as not asking for help when it is needed, cheating, and being disruptive (Kaplan et al., 2002; Murdock et al., 2001; Ryan et al., 1998; Turner et al., 2002).

A classroom *performance goal structure* conveys to students that learning is predominantly a means of achieving extrinsic rewards, and that success is indicated by outperforming others or surpassing normative standards (Ames, 1992). Students' perceptions of their classroom as having a performance goal structure have been associated with a personal performance goal orientation (Midgley et al., 1995) and maladaptive beliefs and behaviors. For example, they tend to use maladaptive coping styles after experiencing failure (Kaplan & Midgley, 1999) and report more negative affect at school (Anderman, 1999a). Additionally, classrooms that are perceived as being performance-focused are likely to have the highest rates of avoidance behaviors, such as not asking for help when it is needed, self-handicapping, cheating, and being disruptive (Anderman et al., 1998; Kaplan, Gheen, and Midgley, 2002; Ryan et al., 1998; Urdan et al., 1998). Furthermore, students whose teachers reported using performance-oriented instructional practices, such as emphasizing the highest test scores and identifying students who scored highest, tended to experience decreases in value for reading and mathematics, even after controlling for prior levels of value beliefs (Anderman et al., 2001).

B. Encouragement Of Task-Related Interaction

Students' involvement in interactions about academic tasks, including asking or answering questions, making suggestions, giving explanations, justifying reasoning, and participating in discussions, is related to their learning and achievement (e.g., Cohen, 1994; Webb & Palincsar, 1996). Additionally, however, students' perceptions that they are given opportunities to participate actively during lessons, and are encouraged to interact with classmates in the pursuit of understanding, are likely to be associated with their motivation. For example, interaction opportunities may foster students' feelings of confidence or efficacy, sustain interest, and support a willingness to persevere with the task when experiencing difficulty or frustration. Students' perception that the teacher encourages them to be actively involved in lessons and participate in discussions is related to their liking and interest of school and specific subject areas (Fraser & Fisher, 1982; Trickett & Moos, 1974).

C. Encouragement Of Mutual Respect

A focus on mutual respect among students involves a perception that the teacher expects all students to value one another and the contributions they make to classroom life, and will not allow students to make fun of others. Classroom environments that are perceived as respectful are likely to be ones in which students can focus on understanding tasks, without having their attention diverted by concern about what others might think or say if they are incorrect or experience difficulty. Respectful environments are also most conducive to student problem-solving, cognitive risk-taking, and conceptual understanding (Cohen, 1994; De Lisi & Golbeck, 1999). Consistent with these expectations, a perception that the teacher promotes respect in the classroom is related positively to increased academic efficacy and more self-regulated learning relative to the previous year (Ryan & Patrick, 2001). Additionally, classrooms perceived by students as most respectful have lowest rates of avoidance behaviors, compared to classrooms perceived as less respectful (Patrick et al., 2003).

D. Role Of Classroom Environment For Exceptional Students' Motivation

As a logical expansion of the research we have presented about classroom environments, it would appear to be valuable for researchers to also consider teachers' instructional practices within, and the motivational and social environments of, classrooms in which exceptional students participate. There is clearly a need to extend the research on the role of the classroom environment for student motivation and engagement to include self-contained special education classes and classrooms that have students with special needs.

Greater consideration of the classroom environment may help researchers to interpret some of the apparent contradictory findings in the special education field. That is, inconsistencies among different studies regarding exceptional students' motivation may reflect to some extent differences in their educational environments, rather than inherent differences 'about the student' that lead them to be, for example, less intrinsically motivated than non-exceptional students. For example, research involving exceptional students has indicated that many of their achievement-related beliefs and behaviors may be attributable to prior experiences, such as the type of feedback they have received from teachers or parents (Olkinuora & Salonen, 1992; Vauras et al., 1992).

In an article published in a learning disabilities journal, Adelman and Taylor (1990), suggested that students' disruptive behavior in class may be related to them experiencing low levels of intrinsic motivation. They suggested that if teachers engaged in practices that promoted students' intrinsic motivation they would experience less misbehavior from those students. Interestingly, as we reported in the previous section, research on classroom goal structures has found a very similar association in a number of studies involving non-exceptional students. That is, students tend to report engaging in less disruptiveness in classrooms they perceive as having a high, compared to low, mastery goal structure (Kaplan et al., 2002; Patrick et al., 2003).

VI. DIRECTIONS FOR FUTURE RESEARCH

It appears that most of the research that has been conducted thus far about the motivation of exceptional students has been largely descriptive and comparative. That is, the research seems to have focused on mean levels of motivational constructs for different groups of exceptionalities, and on comparing them with one another and with non-exceptional students. This research can answer questions regarding in what ways students with different types of disabilities are on average similar to, and different from, other types of students. While informative, it appears time to ask the next level of questions. We need to consider processes that relate motivational beliefs to learning. For example, are the motivational beliefs of exceptional students associated with learning-related behaviors, and with achievement, in the same way as they are for non-exceptional students? What do differences and non-differences in average motivation among groups mean? Is it adaptive for exceptional students to express the same kinds and levels of beliefs as their non-exceptional peers? Should educators be directing their efforts to increasing or decreasing these perceptions or beliefs, to bring them in line with those expressed by regular students? These latter questions are probably best suited to cross-disciplinary research, involving active collaborations of both special education and motivation researchers.

Furthermore, as mentioned in the previous section, research that considers factors associated with classroom motivational environments is sorely needed. Conducting research within theories of motivation that consider both individual differences and educational environments affords a valuable opportunity for greater integration between the fields of special education and educational psychology. Such a focus necessarily integrates the two fields because it focuses on the similarities in motivational needs shared by exceptional and non-exceptional students, while also identifying specific approaches that are beneficial to students with special needs. It directs attention to a concern that *all* students engage in adaptive patterns of motivation, engagement, and achievement when they are in classrooms with optimal motivational environments. In all likelihood, features of classroom environments that are optimally motivating will be similar for students with and without special needs. This is consistent with the critique of research regarding learning disabilities made some while ago by Deci and

Chandler (1986). They suggested that researchers of students with learning disabilities utilize macro-perspectives that identify "general principles of learning and [apply] those same principles to learning-disabled children as well as to all other children" (Deci & Chandler, 1986, p. 588). Furthermore, they argued that the most appropriate macro-approach involves student motivation.

A rare but excellent example of research that integrates both special education and motivation, and individual difference and classroom context perspectives, is a program of research addressing coping strategies and motivation conducted by Vauras and her colleagues (1992). They found that the kinds of feedback that teachers gave to students with learning disabilities was associated with them becoming either more dependent on reassurance from the teacher or more avoidant. They then developed an intervention whereby learning-disabled students received training in adaptive cognitive strategies and coping strategies, with the objective that they would become more mastery-focused and less avoidant or reassurance seeking. Although this training resulted in short-term improvements in the use of cognitive strategies and coping responses to schoolwork, the long-term gains were modest and there was no transfer. The researchers then turned attention to the classroom environment. They developed an experimental intervention that focused on teachers' instructional practices and the psychological environment of the classroom. This involved working with teachers over a four-month period to identify practices and plan and implement lessons that would help to create the most adaptive classroom motivational environments. Students exhibited more adaptive coping and learning strategies in the intervention classrooms, but only when they also received the individual training program. Additionally, the gains they made both persisted over time and transferred to new situations. These results illustrate the necessity of considering both individual and classroom level factors.

Incorporating attention to classroom environments may also involve asking new questions. Rather than focusing on differences between students with and without identified special educational needs, researchers could investigate how well *all* students' needs are met. For example, are students in classrooms with adaptive motivational environments? What is the nature of their relationship with the teacher? What practices lead to the most adaptive levels and types of engagement in school work for all students? There is evidence that many students have educational needs that are not being met well in their regular classes but do not receive special education, perhaps because they do not easily fit diagnostic categories. For example, Anderman and Young (1994) found that the group of students who had the least adaptive motivational profile were students with achievement difficulties who were not receiving assistance; they appeared significantly worse than students with identified disabilities, who did not differ from average achieving students. After comparing students with identified learning disabilities, low achieving students, and students with average achievement, Grolnick and Ryan (1990, p. 183) concluded that "many of the motivational and self-evaluative problems that children with learning disabilities have may be ... apparent in other children who have difficulties in learning." And although Chapman (1988) found that students with learning disabilities maintained a negative motivational and affective profile over the two years they were followed, those students were not receiving any special education services. A focus on classroom motivational environments that integrates both special education and educational psychology would arguably assist all students—those with and without identified disabilities.

REFERENCES

AAMR Ad Hoc Committee on Terminology and Classification (1992). *Mental retardation: Definition, classification, and systems of support* (9th ed.). Washington, DC: American Association on Mental Retardation.

Adelman, H. S., & Chaney, L. E. (1982). Impact of motivation on task performance of children with and without psychoeducational problems. *Journal of Learning Disabilities, 15*, 242–244.

Adelman, H. S., & Taylor, L. (1990). Intrinsic motivation and school misbehavior: Some intervention implications. *Journal of Learning Disabilities, 23*, 541–550.

Ames, C. (1992). Classrooms: Goals, structures, and student motivation. *Journal of Educational Psychology, 84*, 261–271.

Ames, C., & Archer, J. (1988). Achievement goals in the classroom, students' learning strategies, and motivation processes. *Journal of Educational Psychology, 80*, 260–267.

Anderman, E. M., Austin, C. C., & Johnson, D. M. (2002). The development of goal orientation. In A. Wigfield & J. S. Eccles (Eds.), *Development of achievement motivation. A volume in the educational psychology series* (pp. 197–220). San Diego, CA: Academic Press.

Anderman, E. M., Eccles, J. S., Yoon, K. S., Roeser, R., Wigfield, A., & Blumenfeld, P. (2001). Learning to value mathematics and reading: Relations to mastery and performance-oriented instructional practices. *Contemporary Educational Psychology, 26*, 76–95.

Anderman, E. M., Griesinger, T., & Westerfield, G. (1998). Motivation and cheating during early adolescence. *Journal of Educational Psychology, 90*, 84–93.

Anderman, E. M., & Young, A. J. (1994). Motivation and strategy use in science: Individual differences and classroom effects. *Journal of Research in Science Teaching, 31*, 811–831.

Anderman, L. (1999a). Classroom goal orientation, school belonging, and social goals as predictors of students' positive and negative affect following the transition to middle school. *Journal of Research and Development in Education, 32*, 89–103.

Anderman, L. (1999b). Expanding the discussion of social perceptions and academic outcomes: Mechanisms and contextual influences. In T. C. Urdan (Ed.), *Advances in motivation and achievement* (Vol. 11, pp. 303–336). Stamford, Connecticut: JAI Press.

Anderman, L. H., & Anderman, E. M. (1999). Social predictors of changes in students' achievement goal orientations. *Contemporary Educational Psychology, 25*, 21–37.

Anderman, L. H., & Anderman, E. M. (2000). Considering contexts in educational psychology: Introduction to the special issue. *Educational Psychologist, 35*, 67–68.

Bandura, A. (1993). Perceived self-efficacy in cognitive development and functioning. *Educational Psychologist, 28*, 117–148.

Beane, J. A., & Lipka, R. P. (1980). Self-concept and self-esteem: A construct differentiation. *Child Study Journal, 10*, 1–6.

Bear, G. G., Minke, K. M., & Manning, M. A. (2002). Self-concept of students with learning disabilities: A meta-analysis. *School Psychology Review, 31*, 405–427.

Bong, M. (2001). Between- and within-domain relations of academic motivation among middle and high school students: Self-efficacy, task value, and achievement goals. *Journal of Educational Psychology, 93*, 23–34.

Bong, M., & Clark, R. E. (1999). Comparison between self-concept and self-efficacy in academic motivation research. *Educational Psychologist, 34*, 139–153.

Cauce, A. M., Felner, R. D., & Primavera, J. (1982). Social support in high-risk adolescents: Structural components and adaptive impact. *American Journal of Community Psychology, 10*, 417–428.

Chapman, J. W. (1988). Cognitive-motivational characteristics and academic achievement of learning disabled children: A longitudinal study. *Journal of Educational Psychology, 80*, 357–365.

Chen, Y. (1990). Effects of token economy program on decreasing maladaptive behaviors of the moderately and severely retarded children. *Bulletin of Educational Psychology, 23*, 13–48.

Cohen, E. (1994). Restructuring the classroom: Conditions for productive small groups. *Review of Educational Research, 64*, 1–35.

Comaty, J. E., Stasio, M., & Advokat, C. (2001). Analysis of outcome variables of a token economy system in a state psychiatric hospital: A program evaluation. *Research in Developmental Disabilities, 22*, 233–253.

Deci, E. L., & Chandler, C. L. (1986). The importance of motivation for the future of the LD field. *Journal of Learning Disabilities, 19*, 587–594.

Deci, E. L., Koestner, R., & Ryan, R. M. (1999). A meta-analytic review of experiments examining the effects of extrinsic rewards on intrinsic motivation. *Psychological Bulletin, 125*, 627–668.

Deci, E. L., Koestner, R., & Ryan, R. M. (2001). Extrinsic rewards and intrinsic motivation in education: Reconsidered once again. *Review of Educational Research, 71*, 1–27.

Deci, E. L., & Ryan, R. M. (1985). *Intrinsic motivation and self-determination in human behavior.* New York: Plenum Press.

De Lisi, R., & Golbeck, S. L. (1999). Implications of Piagetian theory for peer learning. In A. M. O'Donnell & A. King (Eds.), *Cognitive perspectives on peer learning* (pp. 3–37). Mahwah, NJ: Erlbaum.

Dev, P. C. (1998). Intrinsic motivation and the student with learning disabilities. *Journal of Research and Development in Education, 31*, 98–108.

Eccles, J. (1983). Expectancies, values and academic behaviors. In J. T. Spence (Ed.), *Achievement and achievement motives* (pp. 75–146). San Francisco: Freeman.

Eccles, J. S., & Wigfield, A. (2002). Motivational beliefs, values, and goals. *Annual Review of Psychology, 53*, 109–132.

Elliot, A., & Harackiewicz, J. M. (1996). Approach and avoidance achievement goals and intrinsic motivation: A mediational analysis. *Journal of Personality and Social Psychology, 70*, 968–980.

Elliot, A. J., McGregor, H. A., & Gable, S. (1999). Achievement goals, study strategies, and exam performance: A mediational analysis. *Journal of Educational Psychology, 91*, 549–563.

Felner, R. D., Aber, M. S., Primavera, J., & Cauce, A. M. (1985). Adaptation and vulnerability in high-risk adolescents: An examination of environmental mediators. *American Journal of Community Psychology, 13,* 365–379.

Fraser, B. J., & Fisher, D. L. (1982). Predicting student outcomes from their perceptions of classroom psychosocial environment. *American Educational Research Journal, 19,* 498–518.

Frederickson, N., & Jacobs, S. (2001). Controllability attributions for academic performance and the perceived scholastic competence, global self-worth and achievement of children with dyslexia. *School Psychology International, 22,* 401–416.

Fulk, B. M., Brigham, F. J., & Lohman, D. A. (1998). Motivation and self-regulation: A comparison of students with learning and behavior problems. *Remedial and Special Education, 19,* 300–309.

Goh, S. C., Young, D. J., & Fraser, B. J. (1995). Psychosocial climate and student outcomes in elementary mathematics classrooms: A multilevel analysis. *Journal of Experimental Education, 64,* 29–40.

Goodenow, C. (1993). Classroom belonging among early adolescent students: Relationships to motivation and achievement. *Journal of Early Adolescence, 13,* 21–43.

Gottfried, A. E. (1985). Academic intrinsic motivation in elementary and junior high school students. *Journal of Educational Psychology, 82,* 525–538.

Gottfried, A. E. (1990). Academic intrinsic motivation in young elementary school children. *Journal of Educational Psychology, 77,* 631–645.

Gresham, F. M., & MacMillan, D. L. (1997). Social competence and affective characteristics of students with mild disabilities. *Review of Educational Research, 67,* 377–415.

Grolnick, W. S., & Ryan, R. M. (1990). Self-perceptions, motivation, and adjustment in children with learning disabilities: A multiple group comparison study. *Journal of Learning Disabilities, 23,* 177–184.

Haager, D., & Vaughn, S. (1995). Parent, teacher, peers, and self-reports of the social competence of students with learning disabilities. *Journal of Learning Disabilities, 28* 131., 105–125.

Haertel, G. D., Walberg, H. J., & Haertel, E. H. (1981). Socio-psychological environments and learning: A quantitative synthesis. *British Educational Research Journal, 7,* 27–36.

Hallahan, D. P., & Kauffman, J. M. (1997). *Exceptional learners: Introduction to special education* (7th ed.). Boston, MA: Allyn & Bacon.

Hallahan, D. P., Kauffman, J. M., & Lloyd, J. W. (1996). *Introduction to learning disabilities.* Boston, MA: Allyn & Bacon.

Harackiewicz, J. M., Barron, K. E., Tauer, J. M., & Elliot, A. J. (2002). Predicting success in college: A longitudinal study of achievement goals and ability measures as predictors of interest and performance from freshman year through graduation. *Journal of Educational Psychology, 94,* 562–575.

Harter, S. (1981). A new self-report scale of intrinsic versus extrinsic orientation in the classroom: Motivational and informational components. *Developmental Psychology, 17,* 300–312.

Harter, S., & Pike, R. (1984). The pictorial scale of perceived competence and social acceptance for young children. *Child Development, 55,* 1969–1982.

Hartup, W. W. (1989). Social relationships and their developmental significance. *American Psychologist, 44,* 120–126.

Juvonen, J., & Wentzel, K. R. (1996). *Social motivation: Understanding children's school adjustment.* Cambridge, U.K.: Cambridge University Press.

Kaplan, A., Gheen, M., & Midgley, C. (2002). The classroom goal structure and student disruptive behavior. *British Journal of Educational Psychology, 72,* 191–211.

Kaplan, A., & Midgley, C. (1999). The relationship between perceptions of the classroom goal structure and early adolescents' affect in school: The mediating role of coping strategies. *Learning and Individual Differences, 11*, 187–212.

Krapp, A., Hidi, S., & Renninger, K. A. (1992). Interest, learning, and development. In K. A. Renninger, S. Hidi, & A. Krapp (Eds.), *The role of interest in learning and development* (pp. 3–25). Hillsdale, NJ: Erlbaum.

La Greca, A. M. (1987). Children with learning disabilities: Interpersonal skills and social competence. *Journal of Reading, Writing, and Learning Disabilities International, 3*, 167–185.

Lepper, M. R., Greene, D., & Nisbett, R. E. (1973). Undermining children's intrinsic interest with extrinsic rewards: A test of the "overjustification" hypothesis. *Journal of Personality and Social Psychology, 28*, 129–137.

Maehr, M. L., & Anderman, E. M. (1993). Reinventing schools for early adolescents: Emphasizing task goals. *Elementary School Journal, 93*, 593–610.

Middleton, M., & Midgley, C. (1997). Avoiding the demonstration of lack of ability: An underexplored aspect of goal theory. *Journal of Educational Psychology, 89*, 710–718.

Midgley, C., Anderman, E., & Hicks, L. (1995). Differences between elementary and middle school teachers and students: A goal theory approach. *Journal of Early Adolescence, 15*, 90–113.

Midgley, C., Feldlaufer, H., & Eccles, J. S. (1989). Student/teacher relations and attitudes toward mathematics before and after the transition to junior high school. *Child Development, 60*, 981–992.

Midgley, C., Kaplan, A., Middleton, M., Maehr, M. L., Urdan, T., Anderman, L. H., Anderman, E., & Roeser, R. (1998). The development and validation of scales assessing students' achievement goal orientations. *Contemporary Educational Psychology, 23*, 113–131.

Midgley, C., & Urdan, T. (1995). Predictors of middle school students' use of self-handicapping strategies. *Journal of Early Adolescence, 15*, 389–441.

Moore, S. R., & Simpson, R. L. (1983). Teacher-pupil and peer verbal interactions of learning disabled, behavior-disordered, and nonhandicapped students. *Learning Disability Quarterly, 6*, 273–282.

Moos, R. H., & Moos, B. S. (1978). Classroom social climate and student absences and grades. *Journal of Educational Psychology, 70*, 263–269.

Murdock, T. B., Hale, N. M., & Weber, M. J. (2001). Predictors of cheating among early adolescents: Academic and social motivations. *Contemporary Educational Psychology, 26*, 96–115.

Murphy, P. K., & Alexander, P. A. (2000). A motivated exploration of motivation terminology. *Contemporary Educational Psychology, 25*, 3–53.

Newman, R. S., & Schwager, M. T. (1993). Student perceptions of the teacher and classmates in relation to reported help seeking in math class. *Elementary School Journal, 94*, 3–17.

Olkinuora, E., & Salonen, P. (1992). Adaptation, motivational orientation, and cognition in a subnormally performing child: A systemic perspective for training. In B. Y. L. Wong (Ed.), *Contemporary intervention research in learning disabilities: An international perspective* (pp. 190–213). New York: Springer-Verlag.

Pajares, F., Britner, S. L., & Valiante, G. (2000). Relation between achievement goals and self-beliefs of middle school students in writing and science. *Contemporary Educational Psychology, 25*, 406–422.

Parker, I., Gottlieb, J., Davis, S., & Kunzweiller, C. (1989). Teacher behavior toward low achievers, average achievers, and mainstreamed minority group learning disabled students. *Learning Disabilities Research, 4*, 101–106.

Patrick, H., Anderman, L. H., & Ryan, A. M. (2002). Social motivation and the classroom social environment. In C. Midgley (Ed.), *Goals, goal structures, and patterns of adaptive learning* (pp. 85–108). Mahwah, NJ: Lawrence Erlbaum.

Patrick, H., Hicks, L., & Ryan, A. M. (1997). Relations of perceived social efficacy and social goal pursuit to self-efficacy for academic work. *Journal of Early Adolescence, 17,* 109–128.

Patrick, H., Turner, J. C., Meyer, D. K., & Midgley, C. (2003). How teachers establish psychological environments during the first days of school: Associations with avoidance in mathematics. *Teachers College Record, 105,* 1521–1558.

Pintrich, P. R. (2000a). The role of goal orientation in self-regulated learning. In M. Boekaerts, P. Pintrich, & M. Zeidner (Eds.), *Handbook of self-regulation* (pp. 451–502). San Diego: Academic Press.

Pintrich, P. R. (2000b). Multiple goals, multiple pathways: The role of goal orientation in learning and achievement. *Journal of Educational Psychology, 92,* 544–555.

Pintrich, P. R., Anderman, E. M., & Klobucar, C. (1994). Intraindividual differences in motivation and cognition in students with and without learning disabilities. *Journal of Learning Disabilities, 27,* 360–370.

Pintrich, P. R., & De Groot, E. V. (1990). Motivational and self-regulated learning components of classroom academic performance. *Journal of Educational Psychology, 82,* 33–40.

Pintrich, P. R., & Schunk, D. H. (2002). *Motivation in education: Theory, research, and applications* (2nd ed.). Englewood Cliffs, NJ: Merrill Prentice-Hall.

Reeve, P. T., & Loper, A. B. (1983). Intrinsic vs. extrinsic motivation in learning disabled children. *Perceptual and Motor Skills, 57,* 59–63.

Reid, R., Maag, J. W., Vasa, S. F., & Wright, C. (1994). Who are the children with attention-deficit-hyperactivity disorder? A school-based study *The Journal of Special Education, 28,* 117–137.

Robinson, N. M., Zigler, E., & Gallagher, J. J. (2000). Two ends of the normal curve: Similarities and differences in the study of mental retardation and giftedness. *American Psychologist, 55,* 1413–1424.

Ryan, A. M., Gheen, M., & Midgley, C. (1998). Why do some students avoid asking for help? An examination of the interplay among students' academic efficacy, teacher's social-emotional role and classroom goal structure *Journal of Educational Psychology, 90,* 528–535.

Ryan, A. M., Hicks, L., & Midgley, C. (1997). Social goals, academic goals, and avoiding seeking help in the classroom. *Journal of Early Adolescence, 17,* 152–171.

Ryan, A. M., Hopkins, N. B., & Kiefer, S. M (2004). Young adolescents' social motivation: An achievement goal theory perspective. In P. R. Pintrich & M. L. Maehr (Eds.), *Advances in motivation. Volume 13. Motivating students, improving schools: The legacy of Carol Midgley* (pp. 301–330). Amsterdam, The Netherlands: JAI Press.

Ryan, A. M., & Patrick, H. (2001). The classroom social environment and changes in adolescents' motivation and engagement during middle school. *American Educational Research Journal, 38,* 437–460.

Ryan, A. M., & Pintrich, P. R. (1997). "Should I ask for help?": The role of motivation and attitudes in adolescents' help-seeking in math class *Journal of Educational Psychology, 89,* 329–341.

Ryan, R. M., & Deci, E. L. (2000). Intrinsic and extrinsic motivations: Classic definitions and new directions. *Contemporary Educational Psychology, 25,* 54–67.

Sale, P., & Carey, D. M. (1995). The sociometric status of students with disabilities in a full-inclusion school. *Exceptional Children, 62,* 6–19.

Salend, S., & Henry, K. (1981). Response cost in mainstreamed settings. *Journal of School Psychology, 19*, 242–249.

Salend, S. J., & Lamb, E. A. (1986). Effectiveness of a group-managed interdependent contingency system. *Learning Disability Quarterly, 9*, 268–273.

Schiefele, U., Krapp, A., & Winteler, A. (1992). Interest as a predictor of academic achievement: A meta-analysis of research. In K. A. Renninger, S. Hidi, & A. Krapp (Eds.), *The role of interest in learning and development* (pp. 183–212). Hillsdale, NJ: Erlbaum.

Schmidt, M. (2000). Social integration of students with learning disabilities. *Developmental Disabilities Bulletin, 28*, 19–26.

Schultz, G. F., & Switzky, H. N. (1993). The academic achievement of elementary and junior high school students with behavior disorders and their nonhandicapped peers as a function of motivational orientation. *Learning and Individual Differences, 5*, 31–42.

Silon, E. L., & Harter, S. (1985). Assessment of perceived competence, motivational orientation, and anxiety in segregated and mainstreamed educable mentally retarded children. *Journal of Educational Psychology, 77*, 217–230.

Sisson, L. A., & Dixon, M. J. (1986). Improving mealtime behaviors through token reinforcement: A study with mentally retarded behaviorally disordered children. *Behavior Modification, 10*, 333–354.

Skaalvik, E. M. (1997). Self-enhancing and self-defeating ego orientation: Relations with task and avoidance orientation, achievement, self-perceptions, and anxiety. *Journal of Educational Psychology, 89*, 71–81.

Smith, M. C., Plant, M., Carney, R. N., Arnold, C. S., Jackson, A., Johnson, L. S., Lange, H., Mathis, F. S., & Smith, T. J. (2003). Productivity of educational psychologists in educational psychology journals, 1997–2002. *Contemporary Educational Psychology, 28*, 422–430.

Switzky, H. N. (1999). Intrinsic motivation and motivational self-system processes in persons with mental retardation: A theory of motivational orientation. In E. Zigler & D. Bennett-Gates (Eds.), *Personality development in individuals with mental retardation* (pp. 70–106). New York: Cambridge University Press.

Switzky, H. N. (2001). *Personality and motivational differences in persons with mental retardation.* Mahwah, NJ: Lawrence Erlbaum.

Trickett, E. J., & Moos, R. H. (1973). Social environment of junior high and high school classrooms. *Journal of Educational Psychology, 65*, 93–102.

Trickett, E. J., & Moos, R. H. (1974). Personal correlates of contrasting environments: Student satisfactions in high school classrooms. *American Journal of Community Psychology, 2*, 1–12.

Turner, J. C., Meyer, D. K., Cox, K. E., Logan, C., DiCintio, M., & Thomas, C. T. (1998). Creating contexts for involvement in mathematics. *Journal of Educational Psychology, 90*, 730–745.

Turner, J. C., Midgley, C., Meyer, D. K., Gheen, M., Anderman, E., Kang, Y., & Patrick, H. (2002). The classroom environment and students' reports of avoidance behaviors in mathematics: A multi-method study. *Journal of Educational Psychology, 94*, 88–106.

Urdan, T. C. (1997). Achievement and goal theory: Past results, future directions. In M. L. Maehr & P. R. Pintrich (Eds.), *Advances in motivation and achievement* (Vol. 10, pp. 99–142). Greenwich: JAI Press.

Urdan, T. C., Midgley, C., & Anderman, E. M. (1998). The role of classroom goal structure in students' use of self-handicapping strategies. *American Educational Research Journal, 35*, 101–122.

Urdan, T. C., Ryan, A. M., Anderman, E. M., & Gheen, M. (2002). Goals, goal structures, and avoidance behaviors. In C. Midgley (Ed.), *Goals, goal structures, and patterns of adaptive learning* (pp. 55–83). Mahwah, NJ: Lawrence Erlbaum.

Vaughn, S., Elbaum, B., & Boardman, A. G. (2001). The social functioning of students with learning disabilities: Implications for inclusion. *Exceptionality, 9,* 47–65.

Vauras, M., Lehtinen, E., Kinnunen, R., & Salonen, P. (1992). Socioemotional coping and cognitive processes in training learning-disabled children. In B. Y. L. Wong (Ed.), *Contemporary intervention research in learning disabilities: An international perspective* (pp. 190–213). New York: Springer-Verlag.

Webb, N. M., & Palincsar, A. S. (1996). Group processes in the classroom. In D. C. Berliner & R. C. Calfee (Eds.), *Handbook of educational psychology* (pp. 841–873). New York: Simon & Schuster.

Wentzel, K. R. (1989). Adolescent classroom goals, standards for performance, and academic achievement: An interactionist perspective. *Journal of Educational Psychology, 81,* 131–142.

Wentzel, K. R. (1994). Relations of social goal pursuit to social acceptance, classroom behavior, and perceived social support. *Journal of Educational Psychology, 86,* 173–182.

Wigfield, A. (1994). Expectancy-value theory of achievement motivation: A developmental perspective. *Educational Psychology Review, 6,* 49–78.

Wigfield, A., & Eccles, J. (1992). The development of achievement task values: A theoretical analysis. *Developmental Review, 12,* 265–310.

Wilson, D. R., & David, W. J. (1994). Academic intrinsic motivation and attitudes toward school and learning of learning disabled students. *Learning Disabilities Research and Practice, 9,* 148–156.

Wolters, C. A., Yu, S. L., & Pintrich, P. R. (1996). The relation between goal orientation and students' motivational beliefs and self-regulated learning. *Learning & Individual Differences, 8,* 211–238.

York, J., Vandercook, T., MacDonald, C., Heise-Neff, C., & Caughey, E. (1992). Feedback about integrating middle-school students with severe disabilities in general education classes. *Exceptional Children, 58,* 244–258.

Zimmerman, B. J. (2000). Self efficacy: An essential motive to learn. *Contemporary Educational Psychology, 25,* 82–91.

Loneliness and Developmental Disabilities: Cognitive and Affective Processing Perspectives

MALKA MARGALIT

TEL-AVIV UNIVERSITY

Research findings have documented the social isolation and exclusion among children and adolescents with developmental disabilities (Kramer et al., 1987), and accentuated the importance of social competence for understanding mental retardation and to assist individuals in their efforts to become contributing members in their communities (Siperstein, 1992). This body of research has reported the social difficulties of children with developmental disabilities as measured using sociometric ratings and through assessments from teachers (Gresham, 1986) and parents (Amidzic et al., 2001). Even from an early age, children with developmental disabilities have been often ignored or rejected by their peers and are less often chosen as teammates (Guralnick, 1990; Luftig, 1988). Developing the skills for successful interactions with peers and significant adults (teachers, parents) can be considered one of the most important accomplishments of childhood (Gresham, 1986). The interpersonal, social process begins soon after birth and is influenced by within-individual variables, such as physical abilities and cognitive impairments, and external variables, such as peer and family member involvement and interactions (Elliott & Gresham, 1989).

These contextual conditions and other variables may change during the developmental path of the individual. However, their gradual contribution to the development of the subjective experience of loneliness and social isolation has a consistent impact on the quality of life of individuals with developmental disabilities and their future adjustment opportunities (Siperstein, 1992).

The goals of this chapter are to examine in depth the subjective experience of loneliness reported by children and adolescents with developmental disabilities as reflecting their personal distress and interpersonal difficulties, and to identify factors that predict the positive experience of social connectedness. This chapter will present the theoretical construct of loneliness development within a cognitive-affective model, detailing the meaning of loneliness for children and adolescents with developmental disabilities. The second part of the chapter will be devoted to the description of the *sense of coherence model* and its implications for empowering intervention programs for students with developmental disabilities.

I. DEFINITIONS

Developmental theorists have conceptualized social competence as an organizational construct (Bierman & Welsh, 2000). Loneliness may emerge from different sources: it is commonly accepted that loneliness may represent the unsatisfied need for intimate relationships with good friends and/or unfulfilled expectations for belonging to a desired social group (Weiss, 1973). This model recognizes the contributions that the child's characteristics, interactional partners, and contextual variables play in determining the development, organization, and maintenance of interpersonal relations. Social competence involves the child's ability to generate and coordinate flexible adaptive responses to various interpersonal demands and opportunities (Margalit & Efrati, 2003).

The loneliness experience may be considered a global indicator of dissatisfaction with the quality and/or the quantity of the individual's social inter-relations (Asher et al., 1990). Personal and interpersonal components may contribute to feelings of loneliness (Margalit, 1994). Peplau and Perlman (1982) defined loneliness as the unpleasant experience when individuals perceive a discrepancy between the desired and accomplished patterns of their social networks. This classic definition relates the emotion—unpleasant or negative affect—to the global subjective appraisal of the social situation versus personal expectations.

It should be remembered that loneliness is not a rare human experience. Most children experience loneliness and express their social distress occasionally. Individual differences in loneliness descriptions may range from short-lived feelings of alienation to a chronic and deeply negative experience of being isolated. Research and interventions focus attention towards those children who experience chronic loneliness. Extreme loneliness may include a maladaptive attributional style, in which the child considers being alone as an indicator of personal identity of incompetence and failure (Biovin & Hymel, 1997; Ladd & Burgess, 1999).

Research has shown that children understand the meaning of loneliness. Interviews of preschool children indicated that they knew what the term "loneliness" meant, and could define their experiences as representing two different components of the construct: affective reaction—a negative mood ("feeling sad"), and physical position—solitude ("staying alone") (Asher et al., 1990). Williams and Asher (1992) also showed that the students with developmental disabilities disclosed and shared their comprehension of the concept of loneliness, and used it appropriately for expressing their social distress.

II. THE CONTRIBUTION OF GENETIC AND FAMILY FACTORS

In line with the growing realization of the continuous developmental interplay between genetic and environmental influences, and their dynamic transactions in different contexts, research shows that the same phenotype (expressed and observed behavior) can have multiple underlying genotypes (sources of biological influences) (Berninger, 2001). This approach is beginning to make a significant impact on the conceptualization of development and psychopathology, including the development of loneliness (Emde & Spicer, 2000). McGuire and Clifford (2000) explored the genetic sources of loneliness. Their study was based on data from 275 pairs of siblings (biologically related full-sibling pairs [including dizygotic and monozygotic twins] and biologically unrelated pairs in adoptive families).

A significant genetic contribution predicted individual differences in two measures of loneliness: children's general feelings of loneliness and loneliness in the school. Accumulative genetic contributions together with specific environmental influences appeared to play important roles in the understanding of loneliness

Following this pioneering study of heritable factors in loneliness, three areas of further inquiry should be explored:

1. The heritable aspects in either or both directions of the loneliness experience (the lack of positive connections and/or the negative aspects), alienation, and social isolation;
2. The range of the affective heritable experience—is it across the entire continuum of possible feelings or just at the extreme levels (comparisons between changing moods or chronic feelings of alienation)?
3. The relationship between loneliness and temperament variables—is loneliness related to different heritable temperament variables, or can it be viewed as a unique negative affect (McGuire & Clifford, 2000)?

The examination of environmental contributions to the loneliness experience in the McGuire and Clifford (2000) study revealed that the individuals' genetic characteristics were interacting with the ecological conditions, and the outcomes of these interactions were depicted in differential loneliness expressions for several siblings in the same family. These findings support earlier ecological research that found links between parents' differential treatment of siblings and children's behavioral and emotional adjustment (Dunn et al., 1990; McHale et al., 1995). Reiss and Neiderhiser (2000) related the impact of the genetic sources with family processes, pointing to the central role of the family social processes in mediating genetic influences. The family process may be regarded as a final step in the ongoing transcription of genetic influence into complex behavior and development. Family interactions provide children with their first model of interpersonal relations (Andersson et al., 1987). Thus, the social environment may play both a necessary and specific role in the expression of discrete genetic influences on a wide range of behaviors. Multiple and complex processes have been proposed to account for the interpersonal influences in parent-child relationships, and the sources of influence are not limited solely to parental or child factors but to the ongoing transactions between them (Cook, 2001).

The roots of the loneliness were attributed to the conceptualization of attachment. The study on attachment deals with the early interactive processes in families, reflecting the quality of the emotional ties within the mother and child unit of relations (Josselson, 1992). Studying loneliness as the outcomes of unsatisfactory attachment relations requires consideration of interacting factors over time, and their examination through multiple levels (Wood et al., 2000). This developmental construct is characterized by the dynamic transformation of normative features and individual differences, operating at the different levels of behavioral, emotional, and representational organization (Sroufe & Sampson, 2000).

The presence of a disability within the family dynamically modifies interactions, changing the way the family system operates (Ferguson, 2002). Child-adult interactions are an important determinant in children's development, and the presence of an infant with a developmental delay in the family may be expected to introduce changes not only to family dynamics but also to interactional patterns and attachment style (Fraser, 1986). These changes in parent-infant interactions may stem from the infant's unique needs as a result of the disabilities, and from the parents' emotional and behavioral reactions to the realization of having an infant with special needs. To understand these changes, a transactional-ecological model with ongoing bidirectional influences has to be considered (Maccoby, 1990), wherein children's basic characteristics modify parental behavior and systemic relations within the family, as much as parents influence their children. Within this transactional model, accepting the family as a system which each member affects and is affected by others, research has examined areas that promote or act upon children's social inter-relations and connectedness.

Mothers approach their newborn babies with two types of concerns:

1. the infants' characteristics, needs, and abilities; and
2. their own competencies and priorities to fulfill the maternal roles.

These concerns are reinforced by signals from their babies, indicating to mothers their importance to their infants. If mothers' perceptions of the infant's needs are limited due to the slow development of the children, and if the children's increased needs for attention are not met by the mothers, due to caretaking distress, the child may receive a limited range of shared parent-child activities.

The recognition of the bidirectional nature of the influence, with mothers of temperamentally difficult preschool children reporting more psychosocial difficulties led to understanding that mothers were more prone to anxiety related to their competence as parents. These mothers reported that they felt less emotionally close to their children, and that their parenting role restricted their lives in many ways. In a recent study, Al-Yagon (2003) explored risk factors in predicting adaptive and maladaptive functioning among preschool children with different temperaments. Children with developmental delays and their peers were students in inclusive kindergartens (age range 5 to 6.5 years) in Israel. Risk factors comprised of three groups of measures: (1) child characteristics, (2) maternal and familial ecological variables, and (3) child's attachment style as described by the mothers.

The results of this study indicated different sources for the loneliness experience. Loneliness was predicted by the attachment style only among the group of children with developmental delay. In the group of typically developing children, the role of the attachment style as a factor to predict adaptation or loneliness was not substantiated. Children's temperament contributed directly to an insecure pattern of mother-child attachment, to lower maternal self-confidence, and to a lower level of family cohesion. This study indicated that children's temperament was related to the attachment style, and both factors predicted the development of loneliness, as measured by the Asher et al. questionnaire (1990).

Consistent and similar trends have been identified in several earlier studies with regard to family climate in families with children with mental retardation (Margalit, 1994). The presence of a child with mental retardation in the family was related to increased parental stress and a significant decrease in the social activities of family members (Shulman et al., 1990). In addition, family members reported less cohesive relations among family members and lower levels of open expression of feelings (Margalit & Raviv, 1983). Such a family environment does not support or model close interpersonal relations. This survey of family and genetic factors indicated the importance of personal factors in the loneliness construct.

III. THE LONELINESS CONSTRUCT

The loneliness construct consists of two inter-related dimensions that emerged from different roots (Buchholz & Catton, 1999; Weiss, 1973):

- Emotional loneliness
- Social loneliness

Emotional loneliness refers to a deficiency in developing intimate dyadic relations and interpersonal bonding, and has been conceptualized as emerging from insecure attachment relations. The quality of mother-child inter-relations was considered the source of attachment that predicts emotional loneliness (Bowlby, 1969). The child who experiences emotional loneliness often complains that he/she does not have "a good friend" (Hoza et al., 2000).

Social loneliness reflects frustrations related to the experience of peer rejection and an unsatisfactory peer network, and usually indicates deficits in social comprehension skills and social interaction skills. Children who experience social loneliness often complain that sometimes they are not invited to participate in the peer-group activities.

IV. LONELINESS AND SOCIAL DIFFICULTIES IN DEVELOPMENTAL DISABILITIES

Research results consistently show that students with mental retardation report higher levels of loneliness than their peers without disabilities (Luftig, 1988; Williams & Asher, 1992). It should be clarified that indeed loneliness indicates a subjective stress experience, yet the study of individuals with developmental disabilities suggest that their emotional negative experience is often based on realistic social difficulties, resulting in their poor social network, low social status, and peer rejection (Margalit & Ronen, 1993).

A comparison of loneliness levels among three groups of adolescents with disabilities: (1) students with mental retardation, (2) students with learning disabilities, and (3) students with behavior difficulties, revealed that students with mental retardation reported the highest levels of loneliness (Margalit, 1993).

V. SELF-REPORTS OF SOCIAL COMPETENCE AND LONELINESS

Teachers assessed students with developmental disabilities as revealing various social difficulties and less acceptance by peers (Amidzic et al., 2001). However, several studies have noted a discrepancy between self-reports of social competence and adults' ratings of children's experiences of loneliness. In these studies, children with developmental disabilities consistently evaluated themselves as socially competent as their peers, regardless of the ratings of peer rejection and teachers' assessment of their students' lower social competence. Comparisons of children with and without developmental disabilities revealed that they responded similarly to their non-disabled peers to questionnaires of self-reported social skills (Amidzic et al., 2001; Gresham & Elliott, 1990; Heiman & Margalit, 1998). Two approaches may be considered in explaining these paradoxical results (Spitzberg & Hurt, 1987).

The first approach has tried to minimize the value of the self-reports among students with developmental disabilities, considering students' self-evaluations as a representation of an unrealistic judgment or denial tendency. According to this explanation, these students either revealed their cognitive difficulties through their assessment of their social competence, or due to their emotional distress they tended to overestimate their abilities. An alternative approach focuses attention on the limited information provided by mean scores for understanding the emotional variability expressed by populations of individuals with disabilities.

Two factors support the second approach in explaining the paradox (i.e., the fact that students with developmental disabilities viewed themselves as socially competent as their peers). First, their loneliness scores indicated that they are able to accurately assess and report their social dissatisfaction. Second, observations of students' interactions and teachers' ratings provide validation to the self-reported social skills measures, emphasizing the need to differentiate between styles of interactions such as positive and negative social contacts (Margalit, 1993). Ratings of the negative interactions were negatively and significantly correlated with the following self-reported social skill indices:

- Cooperation (behaviors such as "helping others," "sharing materials in class," and "complying with rules and directions");
- Self-control (behavior that emerged in conflict situation such as "responding appropriately to teasing" and "controlling one's temper"); and
- Assertion (initiating interpersonal behaviors such as "making friends," "asking others for information," and "introducing one's self").

Students who were rated during observations as displaying negative social interactions such as showing verbal and physical acts of aggression (e.g., cursing, annoying others, pushing, and soon) rated themselves as less able to cooperate with adults and peers, initiate fewer positive interactions, and felt themselves to be less in control. Teachers' ratings of the students' behavior difficulties and hyperactivity further validated the self-control skills as reported by the students. Thus, we cannot disregard or minimize the value of the self-reported social skills of these students. We have to consider the lack of significant differences as indicating their diversity, and call for a differential approach in considering their social functioning.

The fourth self reported social skill measure—task orientation—reflectes the conformity of the students to the rules and expectations in the academic setting, was related to academic competence of these students, and is the best predictor of the students' adaptive behavior in the classroom (Margalit, 2000).

VI. DEVELOPMENTAL TRENDS

Several studies examined the developmental trends of loneliness, investigating whether or not levels of loneliness are higher as children age which may reveal inconsistent results. It is commonly accepted that adolescents report increased experiences of loneliness as they develop an identity at this age stage (Brennan, 1982). Research on loneliness in adolescence emphasizes the importance of social experiences for the development of identity (Hamid & Lok, 2000). Lonely youth without disabilities possessed limited social networks, had fewer close friends of both genders, and received less support from their classmates (Prinstein & La-Greca, 2002). Similarly, within their families, their relationships with their parents were less gratifying. They were less trusting of authority figures and less optimistic about the trustworthiness of others (Hamid & Lok, 2000).

Contradictory trends were reported by additional studies, showing that levels of loneliness decreased towards adolescence (Luftig, 1988). This may reflect the growing independence and freedom of older children in forming friendships outside schools. Younger children experience limited autonomy and freedom of mobility, in addition to classmate peer rejection. During adolescence, students are able to join a new social network and to extend their social inter-relations, and thus cope more effectively with their loneliness experiences.

The study of loneliness is related not only to different age stages but also to different social environments. The goals of a comprehensive study of loneliness and depression among students with developmental disabilities (Heiman & Margalit, 1998) were to identify developmental trends within different environmental conditions. This study compared the loneliness of 566 pre-adolescent and adolescent students. The sample included three groups: two groups of students with developmental disabilities in inclusive and special education educational settings, and a comparison group of non-disabled students. The first group consisted of 121 students with mild mental retardation from special education schools. The second group consisted of 189 students with mild mental retardation from self-contained classes in regular schools. The comparison group consisted of 256 non-disabled students. The results of this study provided support to the Luftig (1988) study, indicating that both groups of students with mental retardation reported higher levels of loneliness (using the Asher et al. scale [1990]) and increased scores of depression than their non-disabled peers. The comparison of the students' age groups revealed that younger children considered themselves lonelier.

No significant differences were found for younger children between the two groups of students with developmental disabilities: those students in special schools versus students in self-contained classes in regular schools. Both groups expressed higher levels of loneliness and had increased depressive scores when compared to their non-disabled peers. However, adolescents in self-contained classes reported levels of loneliness and depressions similar to their non-disabled peers, while students in the special schools continued to express their pronounced loneliness. This difference may indicate the critical role of the educational environment as mediated by the developmental stage. The higher levels of loneliness among students in the special schools' setting seems surprising, considering their ability to interact with peers that experience similar difficulties. However, these students continue to experience personal distress due to their severe difficulties. It is not clear if their distress emerged from the growing self-awareness of the gap between themselves and their non-disabled peers. It may also reflect a general dissatisfaction and frustration from their difficulties and their inability to move to an inclusive educational environment. The results of this study revealed that different sources of distress might be expressed by similar emotional expressions, calling for a careful consideration for the predictive factors of social difficulties.

VII. SOURCES OF SOCIAL DIFFICULTIES

Four factors were often identified as predicting social difficulties and loneliness experiences among children with developmental disabilities (Margalit, 1994):

- Knowledge deficit
- Performance deficit
- The role affiliation as lonely and rejected children
- A difficulty to stay alone and engaged in enjoyable activities

A. Knowledge Deficit—the Limited Knowledge Base

Many students with mental retardation have not acquired the age-appropriate knowledge and skills needed to develop satisfactory social relations. Thus, they experience difficulty in initiating, developing, and maintaining satisfactory interpersonal relationships. Several students' immature and sometimes simplistic understanding of complex social concepts, such as friendship, peer collaboration, and conflict resolution, may affect their interpersonal behavior. Social situations are complex and dynamic, and the cognitive limitation as well as limited social learning may affect the capacity of children with mental retardation to comprehend complex interactions.

B. Performance Deficit

Many children do not master the social skills necessary to maintain friendships, and have difficulty in translating age-appropriate social knowledge into effective interpersonal behaviors. They may face difficulties in adapting their knowledge base into age-appropriate behavior. Their peers, who master age-appropriate skills at an earlier age stage, may consider the attempts of students with mental retardation to join a group and collaborate with them in different school projects as immature, childish, and generally inappropriate. Thus, due to peer rejection, students with mental retardation may have fewer opportunities for engaging in social activities.

C. The Children's Role Affiliation as Lonely and Rejected Children

The repeated experiences of loneliness and peer rejection affect the children's interpersonal behavior style. These children adopt the typical behavior patterns of lonely children. They accept the reputation of isolated individuals, and their behavior may reflect their expectations of rejection (Margalit, 1994). Their interpersonal approaches and non-verbal communication reveal their alienated self-concept and their beliefs in their inability to develop and maintain satisfying social relations. These patterns were often presented in their behavior style when they approach peers, or in their reactions to different types of communicating attempts.

D. The Difficulty to Stay Alone

The loneliness experience may also result from the difficulty children with developmental disabilities may have in being alone (Margalit, 1994). The capacity to stay alone matures as children learn to take care of themselves and do not require protective adults to plan and structure their activities (Winnicott, 1965). Children with intellectual disabilities may experience more difficulties in regulating their activities when they are alone, than their peers. Thus, the multiple factors that predicted the loneliness call for the development of a comprehensive model.

VIII. THE AFFECTIVE-COGNITIVE MODEL OF LONELINESS

The concept of loneliness includes embedded cognitive, affective, and behavior components. To fully understand the relative impact of these components, we suggest considering them in the framework of the affective-cognitive multi-process model, designed to explain the various ways in which emotions have an ongoing impact on cognitive functioning (Forgas, 1995). Emotions may serve important functions for children and adults (Keltner & Gross, 1999) by regulating the individual's relations to the external or internal environment.

The "alerting" functions of the emotions were often treated as a disruptive influence on the normative cognition processing in cognitive and developmental studies. Most research in this domain was performed within controlled experimental designs examining the problem solving of typical developing individuals. Neurobiological research (Fox et al., 1996; Nelson & Bloom, 1997) provides support to the impact on cognitive processes, as revealed in various domains such as planning, decision-making, effective information processing, problem solving, judgments, recall, and memory.

The affective-cognitive approach rests upon four basic assumptions:

- Emotions have informational effects
- Emotions have a direct processing role in cognitive processing

- Emotions affect the categorization and organization of knowledge
- Emotional regulation is a critically important in understanding behavior.

A. Emotions Have Informational Effects

Emotions and moods provide a person a global appraisal to situations, and prepare the individual to meet the demands of tasks. Emotions influence the contents of cognitive processes through representations, memories, and behaviors. It has been extensively established in personality research (Forgas, 1991), that individuals evaluate different situations and tasks either as a challenge or a threat to their well-being. This is an individualized appraisal and, thus, it is not surprising that identical tasks may lead to different personal conclusions.

Children with developmental disabilities may view their developmental tasks as a delicate balance between challenges and threats. The inter-relations of their reality construction, appraisal of situations, and outcome expectations affect their learning processes, effort investment, and future adjustment. One child may experience the situation as a challenge worthy of focused efforts to cope with it, exploring different alternative directions, and attempting creative solutions. For another child, a similar task may be perceived as a major threat, initiating negative feelings, anxiety, and fear and leading to retreat approaches and withdrawal coping strategies.

The impact of changing moods further affects the individual's relations with the environment, leading to inconsistent activities. The child may consider an assignment within a specific context of time and place as a challenge worthy of investing effort and engaging in active attempts to meet the task demands. However, within a different contextual condition, the same child may consider the assignment as a threat and a danger, and may react with withdrawal and avoidance behavior.

The situational appraisal process postulates awareness of the constant and dynamic interplay between two major considerations (Damasio, 2003):

- *Appraisal of personal and environmental resources:* the global judgment of two groups of resources: (1) assessment of the self (in terms of personal skills, abilities, and disabilities); and (2) environmental assessment (in terms of the supportive networks and auxiliary agents, such as the availability of help provided by adults and peers).
- *Appraisal of the demands:* individuals adapt their personal investment of efforts according to their assessment of the critical value of the task (considering their positive and negative outcomes) and the probabilities of successful performance.

The balance between these two factors may help to predict the different affective reactions and explain the amount of effort that individuals are willing to invest in tasks or to modify their attempts to reach personal goals. It often represents the co-existing, ongoing interplay of affective, cognitive, and motivational processes during task performance. Children may appraise the situation as a challenge when they consider their prior knowledge (personal resources) or abilities as sufficient or nearly sufficient to meet the situational demands. The appraisal of their environmental resources has been expressed in their confidence that when they face a difficulty, they will get help from adults and/or support from their teachers. An appraisal of the task as a challenge will promote focused efforts and positive outcome expectations.

A threat appraisal may be perceived when the persons appraise themselves as having insufficient resources to meet situational demands (Forgas, 1999). Thus, most efforts will be directed at avoiding the situation or discontinuing the performance of the task. Such a differentiation between threat and challenge may have value for promoting resiliency and mediating efforts, especially among children with difficulties who have experienced failure and frustration.

B. Emotions Have a Direct Processing Role in Cognitive Processing

The relation between affect and cognitive processes is reciprocal and dynamic. Affect can influence processing style, and different information processing strategies can mediate the degree of affect infusion into thinking (Forgas, 1991). Examinations of the differential influences of negative or positive affective states on information processing style revealed their impact on information processing, memorizing facts, and behavior style. Educators should be aware that the cognitive difficulties experienced by students might be more pronounced in different contexts due to affective processing.

Differences between positive and negative mood are not only related to processing style but also to the outcome impact, in terms of prolonged and deeper memory impressions. This focus on processing outcomes further directs the study of the differential impacts of positive and negative experiences on thinking and learning. Baumeister (1999) reported that the impact of a bad mood and negative experience is pronounced, and affects the individual for longer periods than a positive experience. These differentiating influences should alert educators who attempt to mediate the difficult and negative experiences of students with developmental disabilities, and solicit ways to balance negative experiences with positive ones.

C. Representations and Organization of Knowledge

The study of the knowledge acquiring structure may provide an additional research challenge for understanding children with developmental disabilities. The ways in which information has been represented and organized—the categorization and schematic representation of cognitive and self-relevant information (Showers, 1992)—affect learning effectiveness and memory activity. Research on brain activities of expert chess players (Amidzic et al., 2001) showed that effective use of learning is dependent on the organization of memories in chunks. The organization of knowledge structure reflects the joint impact of both affective and cognitive processing (Forgas, 1991). Thus, misconceptions and disorganized learning style among children with developmental disabilities may be attributed not only to cognitive deficits or lack of motivation, but also to the dynamic impact of emotional factors on cognitive structures.

Overall, research has demonstrated that children's and adults' memory is affected by emotional information (Davidson et al., 2001). The model of emotional understanding further clarifies the meaning of emotions for the individual. Children monitor and appraise their world in an effort to detect changes in status of personal goals (Liawag & Stein, 1995). Goals that are either attended to or blocked, may lead to immediate effects on the child's emotional experience. Emotional information increases the level of arousal and attention, and may result in better memory accomplishments. Sometimes, attempts to block painful memories using emotional regulation processes may be considered as adaptive devices for learning activities, without ignoring its impact on memory processing and learning.

D. Emotional Regulation

Emotional regulation studies (Eisenberg et al., 2001) expand our knowledge on developmental considerations and predictive factors. Children's levels of "emotionality," and their ability to regulate their emotional reactions have a clear predictive value for future learning and adjustment in systemic ways (Eisenberg et al., 2001). However, there are ongoing discussions among researchers about what is being regulated. The debate among theoreticians remains whether research should clarify how children regulate the various aspects of their emotional experiences and expressions (i.e., the intensity level, the control of extreme manifestations, and the direction of the emotional expressions). Another possibility is to examine how children use their emotions to regulate their behavior (such as to increase their learning efforts, to struggle with fatigue, and to focus their attention).

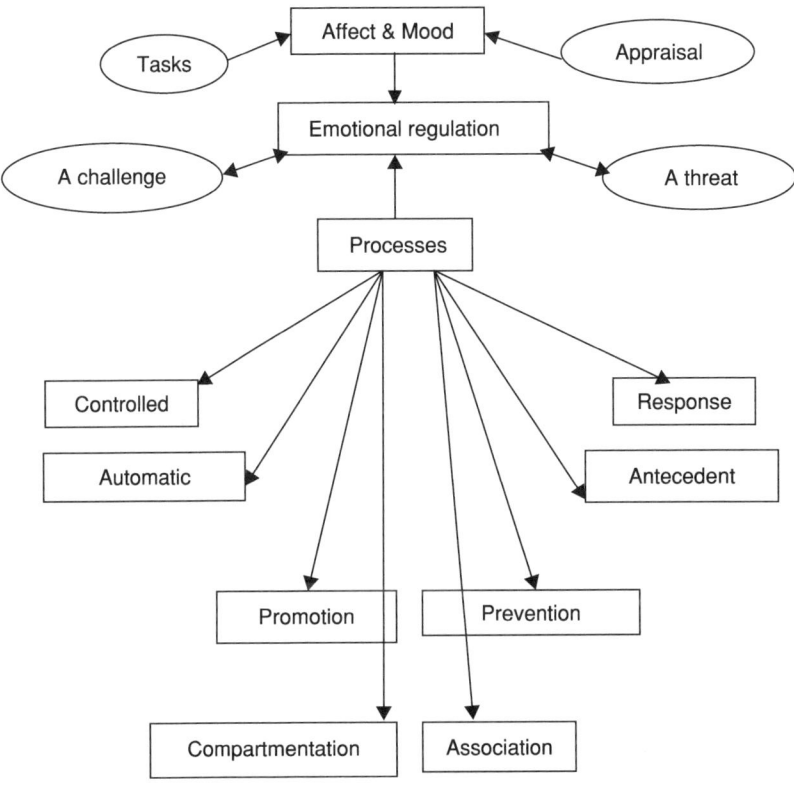

FIG. 1. Emotional regulation.

The identification of different regulative strategies is valuable for intervention planning. Figure 1 presents different strategies for emotional regulation that children often use, such as concentration on specific cues or using directed distraction from annoying cues. Two basic regulatory systems were identified in personality research, as can be seen in Figure 1:

1. Promotive strategies which are concerned with advancement, growth, and accomplishments; and
2. Preventive strategies, which are concerned with security, safety, and responsibility.

Children and adults use different and varied regulating strategies for coping with disturbing information. For example, separation or integrative tendencies (Showers, 1992) refer to the ability of individuals to develop an emotional separation "shield" against the impact of strong negative affect or the help in the compartmentalization of negative mood. Children may say to themselves "I shall not think about it," or they may express their self-evaluation, "I failed in mathematics, but I am very good in swimming." Others will promote a positive mood before task performance by activating positive memories on experiences such as an enjoyable summer vacation. Intervention planning may focus on teaching children the varied regulative strategies to enhance their academic achievement and adjustment.

Situational and contextual variables can impact individuals' approaches to developmental tasks, affecting regulative modes in terms of emotional intensity, directions (positive/negative emotions), and joint impact of interactions between several emotions. The outline of this multi-dimensional model has been used to demonstrate educational possibilities, future research directions, and interventional implications for individuals, families, and educational systems. Yet, the interpersonal perspectives and peer relations have been the major topics in the research of loneliness in children, revealing the impact of popularity and rejection but underscoring the central role of companionship for adjustment.

IX. SOCIAL STATUS AND COMPANIONSHIP

The loneliness experience represents the combined impact of personal conceptions and interpersonal relations. Children with developmental disabilities were more rejected or ignored by peers, had fewer friends, and their companionship provision patterns were different from those of their non-disabled peers (Margalit, 2000). Children's social stuatus is different from measures of friendships. Peer nomination has often been considered the valid measure of children's popularity, and reciprocal nomination was regarded as an indicator of friendship relations. Research has documented that popularity and friendship measures are not identical with lower levels of loneliness. They were moderately related to loneliness reports of children with and without developmental disabilities. Yet, friendship relations appeared to buffer the experiences of individuals from the loneliness episode (Asher et al., 1990). Even having a single friend was reported as predicting decreased loneliness scores.

Research focus on companionship emphasizes the full complexity of interpersonal processes, concentrating on qualitative and quantitative advantages of having a good friend (Gottlieb & Leyser, 1981). If within the peer world, a good friend is expected to attend to one's major relational needs (Parker & Asher, 1993), then the poor quality of friendship may be closely related to alienation and loneliness feelings. Parker and Asher

(1993) listed unique provisions that good peer relations may contribute. Good friends may communicate care and concern to their mates. They can provide help in times of need, share intimate feelings or thoughts ("telling secrets"), and often spend enjoyable time together.

An additional important aspect of friendship relates to conflict and disagreements. The number of conflicts among children provides an important index, and a child's conflict resolution style contributes a crucial perspective to understanding the complicated inter-relations. Unresolved conflicts may increase the experience of social isolation.

Another factor in the loneliness experience, the role of reciprocal negative nominations among peers (having children in your class whom you do not like and who do not like you—"identified enemies"), has also been explored (Margalit et al., 1999). This research examined the social reality of students with learning disabilities. The study revealed the unique negative contribution of having "identified enemies" in class. The results confirmed the hypothesis that within the group of students with learning disabilities, those children who had at least one "identified enemy" in class felt more lonely than children who had no "class enemies." Such significant within-group differences were not found in the analysis of the typically developing groups, revealing the social-emotional vulnerability of children with disabilities to increased and consistent social distress, social rejection, and negative relations.

This research illustrated the functional vulnerability of children with disabilities, who attributed increased importance to peer attitudes, due to their limited social network. Hierarchical multiple regression analysis revealed that the loneliness experience was significantly predicted by the personal measure of resilience, the interpersonal measure of peer reciprocal rejection, and cognitive conception of friendship qualities. Children with learning disabilities who had at least one identified "enemy" in class not only experienced higher levels of loneliness, but also viewed themselves as less socially competent than their non-disabled peers (Margalit et al., 1999). Future research is needed to clarify the predictive role of reciprocal rejection for understanding the loneliness of students with developmental disabilities.

X. COPING AND INTERVENTION

Individuals not only experience social distress in a unique and subjective manner, but also react differently to the painful experience of loneliness. In several studies, in line with the Cassidy and Asher (1992) procedure, students were interviewed to clarify their understanding of loneliness and to determine how they coped with their loneliness (Margalit, 1994). The survey revealed the distinction between active/approach coping strategies and strategies that rely essentially on avoidance/denial. External trends (promoting social skills, generating intimate social inter-relations, and increasing networking with peer groups at school age) and internal trends (cultivating satisfying solitary interests and activities, and enhancing abilities to stay alone without feeling loneliness) were both present within the variety of strategies.

Different categories of activities have been identified, reflecting individual differences in the children's abilities to initiate effective coping activities (Woodward & Kalyan-Masih, 1990). Several children felt helpless and sorry for themselves, and ineffective in their coping style. Others reported that they did not feel very lonely, demonstrating their resilience and effective coping style. The study of different coping strategies among these children, using varying levels of approach and avoidance coping, not only further establishes the existence of their unique and distinct approaches to stressful situations, but also directs the development of individualized interventions.

Without ignoring the complex and dynamic patterns of coping strategies, higher levels of passive and avoidance coping with loneliness were evident among the groups of students with disabilities. In addition, the outcomes of coping efforts may be evaluated according to the proportion of solitary versus social activities exhibited in the children's performance repertoire.

Most diagnostic and intervention efforts for students with various disabilities are based on a clinical model, which identifies and diagnoses the children's causes and expressions of difficulties. Such an approach relies on conceptualizations of disability and pathology as a basic rationale for understanding children's functioning and growth. Garmezy (1983) examined childhood stressors and focused attention on the importance of individual and environmental factors that can predict resilience, growth, and stress-resistance in children (Smith et al., 2001). Thus, the rise in interventions that use concepts such as stress-resistance, ego-resilience, capacities, and invulnerability, in contrast with the usage of terms such as deficits, special difficulties, and pathology, hold unique theoretical significance for understanding the functioning of individuals (Patterson, 2002), with practical implications for developing intervention plans.

Not all children with disabilities experience more loneliness than their non-disabled peers (Margalit, 1994). A small group of youngsters was often identified, who did not view themselves as more lonely than their peers. The search for resilience and adjustment predictors (Richardson, 2002) focuses interest on this unique group of children, who demonstrated age-adequate social skills and average scores on their sense of coherence reports, regardless of their continuous academic difficulties and different disabilities.

Antonovsky (1987) differentiated between the pathogenic approach that seeks to explain why people get sick, and the salutogenic approach (i.e., focusing on the origins of health and coping), which seeks to explain why people do not become ill and stay healthy and active. The pathogenic orientation uses the commonly accepted cause-effect model, dividing people into patients/diseased/disabled and non-patients/healthy categories. Once a disease or disability is defined, a search is made for the causes of maladjustment or a specific illness with the belief that the identification of these causes will lead to taxonomy of the most appropriate efforts for remediation of the maladjustment.

In contrast, the salutogenic orientation focuses on probability models and the continuum model of health/disease. It attempts to identify factors that predict resistance to difficulties, promoting effective coping with stressful situations and buffering pressures and disappointment. Antonovsky's (1987) sense of coherence construct provides a global estimation of self perception, unique in its emphasis on the individual-environmental perspective and on a positive approach to coping with stress.

The sense of coherence construct (Antonovsky, 1987) can be defined as a global orientation, a generalized world view, that expresses the extent to which one has an enduring feeling of confidence:

1. That the individual's internal and external environments are structured and predictable;
2. That inner and outer resources are available to meet demands, and that there is a high probability that things will work out as well as can be expected; and
3. That these demands are viewed as challenges worthy of energy investment.

A strong sense of coherence relates to the availability of a wide and varied repertoire of coping strategies, and to the flexibility in selecting the particular coping strategy that seems most appropriate at a certain time with a given environmental condition. Antonovsky and Sourani (1988) considered the sense of coherence construct not as a specific coping style, but rather as a characteristic of flexibility in selecting appropriate coping behaviors. An individual who demonstrates a high sense of coherence would succeed in transforming his/her potential resources into reality and, thus, will be more adequately able to cope with life stressors.

Within this concept, three main inter-related components were identified: (1) comprehensibility; (2) manageability; and (3) meaningfulness.

Comprehensibility refers to the extent to which the child perceives environmental information as ordered, consistent, structured, and clear. *Manageability* defines the extent to which the child usually feels that the resources that are at his/her disposal are adequate to meet substantial demands. *Meaningfulness* represents the emotional and motivational element of this concept. It defines the extent that the child feels that life makes sense emotionally, and demands can be viewed as challenges worthy of commitment.

Children with disabilities who are able to understand (even in a simplistic way) most demands and expectations within their environments, who can cope (even with adults' help) with most developmental tasks, and who are ready to focus efforts, viewing most demands as challenges and worthy of personal involvement, will feel more coherent and resilient than their peers. It is not surprising that lower sense of coherence scores were repeatedly found among children with various disabilities when compared to typical developing peers (Margalit, 1994). Those resilient individuals whose social competence and sense of coherence did not differ from comparison groups call for indepth examination.

Empowerment has often been viewed as the process that facilitates the individual's identification and recognition of needs and the ability to use existing personal competencies to obtain resources to meet these needs. Intervention goals may be directed toward changing the child and/or changing the environment in terms of family and school, integrating both the systemic and skill-deficit models to promote personal empowerment, and satisfying social interactions to decrease the loneliness experience. Resilience research supported this approach and demonstrated that feelings of control and positive self-concept predict resilient coping (Cichetti & Rogosch, 1997). Within the salutogenic perspective (Antonovsky, 1987), the empowerment approach has been using enabling experiences to promote children's competence and sense of control. The systemic climate creates opportunities for competencies to be experienced.

This systemic approach directs intervention efforts not only toward children who demonstrate interpersonal dissatisfaction, but also targets their peers and significant adults. Parents and teachers can structure environments to promote companionship and satisfactory peer inter-relations. Developing a knowledge base about the social life of their children, and becoming aware of different developmental aspects of interpersonal relations, such as expressions of aggressiveness and shyness, may enable these adults to support their children-adaptive interpersonal relations. Parents and teachers can be effective in helping children to cope with loneliness by creating opportunities and promoting adaptive social behaviors and skills, initiating satisfactory solitary and social play activities, and helping children deal with their emotions (Ladd, 1988). To help them in developing effective interventions, two related aspects should be examined in depth: skill selection and procedure selection.

Different procedures were found to be effective in social skill training programs, such as modeling, peer tutoring, role-playing, and problem-solving sequences. Adult- and peer-mediated approaches were applied in order to initiate change not only within the child who feels lonely and needs training in friendship-making skills and friendship-maintenance strategies, but also in the environment in order to encourage and promote companionship opportunities (Rizzo, 1988).

The commonly accepted interventions for loneliness are based on the social skills deficit construct within the model of effective information processing (Kramer, Piersel, & Glover, 1987). It was assumed that as a result of these children's chronic cognitive difficulties in accurately processing environmental information, actively exploring social interactions, and effectively solving social problems in a rewarding manner, deficient social skills and behavioral difficulties often emerge, manifested either in aggressive or passive tendencies (Taylor et al., 1987). Thus, social skills training with a focus on the child's social information processing may foster the development of social skills and peer acceptance and may decrease peer rejection and loneliness (Asher et al., 1990).

The goal of most social learning programs is to help the individual to develop the skills necessary for changing children, the environmental context, or both (Andrasik & Matson, 1985). The majority of studies on social skills have involved standard social skill training packages (Matson & DiLorenzo, 1986). The basic package includes a number of component techniques such as: (1) clear instruction procedures; (2) modeling how to perform the skill; (3) role-playing, rehearsal, and experimenting; and (4) performance feedback and transfer to different environments. The packages were used for promoting adjusted behavior within different social settings, and were evaluated by sociometric measures and teachers' ratings. For example, the computer-assisted social skills program "I Found a Solution" (Margalit, 1995), presented students with computerized social simulations and adventure games within a controlled and structured mini-environment (i.e., computer environment) in which the child is encouraged to experiment with different solutions for conflictual social situations.

Group discussions, role-playing exercises, and homework tasks were included as part of the training to enable experimentation with and rehearsal of effective problem-solving strategies. Within the program, the strategy training focused on instruction in planning (i.e., how to devise and monitor solution plans and evaluate their efficiency from the student's point of view) and self-monitoring (i.e., how to develop self-regulation through practice with self-instructional training procedures such as self-directed commands, suggestions, and rewards). In line with recommendations from Deshler, Schumaker, Harris, and Graham (1999), the intervention's strategy training emphasized the modeling, explaining, and rehearsing of desired social skills strategies (e.g., assertion, cooperation, self-control), while continuously pointing out the advantages of applying these behaviors. In several studies (Margalit, 1991; Margalit & Weisel, 1990), the impact of this program was demonstrated through case studies, observations, and assessments of social skills.

It was hypothesized that following social skills training, individuals in the trained group would improve their social skills, decrease their disruptive behavior, be rated by their peers as more skilled, and accepted socially. It was also expected that, following the intervention, the children in the experimental group would also feel less lonely than the children in the comparison group. The results of the several studies (Margalit, 1995) demonstrated that the trained group of students with mental retardation increased their different measures of social competence, and the differences between them and the matched control groups were significant following the intervention procedures. However, if no specific training for teachers and students was scheduled, no significant differences in the loneliness experience was found. Following these results, the loneliness regulation module was entered among the specified targets of the intervention program, including mood awareness and emotional regulation, and then the students and teachers rated lower levels in loneliness (Margalit, 1995).

These results emphasized the importance of the loneliness construct for children with mental retardation. Following successful social skill intervention programs, when students and teachers reported better social competence, and even their peers viewed them in more accepting ways, the students may continue to consider themselves more lonely than non-disabled peers. Research has suggested that once a person assumes a particular social role, reciprocal interaction patterns may perpetuate behavior that is consistent with that social role (Vitkus & Horowitz, 1987). They may continue accepting the role of the lonely individual, and not be able to change this role without directed intervention. However, direct training empowers their abilities to cope with loneliness (Margalit, 1995).

Personal and social change following successful interventions rely extensively on different methods of empowerment (Bandura, 1988) such as providing individuals with knowledge, skills, and resilient self-beliefs of efficacy to alter aspects of their lives over which they have control. Personal beliefs and perceived self-efficacy about one's capabilities to organize and implement the actions necessary for attaining designated levels of performance in different areas have been found important in mediating behavioral change. Self-judgments of personal efficacy affect the individual's choice of activities and selection of environments (Ozer & Bandura, 1990).

Recent research presented the need to move from a skill training approach to competence promotion (Simon & Bjork, 2001). For long-term retention, contextual-inference practice (practicing skills that are mixed with other tasks) results in better learning than isolated and blocked training practice. The advantage of blocked practice, sometimes within laboratories and clinics, lies in the promotion of the experience of achievements and mastery within an isolated and controlled environment. However, the temporary boosts that blocked practice provide, allows students and, sometimes, their teachers to overestimate how well children have mastered the skills they have practiced. Blocked practice leads to better and measurable short-term performance, but poorer long-term learning, especially within realistic environments. It was hypothesized that blocked practice differentiates between the required skills encouraging the on-task students to make a mental trial-by-trial adjustment, which enhance current practice. However, only contextual-based practice induces retrieval processes and the conceptual categorization that enhances a better future performance.

In addition, planning requires the consideration of the cost of multitasking (doing several tasks together) for children's mental resources (Rubinstein et al., 2001). For each aspect of human performance—perceiving, thinking, and acting—people have specific mental resources whose effective use requires inner supervision through executive mental control. Studies demonstrate that the time cost was greater when the subjects had to switch to complex tasks and to unfamiliar tasks. Intervention planning requires a multilevel consideration of the most efficient conditions for task learning and retention. The contribution to performance of the positive mood has been related to feelings of control and mastery during skill learning.

XI. LONELINESS AND TECHNOLOGY

The entrance of technology into educational systems and homes has initiated reconsideration of the established concepts of interpersonal relations, realizing the new opportunities related to distance communications and virtual social inter-relations (Margalit & Efrati, 2003). The ability to contact unknown people, regardless of distance barriers, challenges our established conceptualization of social relations, connectedness, and alienation. To identify the model of loneliness within the computer age, 756 students (grades 2 to 4) participated in a study including 368 students with learning disabilities (196 boys and 172 girls) and 388 students with average achievements (214 boys and 174 girls) (Margalit & Weissberg, 2001). The study simultaneously examined several predictors of loneliness, using a structural equation modeling analysis and a common loneliness model was identified for students with and without disabilities.

The results showed that in addition to the demographic variables: age, gender and disability status (learning disabled), three factors predicted the loneliness experience: (1) personal—expressed by the sense of coherence measure; (2) interpersonal—expressed by peer nominations; and (3) instrumental—the attitudes towards computers that mediated the aversive loneliness experience. Separate analysis of the model for each group revealed that for the group of typical achieving students, all five predictors were significant. Each one of the following variables predicted the loneliness experience: age, gender, and personal and interpersonal variables. For a group of students with learning disabilities, the analysis revealed that only two measures remained significant: their personal self-perceptions in terms of the sense of coherence, and their attitudes towards computers. The results of this study pointed to the significant role of computers in predicting lower levels of loneliness for students with learning disabilities. The instrumental mediation for the loneliness experience—the computers—needs in-depth examination to clarify if the future role of technology in children's lives indeed may challenge the traditional loneliness and companionship conceptualizations for students with developmental disabilities. Detailed examinations of how e-friends and web-peers may mediate the loneliness experience will clarify the possible direct impact (in terms of expending social networks) and indirect impact (in terms of self-perceptions and social place in different environments). We also need to examine the impact of computers' involvement as out-of-school activities and enhancing the ability of children for solitude and independence.

In summary, the existing research demonstrated the examination of loneliness within the intellectual disability perspective and should be treated from a comprehensive multidimensional (cognitive and affective) position. In addition, the identification and examination of contextual protective factors may provide a better understanding for their buffering and mediating role, resiliency, and direct planning intervention. In line with the resiliency approach, future research should examine the adaptability of these approaches for in-depth examinations of the learning and coping processes among children with developmental disabilities.

Finally, the model of empowering focuses intervention efforts toward promoting change in the processes and outcomes that are directed at children's experiences of themselves, their peers, and adults from early developmental stages (Brooks-Gunn, 2003). In comprehensive intervention approaches, social skill training programs have to be thoroughly re-examined; there is a need for introducing revised conceptualizations and innovative procedures. The empowering approach attempts to activate the individual's search for individualistic answers to social needs and may foster his/her sense of coherence and ability to develop both meaningful connections and areas of interest for enjoyable solitary activities. It should be recognized that throughout life, individuals with and without disabilities consistently attempt to control and regulate their social life by moving from periods of intensive social inter-relations, in which they prefer to spend time with other people, to solitude periods, when they want to be left alone. Empowerment approaches acknowledge the different routes to helping children in coping with loneliness, and the importance of multiple interventional methods in promoting competency and social growth.

REFERENCES

Al-Yagon, M. (2003). Children at-risk for developing learning disorders: Multiple perspectives. *Journal of Learning Disabilities Journal of Learning Disabilities, 36*(4), 318–328.

Amidzic, O., Riehle, H. J., Fehr, T., Wiebruch, C., & Elbert, T. (2001). Pattern of focal y-bursts in chess players. *Nature 412,* 603.

Andersson, L., Mullins, L. C., & Johnson, D. P. (1987). Parental intrusion versus social isolation: A dichotomous view of the sources of loneliness. In M. Hojat & R. Crandall (Eds.), Loneliness: Theory, research, and applications [Special issue]. *Journal of Social Behavior and Personality, 2,* 125–134.

Andrasik, F., & Matson, J. L. (1985). Social skills training for the mentally retarded. In L. L'Sbate (Ed.), *Handbook of social skills training and research* (pp. 418–453). New York: John Wiley.

Antonovsky, A. (1987). *Unraveling the mystery of health.* San Francisco: Jossey-Bass.

Antonovsky, A., & Sourani, T. (1988). Family sense of coherence and family adaptation. *Journal of Marriage and the Family, 50,* 79–92.

Asher, S. R., Parkhurst, J. T., Hymel, S., & Williams, G. A. (1990). Peer rejection and loneliness in childhood. In S. R. Asher & J. D. Coie (Eds.), *Peer rejection in childhood* (pp. 253–273). Cambridge, England: University Press.

Bandura, A. (1988). Self-efficacy conception of anxiety. *Anxiety Research, 1,* 77–98.

Baumeister, R. F. (1999, August). *Bad is stronger than good.* Paper presented at the Annual convention of the American Psychological Association, Boston.

Berninger, V. W. (2001). Understanding the nature-nurture interactions in language and learning disabilities. *Learning Disability Quarterly, 24*(3), 139–140.

Bierman, K. L., & Welsh, J. A. (2000). Assessing social dysfunction: The contributions of laboratory and performance-based measures. *Journal of Clinical Child Psychology, 29*(4), 526–539.

Biovin, J., & Hymel, S. (1997). Peer experience and social self-perceptions: A sequential model. *Developmental Psychology, 33,* 135–145.

Bowlby, J. (1969). *Attachment and loss: Vol. 1.* Attachment. New York: Basic Books.

Brennan, T. (1982). Loneliness at adolescence. In L. A. Peplau & D. Perlman (Eds.), *Loneliness: A sourcebook of current theory, research and therapy* (pp. 269–290). New York: Wiley.

Brooks-Gunn, J. (2003). Do you believe in magic? What we can expect from early childhood intervention programs *Social Policy Report, 17*(1), 3–14.

Buchholz, E. S., & Catton, R. (1999). Adolescents' perceptions of aloneness and loneliness. *Adolescence, 34,* 203–213.

Cassidy, J., & Asher, S. R. (1992). Loneliness and peer relations in young children. *Child Development, 63,* 350–365.

Cicchetti, D., & Rogosch, F. A. (1997). The role of self-organization in the promotion of resilience in mal-treated children. *Development and Psychopathology, 9,* 799–817.

Cook, W. L. (2001). Interpersonal influence in family systems: A social relations model analysis. *Child Development, 72*(4), 1179–1197.

Damasio, A. (2003). *Looking for Spinoza: Joy, sorrow, and the feeling brain.* Orlando: Harcourt.

Davidson, D., Luo, Z., & Burden, M. J. (2001). Children's recall of emotional behaviors, emotional labels and nonemotional behaviors: Does emotion enhance memory? *Cognition and emotion, 15*(1), 1–26.

Deshler, D. D., Schumaker, J., Harris, K. R., & Graham, S. (1999). *Teaching every adolescent every day.* Cambridge, Ma: Brookline.

Dunn, I., Stocker, C., & Plomin, R. (1990). Nonshared experience within the family: Correlates of behavior problems in middle childhood. *Developmental and Psychopathology, 2,* 113–126.

Eisenberg, N., Cumberland, A., Spinrad, T. L., Shepard, S. A., Reiser, M., Murphy, B. C., Losoya, S. H., & Guthrie, I. A. (2001). The relations of regulation and emotionality to children's externalizing and internalizing problem behavior. *Child Development, 72*(4), 1112–1134.

Elliott, S. N., & Gersham, F. M. (1989). *Preschoolers' social behavior and family background: Teachers' and parents' assessments.* New Orleans, LA.: The American Psychological Association.

Emde, R., & Spicer, P. (2000). Experience in the midst of variation: New horizons for development and psychopathology. *Development and Psychopathology, 12,* 313–331.

Ferguson, P. M. (2002). A place in the family: An historical interpretation of research on parental reactions to having a child with a disability. *Journal of Special Education, 36*(3), 124–130.

Forgas, J. P. (1991). *Emotion and social judgment.* Oxford: Pergamon.

Forgas, J. P. (1995). Mood and judgment: The affect infusion model (AIM). *Psychological Bulletin, 116,* 39–66.

Forgas, J. P. (1999). Feeling and speaking: Mood effects on verbal communication strategies. *Personality and Social Psychology Bulletin, 25*(7), 850–863.

Fox, N. A., Schmidt, L. A., Calkin, S. D., Rubin, K. H., & Coplan, R. J. (1996). The role of frontal activation in the regulation and dysregulation of social behavior during preschool years. *Development and Psychopathology, 8*(1), 89–102.

Fraser, B. C. (1986). Child impairment and parent/infant communication. *Child: Care, Health and Development, 12,* 141–150.

Gottlieb, J., & Leyser, Y. (1981). Friendship between mentally retarded children. In S. R. Asher & J. M. Gottman (Eds.), *The development of children's friendships* (pp. 150–181). New York: Cambridge University Press.

Garmezy, N. (1983). Stressors of childhood. In N. Garmezy & M. Rutter (Eds.), *Stress, coping and development in children* (pp. 43–84). New York: McGraw-Hill Books.

Gresham, F. M. (1986). Conceptual and definitional issues in the assessment of children's social skills: Implications for classification and training. *Journal of Clinical Child Psychology, 15,* 3–15.

Gresham, F. M., & Elliott, S. N. (1990). *Social skills rating system manual.* Circle Pines, MN: American Guidance Services.

Guralnick, M. J. (1990). Social competence and early intervention. *Journal of Early intervention, 14,* 3–14.

Hamid, P. N., & Lok, D. P. P. (2000). Loneliness in Chinese adolescents: A comparison of social support and interpersonal trust in 13 to 19 years olds. *International Journal of Adolescence and Youth, 8*(1), 45–63.

Heiman, T., & Margalit, T. (1998). Loneliness, depression and social skills among students with mild mental retardation in different educational settings. *The Journal of Special Education, 32*(3), 154–163.

Hoza, B., Bukowski, W. M., & Beery, S. (2000). Assessing peer network and dyadic loneliness. *Journal of Clinical Child Psychology, 29*(1), 119–128.

Josselson, R. (1992). *The space between us.* San Francisco: Jossey-Bass.

Keltner, D., & Gross, J. J. (1999). Functional accounts of emotions. *Cognition and emotion, 13*(5), 467–480.

Kramer, J. J., Piersel, W. C., & Glover, J. A. (1987). Cognitive and social development of mildly retarded children. In M. C. Wang & M. C. Reynolds (Eds.), *Handbook of special education research and practice: Mildly handicapped conditions* (Vol. 2, pp. 43–58). Oxford: Pergamon Press.

Ladd, G. W. (1988). Friendship patterns and peer status during early and middle childhood. *Developmental and Behavioral Pediatrics, 9,* 229–238.

Ladd, G. W., & Burgess, K. B. (1999). Changing the relationship trajectories of aggressive, withdrawn and aggressive/withdrawn children during early grade school. *Child Development, 70,* 910–929.

Liawag, M. D., & Stein, N. I. (1995). Children's memory for emotional events: The importance of emotional related retrieval cues. *Journal of Experimental Child Psychology, 60,* 2–31.

Luftig, R. L. (1988). Assessment of perceived school loneliness and isolation of mentally retarded and nonretarded students. *American Journal of Mental Retardation, 92,* 472–475.

Maccoby, E. E. (1990). Gender and relationships: A developmental perspective. *American Psychologist, 45,* 513–520.

Margalit, M. (1991). Promoting classroom adjustment and social skills for students with mental retardation within an experimental and control group design. *Exceptionality, 2,* 195–204.

Margalit, M. (1993). Social skills and classroom behavior among adolescents with mild mental retardation. *American Journal on Mental Retardation, 97*(6), 685–691.

Margalit, M. (1994). *Loneliness among children with special needs: Theory, research, coping and intervention.* New York: Springer-Verlag.

Margalit, M. (1995). Technology and social skills training for students with special needs in Israel: "I found a solution." *DISES Monograph, 3,* 23–36.

Margalit, M. (2000, November). *Strategic planning in the education of students with developmental disabilities: The joint impact of cognitive and emotional approaches.* Paper presented at the MIND's Millennium Symposium on Intellectual Disability, Singapore.

Margalit, M., & Efrati, M. (2003, April). *Self-perception and mood of students with learning disabilities (LD).* Presented at the SRCD Biennial Meeting at the symposium: "Self perceptions of children and adolescents with LD." Tampa, FL.

Margalit, M., & Raviv, A. (1983). Mothers' perceptions of family climate in families with a mentally retarded child. *The Exceptional Child, 30*(2), 163–169.

Margalit, M., & Ronen, T. (1993). Loneliness and social competence among preadolescents and adolescents with mild mental retardation. *Mental Handicap Research, 6*(2), 97–111.

Margalit, M., Tur-Kaspa, H., & Most, T. (1999). Reciprocal nominations, reciprocal rejections and loneliness among students with learning disorders. *Educational Psychology, 19,* 79–90.

Margalit, M., & Weisel, A. (1990). Computer-assisted social skills learning for adolescents with mild disabilities and social difficulties. *Educational Psychology, 10,* 343–354.

Margalit, M., & Weissberg, L. (2001, June). *The role of computers in the loneliness developmental model for students with learning disabilities.* Paper presented at the International Academy of Research in Learning Disabilities 25th Anniversary Conference, Antwerp, Netherlands.

Matson, J. L., & DiLorenzo, T. M. (1986). Social skills training and mental handicap and organic impairment. In C. R. Hollin & P. Trower (Eds.), *Handbook of social skills training* (Vol. 2, pp. 67–90). New York: Pergamon.

McGuire, S., & Clifford, J. (2000). Genetic and environmental contributions to loneliness in children. *Psychological Science, 11*(6), 487–491.

McHale, S. M., Crouter, A. C., McGuire, S., & Updegraff, K. A. (1995). Congruence between mothers' and fathers' differential treatment of siblings: Links with family relations and children's well-being. *Child Development, 66,* 116–126.

Nelson, C. A., & Bloom, F. E. (1997). Child development and neuroscience. *Child Development, 68*(5), 970–987.

Ozer, E. M., & Bandura, A. (1990). Mechanisms governing empowerment effects: A self-efficacy analysis. *Journal of Personality and Social Psychology, 58,* 472–486.

Parker, J. G., & Asher, S. R. (1993). Friendship and friendship quality in middle childhood. *Developmental Psychology, 29*(4), 611–621.

Peplau, L. A., & Perlman, D. (1982). Perspectives on loneliness. In L. A. Peplau & D. Perlman (Eds.), *Loneliness: A sourcebook of current theory, research and therapy* (pp. 1–18). New York: Wiley.

Prinstein, M. J., & La-Greca, A. M. (2002). Peer crowd affiliation and internalizing distress in childhood and adolescence: A longitudinal follow-back study. *Journal of Research on Adolescence, 12*(3), 325–351.

Reiss, D., & Neiderhiser, J. M. (2000). The interplay of genetic influences and social processes in developmental theory: Specific mechanisms are coming into view. *Development and Psychopathology, 12,* 357–374.

Richardson, G. E. (2002). The metatheory of resilience and resiliency. *Journal of Clinical Psychology, 58*(3), 307–321.

Rizzo, T. A. (1988). The relationship between friendship and sociometric judgements of peer acceptance and rejection. *Child Study Journal, 18,* 161–191.

Rubinstein, J. S., Meyer, D. E., & Evans, J. E. (2001). Executive control of cognitive processes in task switching. *Journal of Experimental Psychology: Human Perception and Performance, 27*(4), 763–797.

Showers, C. (1992). Compartmentation of positive and negative self-knowledge: Keeping bad apples out of the bunch. *Journal of Personality and Social Psychology, 62,* 1036–1049.

Shulman, S., Margalit, M., Gadish, O., & Stuchiner, N. (1990). The family system of moderately mentally retarded children. *Journal of Mental Deficiency Research, 34,* 341–350.

Simon, D. A., & Bjork, R. A. (2001). Metacognition in motor learning. *Journal of Experimental Psychology: Learning, Memory and Cognition, 27*(4), 250–283.

Siperstein, G. N. (1992). Social competence: An important construct in mental retardation. *American Journal on Mental Retardation, 96*(4), 3–4.

Spitzberg, B. H., & Hurt, H. T. (1987). The relationship of interpersonal competence and skills to reported loneliness across time. In M. Hojat & R. Crandall (Eds.), Loneliness: Theory, research and applications [Special issue]. *Journal of Social Behavior and Personality, 2,* 157–172.

Sroufe, L. A., & Sampson, M. C. (2000). Attachment theory and systems concept. *Human Development, 43,* 321–326.

Taylor, A. R., Asher, S. R., & Williams, G. A. (1987). The social adaptation of mainstreamed mildly retarded children. *Child Development, 58,* 1321–1334.

Vitkus, J., & Horowitz, L. M. (1987). Poor social performance of lonely people: Lacking a skill or adopting a role? *Journal of Personality and Social Psychology, 52,* 1266–1273.

Weiss, R. S. (1973). *Loneliness: The experience of emotional and social isolation.* Cambridge: MIT Press.

Williams, G. A., & Asher, S. R. (1992). Assessment of loneliness at school among children with mild mental retardation. *American Journal of Mental Retardation, 96,* 373–385.

Winnicott, D. W. (1965). The capacity to be alone. In D. W. Winnicott (Ed.), *The maturation processes and the facilitating environment* (pp. 29–36). New York: International Universities Press.

Wood, B. L., Klebba, K. B., & Miller, B. D. (2000). Evolving the biobehavioral family model: The fit of attachment. *Family Process, 39*(3), 319–344.

Woodward, J. C., & Kalyan-Masih, V. (1990). Loneliness, coping strategies and cognitive styles of the gifted rural adolescent. *Adolescence, 25,* 977–988.

The Motivation to Maintain Subjective Well-Being: A Homeostatic Model

ROBERT A. CUMMINS

DEAKIN UNIVERSITY

ANNA L. D. LAU

HONG KONG POLYTECHNIC UNIVERSITY

Measuring quality of life through self-evaluation is a recent idea capturing much attention from both researchers and practitioners. Researcher interest stems from the formalization of subjective well-being (SWB) as a definable, measurable construct with theoretical characteristics that are slowly becoming understood. Practitioner interest stems from SWB offering an alternative to descriptions of economic conditions, physical health, or living conditions as a measure of life quality.

With this noted, it is also universally acknowledged that the field is in its infancy. Very few issues of definition, measurement, or conceptual structure have the status of general agreement. Therefore, this chapter will commence with a general discussion of nomenclature and instrumentation with a view to defining the descriptive terms and measurement procedures that underpin the subsequent discussion. This will be followed by an introduction to the idea that SWB is not free to vary in response to changing external conditions, but is held within an idiosyncratic range by a system of homeostasis.

A model for homeostasis will be proposed that comprises personality, a set of cognitive buffers, met and unmet needs, and adaptation. Motivation arises from conditions that challenge the maintenance of SWB and is strongly linked with two aspects of the model: personality and needs. It is linked to personality since this is responsible for the level at which SWB is normally maintained for each individual. Thus, people who normally have high levels of SWB will also have high levels of motivation to engage in personally enhancing activities. Unmet needs represent the cognitive manifestation of motivation in the model.

While the following text will make reference to the literature on intellectual disability wherever possible, most material will be drawn from other sources. This strategy reflects the authors' belief that the mechanisms for the maintenance of SWB do not operate differently for people with an intellectual disability than for any other group. Additionally, the literature within the area of disability is far too limited to provide unassisted support for understanding such a complex issue as the homeostatic control of well-being. The issue of well-being maintenance, however, is of vital importance to the disability field since the people concerned are at a higher than normal risk of experiencing a poor life quality. The reasons for this will become apparent as our description of the homeostatic system unfolds. But before embarking on this journey, we need to clarify issues of nomenclature.

I. ISSUES OF NOMENCLATURE AND MEASUREMENT

Anyone reading the quality-of-life literature will be struck by the inconsistent use of terminology. The words *quality of life* are used with such abandon that readers must delve into the text to ascertain the intended meaning. Other terms such as *happiness* and *well-being* are likewise afflicted. For this reason, it is necessary to explicitly define our own choice of nomenclature, as presented in the following text. We judge this taxonomy to be based on the majority opinion within the literature at this time.

It is widely acknowledged that, in agreement with Campbell et al. (1976), perceived well-being comprises both affect and cognition. The term SWB is used to describe this combined sensibility. Other terms describe a focus onto one process or the other. To take affect first, the most general term is *happiness* and can be measured either by the use of a simple question ('How happy are you with your life as a whole?') or by the use of more complex scales. The generation of such scales has traditionally been based around the subdivisions of *positive and negative affect*. However, recent literature illustrates this simple dichotomy as inadequate. Using the conceptualization represented by a circumplex model, affect has emerged as a two-dimensional structure. One dimension is emotional valence (positive or negative) while the other is activation (strong or weak) (Larson & Diener, 1992; Russell & Carroll, 1999; Watson & Tellegen, 1985). This understanding casts fresh doubt on the multitude of studies that have employed single-dimensional scales, such as the Positive and Negative Affect Scale (Watson et al., 1988) and the Affect Balance Scale (Bradburn, 1969). However, currently no commonly used bidimensional scale has emerged, although Huelsman et al. (1998) have generated a list of terms that could be used for this purpose.

In terms of the cognitive component, it is generally recognized that this part of SWB involves some form of internal comparison process. The precise nature of such comparisons is not entirely certain but the most complete description of possible contenders has been provided by the Multiple Discrepancies Theory (Michalos, 1985). This theory proposes comparisons with the self in the past, other people, and so on, and has received considerable support (e.g., Mellor et al., 1999). As one consequence, it is generally accepted that this cognitive component of well-being can be measured through questions of 'satisfaction'.

At the simplest level, this cognitive component can also be measured by a single question: 'How satisfied are you with your life as a whole?' This yields a measure of *life satisfaction*. In addition, it is now widely recognized that life satisfaction can be divided into a number of 'domains', representing the component areas of life experience, and that domain satisfaction, in aggregate, reflects life satisfaction (Campbell et al., 1976; Diener, 1984). How to precisely characterize such domains has yielded a wide variety of opinion. However, this situation has become less contentious in recent years, with many authors agreeing on the character of some central domains, such as those involving health, wealth, and relationships (e.g., Felce & Perry, 1995; Flanagan, 1978; Headey & Wearing, 1992). Two recent documents have consolidated such views. The International Association for the Scientific Study of Intellectual Disability (Schalock et al., 2000) and the International Society for Quality of Life Studies (Hagerty et al., 2001) have both reviewed quality-of-life measurement. They have separately agreed that domains should exhibit a number of defining characteristics. These include being both objectively and subjectively described, being parsimonious, and being descriptive of generic life areas.

One instrument that is consistent with these views is the Comprehensive Quality of Life Scale (ComQol) (Cummins, 1997a,b) which employs seven domains as material well-being: health, productivity, relationships, safety, community, and emotional well-being. (For a more detailed argument justifying these domains, see Cummins, 1996, 1997c). The aggregate of satisfaction across life domains yields Subjective Quality of Life (SQOL).

For a recent review of the ComQol scale and other instruments designed to measure the SWB of people with an intellectual disability, see Cummins (1997d). For a listing and brief description of available instruments to measure SWB for people in other population groupings and general population samples consult the *Directory of Instruments to Measure Quality of Life* (Cummins, 2001a), published on the web-site of the Australian Centre on Quality of Life (http//acqol.deakin.edu.au).

II. GENERIC VERSUS SPECIFIC INSTRUMENTATION

A glance through the above-referenced Directory will reveal over 600 instruments, many of which have been designed to measure the SWB of particular population subgroups. Notably, however, there is an absence of measures designed for subgroups who are relatively advantaged, such as 'people who own private yachts' or 'Olympic athletes'. Instead, specific instruments are inevitably designed to measure the SWB of people who are disadvantaged, due to some medical condition, low income, or congenital condition such as an intellectual disability. This has a number of unfortunate consequences. One is that such scales have a deficit orientation, such that a high score indicates a relative lack of disability, rather than a high quality of life. For example, the medical literature in this area is dominated by a poorly defined construct called 'health-related quality of life'. Depending on the scale that is employed, the measures involve disease symptoms, functional status, standards of care, patient perceptions of their health, and so on, often combined into a single scale. But such scales have little in common with SWB, even when they involve patient perceptions. A 'cancer' quality-of-life scale, for example, may inquire whether the respondent experiences nausea (e.g., see the European Organization for Research and Treatment of Cancer Quality of Life Questionnaire; Aaronson et al., 1993). Therefore, the absence of nausea contributes to a high quality of life as recorded by the scale. This brings into sharp focus the difference between such instruments and true SWB scales. The former have a deficit approach to quality of life, such that the maximum score indicates only that the respondent's well-being is not being compromised by their medical condition. True SWB scales, on the other hand, yield a score that can be referred to the normative distribution of SWB within the general population.

A similar state of affairs occurs within the area of intellectual disability. A recent review of scales designed to measure SWB through self-report (Ager & Hatton, 1999; Cummins, 1997d, 2001b) lists many scales that suffer the same interpretive limitations as the health-related quality-of-life scales. That is, they include items with a deficit orientation, such as the degree of autonomy or choice, which rarely feature in scales designed for the general population. Thus, in order to be valid, SWB scales for people with an intellectual disability must also be relevant to the general population. This allows the resultant scores to be compared against general population normative data, as has been demonstrated for the ComQol (Cummins, 1996, 1999).

III. NORMATIVE VALUES

One of the surprising features of both life satisfaction and SQOL is that their values can be described in terms of an empirical normative standard. This has been determined through a series of studies demonstrating that Western population mean scores for SQOL predictably lie within the range 70% to 80% of the scale maximum (%SM) (Cummins, 1995, 1996, 1998, 2003). The statistic %SM describes the conversion of Likert scale data to a range from 0 to 100. This conversion is simply made by a two-step process which allows the 'percentage' calculation to be based on the principle of a ratio scale commencing with 0. The steps are: (1) re-code the Likert scale scoring to commence with 0, thus, a scale scored 1 to 5 is recoded 0 to 4; and (2) a percentage is then calculated against the maximum scale score. For example, a score of 3 is calculated as $3/4 \times 100 = 75$ %SM.

When the mean values from general population surveys are recoded in this manner, and then combined as data, their mean and standard deviation can be described as 75 ± 2.5 %SM. Hence, the range 70 to 80 %SM describes two standard deviations around the mean and, thus, approximates the normative range for general population sample mean scores (Fig. 1). This

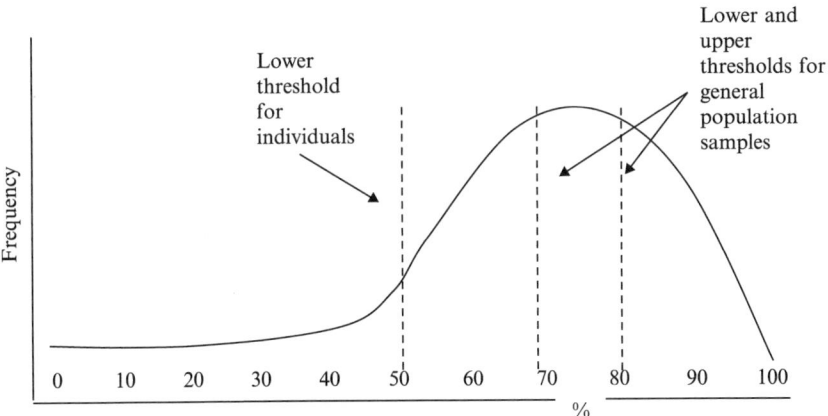

FIG. 1. The normal distribution of subjective quality of life.

distribution has been demonstrated for life satisfaction and SQOL measured by the Comprehensive Quality of Life Scale (Cummins, 1997a,b). While all other SWB scales seem to yield general population mean values that lie between 60 to 90 %SM (personal observation, Cummins), the distribution of only one other scale has been systematically studied. The Satisfaction With Life Scale (Diener et al., 1985) yields values 5 to 10 %SM below the 70 to 80 %SM range, and the reasons for this lie within the items comprising the scale (Pallant & Cummins, 2002).

The hypothesized range of 70 to 80 %SM for SQOL population mean scores has been confirmed by a variety of data. At the top end of the range, no samples yet discovered have a mean value that lies significantly above 80 %SM. For general population samples, the life satisfaction values for the Nordic countries, which are higher than all of the other countries, do not exceed this value (Cummins, 1995). In terms of population subgroups, one of the highest recorded levels of life satisfaction has been derived from people who are very rich, and their values also average to around 80 %SM (Cummins, 2000a). In an entirely different sphere of comparison, 'Back-to-the-Landers' in the U.S., the other subgroup with very high levels of life satisfaction, also has a mean value that approximates 80 %SM (Jacob & Brinkenhoff, 1999). The implication of such data is that group mean values for SQOL cannot be reliably held above 80 %SM. This has received quite explicit confirmation from Groot and VandenBrink (2000) who found that additional income made no difference to life satisfaction for people with minimum value of 80 %SM.

The lower threshold of 70 %SM has been verified through a detailed analysis of sample variance (Cummins, 2003). From Fig. 1 it can be predicted that as the mean value of samples descends below the threshold at 70 %SM, an increasing proportion of the sample has SQOL scores that lie in the lower distributional tail. The inclusion of these scores systematically increases the sample variance. This pattern of change in sample variance around 70 %SM has been confirmed (Cummins, 2003).

The values discussed so far represent calculations based on sample mean scores. The values for individuals show a broader distribution which appears sensitive to the measurement instrument. Life satisfaction as measured by a single question, shows a normative, within sample distribution, of 75 ± 18 %SM or a range of about 40 to 100 %SM (Cummins, 2003). The SQOL, as measured through the ComQol scale, shows a normative distribution of 75 ± 12 %SM, or a range of about 50 to 100 %SM (Cummins, 1999). This has been depicted in Fig. 1 by the vertical line at approximately 50 %SM demarcating two standard deviations (± 12 %SM) from the mean (75 %SM). Thus, in approximate terms, individual people generally maintain their SQOL within the positive sector of the %SM range.

From the data that have been presented, it can be seen that levels of SWB are predictable within the normative ranges described. Therefore, it is not surprising that authors have reported a high level of stability in SWB over time. For example, Bowling (1996) reported correlations of 0.46 to 0.65 in the life satisfaction of elderly people over a three-year period; Suh and Diener (1996) reported correlations of 0.56 and 0.61, respectively, for positive and negative affect in college students over a two-year period; Headey and Wearing (1989) report coefficients of 0.64, 0.51, and 0.52 when using their Life Satisfaction Index on a general population sample at two, four, and six years; while Costa and McCrae (1989) report correlations of 0.47 to 0.63 using a battery of SWB instruments over a two-year period.

These data, together with the predictable ranges of SQOL values, constitute converging evidence that SWB is not simply free to vary at the whim of personal circumstances, but it is managed. This idea, that SWB is under active internal control, is termed SWB homeostasis.

IV. SWB HOMEOSTASIS

The general idea of the proposed homeostatic system is that SWB is managed, for each individual, within a 'set-point-range' (Cummins, 2000b). That is, each person has an built-in 'set-point' for their normal level of SWB, as proposed by Headey and Wearing (1992), and their perceived SWB is normally held within a narrow range around this setting. This idea also involves the concept of threshold, as previously discussed, which we propose exists at the margins of the set-point-range. That is, as SWB approaches these margins, the homeostatic system resists further change and, if the threshold is exceeded, the homeostatic system fails and SWB comes under the control of the challenging agent. Over time, however, the homeostatic system works to regain control of SWB and to bring levels back to within the normal range for the individual person.

Empirical evidence for this proposition is available at the level of sample means. As has been described, Cummins (2003) found a systematic increase in variance as sample means fell below 70 %SM, the hypothesized lower threshold. In addition, 80 %SM appears to be the highest value that can be sustained by a representative sample.

At the level of individuals, homeostasis predicts that people who suffer some event that depresses their SWB below the threshold should improve their levels of SWB over time. This has been widely reported, for example, by people who have received a diagnosis of cancer (Bloom et al., 1991), who have received burns (Andreasen & Norris, 1972), and who have become paraplegic/tetraplegic (Bach & Tilton, 1994). However, all homeostatic systems have their limitations, and so it would also be expected that SWB recovery would be contingent on the residual discomfort or lost functional status not being overly severe. This limitation is exemplified by the variable degree of recovery shown by people with paraplegia/tetraplegia as reported in the preceding text. In fact, such recovery was restricted to people left with autonomous breathing. If they remained ventilator-assisted no significant SWB recovery occurred (Bach & Tilton, 1994).

This understanding, that the temporal stability of SWB depends on the severity of the challenging agent, allows a further prediction: that the stability of SWB, mentioned earlier, should be restricted to two broad groups. The first is those who have levels of SWB within their homeostatic range, and who experience no major event sufficient to disrupt homeostasis. The second is those who experience homeostatic defeat due to some chronic condition, like extreme poverty, to which they cannot adapt. The least stability should be evidenced by people who, at the time of initial measurement, were experiencing homeostatic defeat due to either a transitory event or to circumstances that could be accommodated over time by the processes of homeostasis.

Data consistent with these predictions have been reported by Landua (1992) in a large, longitudinal population study. He measured life satisfaction on a 0 to 10 scale, but then created response categories as 0 to 4, 5 to 6, 7 to 8, and 9 to 10. Measures were made at baseline and then four years later, when it was found that the following percentages of people had remained in their initial category: 11% (0 to 4), 50% (5 to 6), 63% (7 to 8), and 61% (9 to 10). Thus, as predicted, the greatest stability was recorded by people with an initial SWB of at least 70 %SM and the lowest stability by people who initially scored <40 %SM. These data are consistent with the idea that this low scoring group initially comprised a high proportion of people who were suffering homeostatic defeat due to either transitory events or circumstances that were amenable to adaptation. Thus, over the four-year interval, many of these people were able to re-establish homeostatic control, with the result that their life satisfaction moved above 40 %SM and out of the lowest response category.

A further set of predictions arises from a consideration of the thresholds depicted in Fig. 1. These allow the prediction that the correlation between SWB and extrinsic indicators will increase as SWB moves outside its normative set-point-range. Extrinsic in this context refers to perceptions that arise outside the homeostatic system. These may have their origins either external to the person, in terms of objective indices or life events, or within the person, such as in perception of pain.

Provided that the homeostatic system is not overly challenged by such extrinsic influences and the homeostatic system can adapt to their presence, they will have little discernable influence on SWB. However, as the strength of an extrinsic influence increases, at some value it will exceed the adaptive

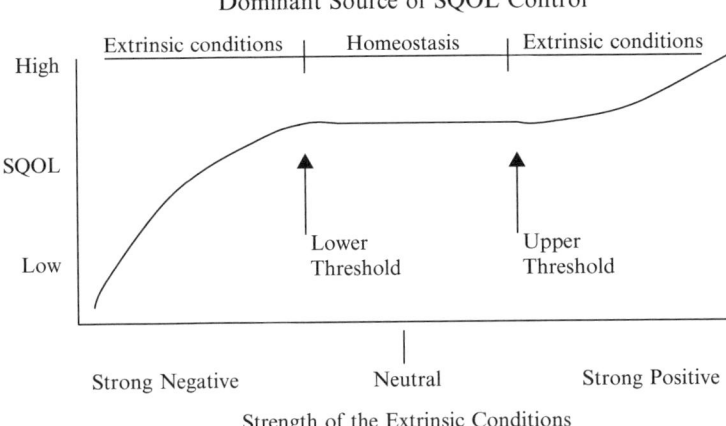

FIG. 2. The relationship between subjective and objective quality of life.

capacity of the homeostatic system, and the control of SWB will fall under the influence of the extrinsic agency. In other words, the plot of the relationship between the strength of the extrinsic agent and the value of SWB is curvilinear around each threshold, as depicted in Fig. 2.

Figure 2 describes the changing relationship between the strength of the external agencies and SQOL. It indicates that provided the strength of extrinsic agents remains at subthreshold (i.e., above the lower threshold and below the upper threshold), their variation will exert little systematic influence on SWB, which is held within its set-point-range. This will change, however, if the strength of the agents exceeds the homeostatic threshold. Once this happens, the extrinsic agents begin to wrest control of SWB away from the homeostatic system, causing SWB to rise or fall. As this occurs, the agencies and SQOL start to co-vary.

This theoretical understanding allows the following specific predictions:

1. Under maintenance conditions, where no threat to homeostasis can be recognized, there should be no systematic relationship between the objective circumstances of people's lives and their SWB. This is because homeostasis, not the extrinsic conditions, are controlling levels of SWB. This lack of relationship has been confirmed in an empirical review (Cummins, 2000c).

2. Under non-maintenance conditions where the homeostatic system is facing defeat, the relative strength of the relationship between extrinsic conditions and SWB changes. Here, the extrinsic conditions are the dominating force, defeating homeostasis and, thereby, wresting control of SWB by causing it to rise or fall. Under these conditions, the correlation

between SWB and the extrinsic condition is much enhanced, while the correlation between SWB and all aspects of the homeostatic system (to be described) consequentially fall.

Some evidence for this has also been presented in the review by Cummins (2000c) which demonstrated a generally higher correlation between SWB and objective variables under conditions of extrinsic threat. Further evidence can be deduced from studying the relationship between perceived health and physical health. Perceived health, as a component of SWB, is generally unrelated to physical health in general population samples due to the influence of homeostasis. Duckitt (1983), on the other hand, reported a high correlation between objective health and perceived health among elderly women. Such data are consistent with these women being under homeostatic threat from the compromised state of their physical health.

3. There will be a law of diminishing returns in the ability of improved objective conditions to cause an increase in SWB. That is, in conditions of marked deficit, many of the objective indicators will have the power to control SWB (e.g., chronic poverty, friendlessness, lack of safety, and so on). However, if such circumstances are improved to the point that they are no longer instrumental in causing homeostatic defeat, further improvements are predicted to have little further effect on SWB for two reasons. First, control has been returned to the homeostatic system, and so further improvements will be absorbed by the system, effectively holding the SWB output constant. Second, if a sudden, marked improvement occurs that exceeds the upper threshold, the processes of adaptation, to be described in Section IX, will quite rapidly diminish the impact of this new experience and, once again, return control to homeostasis.

An example of this latter phenomenon has been provided by Groot and VandenBrink (2000). They divided a large population sample into deciles on the basis of life satisfaction. True to prediction, they found that in the two deciles above 80 %SM, income had lost its ability to further increase life satisfaction.

This understanding has enormous implications for the use of SWB as a measure of outcome for people with an intellectual disability. It means that an intervention that succeeds in improving extrinsic conditions may or may not cause a concomitant increase in SWB. If the initial level of SWB represented a condition of homeostatic defeat then such an intervention could be expected to also raise SWB. On the other hand, if the initial level of SWB fell within the normal range of values, improved extrinsic circumstances will not be reflected in higher levels of SWB. For this reason, outcome measurement for interventions involving people with an intellectual disability should always include both objective and subjective measures.

In summary, a considerable body of data is consistent with the idea of a homeostatically controlled level of SWB. Not only does SWB appear to be held within a range characterized by upper and lower thresholds, but also deviations from this narrative range are characterized by instability and a heightened correlation between SWB and the responsible extrinsic agent. What is now required, in order to understand these ideas further, is an indication of the psychological processes that might comprise such a homeostatic system. Our model will now be described.

V. A MODEL FOR HOMEOSTASIS

The idea that SWB is maintained by the brain in some form of dynamic equilibrium has been proposed by several other authors (Headey & Wearing, 1989; Nieboer, 1997; Ormel, 1983; Ormel & Schanfeli, 1991). However, apart from a shared view that personality must be somewhere involved in such maintenance, these theorists have not attempted to explain the mechanisms that are responsible for such an equilibrium state. We will now attempt to fill this gap by outlining a model for the homeostatic control of SWB. This model is represented diagramatically in Fig. 3.

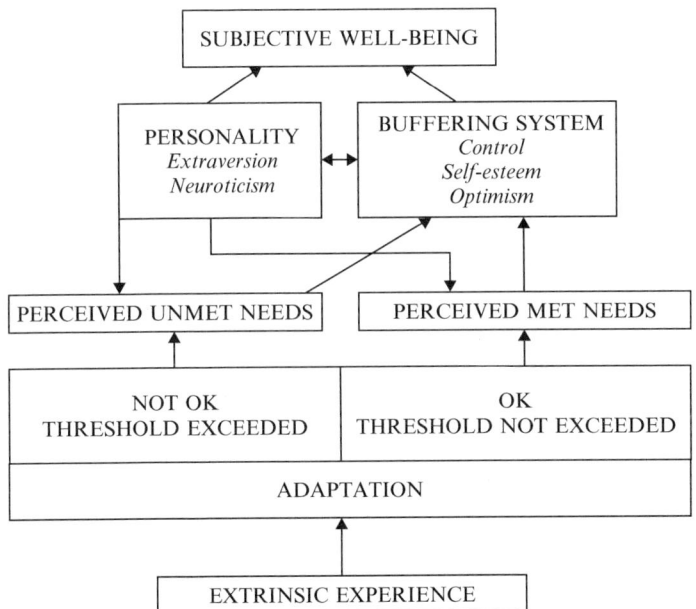

FIG. 3. A homeostatic model for subjective well-being.

This model proposes three levels of processing between some perceptual input that is extrinsic to the system and SWB, which is depicted as the output. The first level of processing constitutes the unconscious processes of adaptation and habituation. The second involves the conscious awareness of met and unmet needs. The third involves a system of cognitive 'buffers', designed to absorb the impact of changing need states in order to maintain a steady-state output, which is SWB. It also proposes that the second and third levels are strongly influenced by personality, which provides the affective balance underpinning conscious awareness. Thus, SWB is depicted as an output under the influence of personality, which provides the affective component, and the buffers, that provide the cognitive component.

Each of these processes will now be described in more detail. This description will commence with personality since this is proposed to influence the whole system, including responsibility for the set-point-range in SWB previously discussed.

VI. PERSONALITY

Within the literature there is strong, convergent evidence that personality is a major determinant of how happy or sad people feel with their lives. On the basis of his longitudinal studies involving people with an intellectual disability, esteemed ethnographer Robert Edgerton (1990) concluded:

> "The pattern that emerges again and again is that people who were happy and hopeful 10, 20, or even 30 years ago remain so no matter what ill-fortune they suffer; and those who were sad or negative about life do not change even though their environment improves significantly. The data clearly indicate that major life stressors or major gratifications can bring about changes in affect and expressed life satisfaction, but these changes are short-lived.
>
> Counterintuitive as this finding may seem to those like myself who believe in the causal power of environmental factors, these data support that internal dispositions—call them temperament for want of a better term—are better predictors of people's satisfaction with the quality of their lives than are objective environmental variables" (p. 156–157).

Quantitative data have overwhelmingly confirmed this view, most particularly with respect to the two personality dimensions of extraversion and neuroticism. Practically all of the many studies that have looked at the relationship between these dimensions and SWB have found a robust correlation. This has led to the 'top-down' hypothesis, such that SWB is substantially influenced by personality (e.g., Mallard et al., 1997).

As a consequence of this understanding and other research to be cited later, Fig. 3 depicts personality as underpinning the model by delivering a constant, background level of affect to the system (Carver, 2000). This acts at three levels. First, it constitutes a direct effect on SWB. Second, it creates a set-point-range for the operation of the cognitive buffers which, in turn, maintain SWB within this range despite fluctuations in needs (Fig. 3). Third, it impacts on the need to influence the level of arousal and, hence, motivation. However, before considering the nature of these links it is important to clarify the relationship between personality and affect, most particularly in relation to the construct of motivation.

It can also be noted at this point, that Fig. 3 indicates an influence of the homeostatic system on personality. While this is clearly against the conventional view (e.g., McCrae & Costa, 1995) that personality traits are stable in adulthood due to their strong degree of genetic determination (e.g., Jang et al., 1996; Macaskill et al., 1994; Saudino et al., 1999), it reflects the outcome of a recent meta-analysis reported by Roberts and DelVecchio (2000). These authors concluded that while traits are mostly consistent in adulthood they do retain a dynamic quality and, therefore, are not immutable. The extent of this influence is, however, not reliably determined at this stage.

A. Personality and Affect

The dimensions of personality that seem crucial to an understanding of the homeostatic system are neuroticism and extraversion. Both dimensions are intimately linked with affect and, for the purpose of this discussion, neuroticism will be considered roughly equivalent to negative affectivity, while extraversion will be considered roughly equivalent to positive affectivity (Fogarty et al., 1999; Watson & Clark, 1992; Wilson & Gullone, 1999).

A good description of negative affectivity has been provided by Brief, Butcher, George, and Link (1993) as

"a mood-dispositional dimension that reflects pervasive individual differences in negative emotionality and self-concept" (p. 647).

In particular, people high on negative affectivity are nervous, apprehensive, irritable, overly sensitive, and emotionally labile (Watson & Pennebaker, 1989), as well as having a more negative worldview, rating peers less favorably, and experiencing a wide variety of negative emotions in the absence of known stressors (Elliott et al., 1994). They also have a tendency to experience anxiety, dysthymia, and depression. In confirmation of the unidimensional nature of these negative affective states, they all tend to covary (e.g., Abbey & Andrews, 1985; Depue & Montoe, 1986; Hunt et al., 1967; Watson & Pennebaker, 1989; Watson et al., 1995). Thus, for the purpose of this discussion, neuroticism will be considered as the source of constitutional negative affect influencing the homeostatic system.

Extraversion, as the source of constitutional positive affect, appears as the natural opposing force to neuroticism, and it seems reasonable to suggest that it is the balance between these two personality dimensions that provides the set-point-range for SWB. It can also be seen from Fig. 3 that personality is depicted as having both a direct and an indirect influence on SWB (see the following text). This is consistent with the hierarchical view of the relationship between personality, affect, and 'mood' proposed by Wakefield (1989). In this scheme, extraversion and neuroticism are considered primary traits, positive and negative affectivity as secondary traits, and 'mood' is considered as a state (also see Nemanick & Munz, 1997). Thus, SWB is seen as being under the influence of both personality, which provides the affective component, and the cognitive buffers, which reflect the self in interaction with extrinsic factors.

B. Direct and Indirect Links With SWB

There is general agreement in the literature that extraversion is positively correlated with happiness (e.g., Argyle & Lu, 1990; Diener et al., 1992; Francis, 1999) and life satisfaction (e.g., Doyle & Youn, 2000). There is also agreement that neuroticism is negatively correlated with happiness (e.g., Francis, 1999; Lu & Shih, 1997) and life satisfaction (e.g., Brief Butcher et al., 1993). These relationships are consistent with the affectivity link mentioned earlier. However, Fig. 3 also depicts an indirect link between personality and SWB, mediated by the buffering systems of perceived control, self-esteem, and optimism. The evidence for this indirect link will now be examined.

Two studies provide such evidence in relation to neuroticism. In the first, Brief et al. (1993) found an indirect effect (and no direct effect) of negative affectivity on life satisfaction, mediated by perceived health, which included 'the extent of physical discomfort or limitation'. The second, by Lu and Shih (1997), found an indirect effect (and a direct effect) of neuroticism on happiness mediated by mental health, which included the reporting of somatic symptoms. Thus, if it is assumed that both perceived physical limitations and the presence of somatic symptoms contain elements of perceived control, then an interpretation of both of these studies is that the buffer of perceived control is influenced by neuroticism. This will be discussed further in Section VII.

Another indicator that personality exerts an indirect effect on SWB is that high levels of neuroticism attenuate the influence of positive experiences on overall mood. Just such an indirect influence was reported by Elliott et al. (1994) who found that, among individuals high in negative affectivity, social support (a met need) had an attenuated ability to relieve depression. Such attenuation, coupled with the dominating influence of neuroticism, can be hypothesized to make such people highly susceptible to stressful influences. Thus, as described by Flynn and Cappeliez (1993), this negativity bias, or loss of the normal positivity bias, actually makes it more difficult for people to recover normal homeostatic functioning because they enter a downward spiral. The loss of positivity bias leads to a heightened state of reality awareness within the cognitive buffers. As a consequence people perceive more clearly not only their inability to meet the demands of the situation, but also that the situation is unlikely to improve. In turn, this engenders self-denigration, social-withdrawal, and further dysphoria, eventually leading into depression.

The indirect link between positive affectivity and SWB can also be demonstrated. Here it is proposed that extraversion acts on the buffers and the perception of met needs, thereby constituting what Flynn and Cappeliez (1993) term 'protective factors' for the person's well-being. These factors are high self-perceived social competence, high learned resourcefulness, a perceived high frequency of pleasant events, and the perceived availability of a close and immediate confidant. Thus, it might be expected that such protective factors would reinforce one another, and so co-vary, in much the same manner as described for the components of negative affectivity. This is, indeed, the case. For example, internal control and social performance correlate positively (Abbey & Andrews, 1985) while in a meta-analysis. DeNeve and Cooper (1998) report an average correlation >0.3 between the following traits: trust, emotional stability, desire for control, hardiness (the tendency to cope positively with life events), and positive affectivity.

In summary, and as also argued by Fyrand et al. (1997), on the basis of structural modelling, the personality traits of neuroticism and extraversion seem likely to be causally related to levels of SWB through both direct and indirect links involving the cognitive buffers and met needs.

C. Strength of Relationship Between Personality and SWB

To what extent can personality predict SWB? No consensus has yet emerged. Estimates range from very low and ambiguous degrees of relationship (Diener & Larsen, 1984) to strong correlations. For example,

Sandvik et al. (1993) concluded that, among their sample of college students, about one-half of the variance in SWB could be attributed to personality and stable environmental conditions. The reason for such wide differences of opinion is that such an estimation is likely dependent on many other considerations:

1. The similarity of the SWB measure to trait affect (for example, see the review by DeNeve, 1999). For example, positive affect can be expected to show a stronger correlation with extraversion than with life satisfaction. Indeed, in studies where extraversion and neuroticism are used as covariates, they appear to negate the influence of positive and negative affect on some other measure of well-being. This was demonstrated by Fogarty et al. (1999) in relation to job satisfaction.

2. The degree to which the personality variables reflect extraversion or neuroticism as opposed to the other factors of personality. For example, Edwards (1998) reports that within a meta-analysis involving a very heterogeneous collection of 137 'personality' traits, they found an average correlation with SWB of 0.19. Clearly this is less than would be expected using either measures of extraversion or neuroticism as the correlates. In a similar vein, Fogarty et al. (1999) found strong correlations between job satisfaction and both extraversion and neuroticism, but weak correlations with the personality factors of openness, agreeableness, and conscientiousness.

3. Homeostasis theory predicts that the correlations should be maximal in samples with normal levels of SWB where no obvious source of threat to well-being is in operation. This is because, under such conditions, the level of SWB should be minimally affected by extrinsic influences, and so its value should most closely reflect the set-point-range managed by personality. Under extrinsic threat conditions, on the other hand, the control of SWB is predicted to shift, first, to the homeostatic system of buffers, and then when homeostasis is defeated, to the threatening agent itself, as it causes SWB to fall below its normal range (Fig. 2).

Evidence for such a shift in the control of SWB can be deduced from the study by Duckitt (1983) on elderly women. Consistent with the expectation that this sample would be under homeostatic threat due to poor medical health, a high correlation was found between objective and perceived health. Moreover, personality did not correlate with perceived health after objective health had been partialled out, thus further emphasizing the dominance of objective health over SWB. It was also found that life satisfaction and life events remained correlated with perceived health even after objective health had been partialled out. This indicates the continued association between measures of SWB (life satisfaction and perceived health) as expected from a 'bottom-up' model. Moreover, the continual influence of life events on perceived health after partialling out objective health, can also be explained in terms of the model as follows: because the homeostatic buffers had been defeated by poor objective health, the system had little capacity to absorb the impact of other negative events so that they also exerted a direct effect to reduce life satisfaction.

So, in the light of all of this it seems that the strength of the relationship between personality and SWB will be situationally variable and will depend on the nature of the measures employed. In corroboration of this view, Diener et al. (1999) conclude from their review of this area, that while it is clear that personality and SWB are linked, no simple general estimate of the strength of this linkage can be made. However, it is possible that if samples were separated on the basis of their relative degree of homeostatic threat, more consistent estimates may be possible.

D. Personality, Needs, and Motivation

The issue of motivation in the field of intellectual disability has been generally neglected (Switzky, 2003). Yet, as this author states:

"Personality and motivational self-system processes are the fulcrum around which all other psychological, educational, and self-regulatory processes rotate to energize behavior and performance in mentally retarded persons" (Switzky, 1999, p. 70).

The above quotation, which leads to a major review of this topic (Switzky, 1999), clearly places personality at the center of operations. This view is consistent with the role of personality depicted in Fig. 3 and, most importantly from a motivational viewpoint, it is consistent with the proposed influence of personality on the strength of met and unmet needs. The evidence for such a genetic link appears to be strongest in relation to perceived social support (e.g., Bergeman et al., 1991). This link has special significance in terms of the model since it may represent the simplest connection between personality and motivation, as can be seen from the powerful study by Lucas et al. (2000).

These authors studied extraversion with particular attention to the facet of 'sociability', as the enjoyment of social activities, preference for being with others, and 'reward sensitivity'. This latter term depicts an underlying motivational system characterized by a strong Behavioural Activating System (Gray, 1970) which regulates reactions to positive stimuli. According to Depue and Collins (1999), the operation of this system can be described in the following terms:

"Exposure to ... incentive stimuli (or activation of their central representation) elicits an incentive emotional state that facilitates and guides approach behaviour to a goal. In humans, incentive motivational states are associated with strong positive affect characterized by feelings of desire, wanting, excitement, energy, potency, and self-efficacy" (p. 495).

Thus, it can be seen that the role of the Behavioural Activating System is to motivate and guide goal directed behavior. This is consistent with the general view, offered by many authors (e.g., Avia, 1997; Izard, 1993), that one of the main functions of the emotional system is to motivate specific response patterns which are related to feelings of positive affect.

Lucas et al. (2000) provide compelling evidence that the sociability facets of extraversion form a higher-order factor of reward sensitivity. The facets they identified are: affiliation (enjoying and valuing close interpersonal bonds, being warm and affectionate); ascendance (feeling dominant or being an exhibitionist); venturesome (feelings of excitement seeking and desire for change); and social interaction (preference for social interaction). Thus, it is proposed that these facets of extraversion form an aspect of motivation (reward sensitivity) which reflects the degree to which people are motivated by the prospect of a reward.

They then ask why reward sensitivity is linked to the enhanced sociability of extraverts, and provide an interesting answer: social situations involving warmth, affection, and close emotional bonds, are especially rewarding. Thus, the increased sociability of extraverts (e.g., Argyle & Lu, 1990) is simply a by-product of greater sensitivity to rewards. This is not to say, however, that such increased sensitivity is confined to social situations. As these authors also note, extraverts tend to feel more positive affect even when they are alone (e.g., Diener et al., 1992), but there does appear to be some special motivational power attributable to social rewards.

They offer an interesting piece of confirmatory evidence which draws on cross-cultural data. As Lucas et al. (2002) note, social contact may serve different purposes in different cultures. For example, while within individualistic cultures people are more likely to seek social interaction because it is rewarding, in collectivistic cultures a more central goal may be group harmony. In confirmation of social reward sensitivity, while extraversion and positive affect correlated in samples from both cultures, the relationship was less in collectivist samples. Thus, they conclude:

"sensitivity to rewards, rather than sociability, forms the core of extraversion" (p. 466).

It seems possible that this differential reward sensitivity may also explain why extraverts appear to experience more positive events (Headey et al., 1985) and more adverse events (Headey & Wearing, 1989). That is, people who are sensitive to rewards seek more interaction with their environment and, subsequently, experience more 'events'. The fact that these authors found that favorable and adverse events kept happening to the same people over time is further evidence that reward sensitivity represents a stable personality characteristic, linked to met and unmet needs. The influence of reward sensitivity can also be linked, via personality, to SWB. Assuming that such sensitivity facilitates a search for affiliation, then such activity has been reported to produce a positive feedback cycle in which the searching behavior and SWB are mutually reinforcing to one another (Filipp & Klauer, 1991). Thus, as also concluded by DeNeve (1999), relationship-enhancing traits are important for SWB maintenance.

The linkage between neuroticism and needs is less established. However, such a connection has been supported by Fyrand et al. (1997) who found a strong correlation, among people with arthritis, between depression and the lack of social support (an unmet need). However, the relationship virtually disappeared after the effects of neuroticism were removed. The authors conclude that neuroticism therefore, may have caused the perceived lack of social support.

In summary, a case can certainly be made that the two personality dimensions of extraversion and neuroticism are intimately related to levels of SWB. The nature of the relationship has been argued to be both direct and indirect. The direct link involves a constant background level of affect. The indirect links with SWB are made through the cognitive buffers (discussed in the next section) and met/unmet needs. These links, together with the direct supply of affect, are argued to create the stable set-point-range for individual levels of well-being. The case has also been argued that extraversion is strongly implicated in the creation of motivation, most particularly by way of generating a sensitivity to social rewards. Thus, personality has a powerful role in the maintenance of SWB through the supply of a steady level of affect and the generation of reward motivation.

VII. THE COGNITIVE BUFFERING SYSTEM

In a recent review, DeNeve (1999) found overwhelming evidence that the way people think about and explain what happens in their lives is intimately tied to levels of SWB. We have attempted to operationalize this pathway to SWB by proposing a tripartite system of cognitive buffers that involves perceived control, self-esteem, and optimism (Cummins & Nistico, 2002). Each of these components will now be considered.

A. Perceived Control

There is a broadly held view that perceived control is central to the life quality of people with an intellectual disability (e.g., Brown, 1996; Romney et al., 1994; Tonkens & Weijers, 1999) and the most common classification system for perceived control is its division into internal and external locus of control (Rotter, 1966). Internal control describes a perception that control over an event rests with the person. External control attributes such control to an external agency, such as luck or some powerful other person or force. At least within Western culture, it is generally assumed that people prefer internal control, and so the presence of external control is indicative that the person is attempting to cope with events that lie outside their sphere of actual control. Kaplan De-Nour (1981), for example, reported higher levels of external control among people on dialysis than the general population.

Perceived control is proposed to operate as a cognitive buffer in the following manner. Under normal conditions, where the person believes their environment is under their control, they will evidence internal control. This, in turn, reinforces SWB. Thus, Phares (1978) in a review on this topic describes:

> "the typical internal to be one who actively comes to grips with the world. Compared to the external, the internal is resistant to social pressure and dedicated to the pursuit of excellence" (p. 295).

However, the extrinsic environment cannot always be perceived as under one's personal control, such as when negative life events must be endured. This is when the perception of external control can act as a buffer. That is, if negative life events were simply accepted as evidence of a complete loss of control this would be indicative of helplessness and very damaging to SWB. On the other hand, if such events can be understood as simply bad luck (the event is unlikely to recur) or the will of God (there is a higher, but not understood purpose underlying the event), then the negative feelings associated with the event can be reduced, and the impact on SWB diminished. This is the proposed role of external control, not to directly enhance SWB but to buffer the potential negative impact of negative life events.

The capacity of the buffer, however, is limited in this regard, and this capacity will be exceeded by either a strong or protracted negative event. As a consequence, high levels of external control will most commonly be linked to a measurable reduction in SWB, even though the model predicts such a reduction to be less than would be the case in the absence of the external control buffer.

These predictions can be readily confirmed. For example, a high internal locus of control has been linked to happiness (Kopp & Ruzicka, 1993; Mullis, 1992) and life satisfaction (Cvetanovski & Jex, 1994; Lewinsohn et al., 1991; Sloper et al., 1991). Conversely, a low internal locus of control has been linked to anxiety (Cvetanovski & Jex, 1994; Lefcourt, 1976; Rawson, 1992) and general malaise (Sloper et al., 1991).

A low internal locus of control has also been linked to depression (e.g., Cvetanovski & Jex, 1994; Lefcourt, 1976; Rawson, 1992). This is consistent with the pattern of relationships between variables that has been described, and also the view of a fragile buffer system that has lost much of its resilience to external challenge, a view also proposed by Lefcourt (1976).

Such data have particular relevance to people with an intellectual disability. These people are more likely to experience low levels of control due to institutionalized living conditions (e.g., Iahoda & Cattermole, 1995), low autonomy within their family environment (Brown & Timmons, 1994), or poor coping skills for life within the general community (Tymchuk, 1991). As a consequence of this unmet need, people with disabilities commonly regard their level of independence as a major issue in their lives (Disability Services Victoria, 2000) and this chronically experienced lack of control threatens the integrity of the homeostatic system, as has been described in the preceding text.

B. Control and Personality

According to the model, perceived control is heavily influenced by personality and yet distinct from the personality factors. Evidence for this comes from the review by Lefcourt (1976) who concluded that, while locus of control can be changed by intervention or circumstances, there is little evidence for the persistence of such changes. This is consistent with a role for personality in setting the resting level of perceived internal control, and returning control to such levels following homeostatic defeat, an analogous argument to that mounted with respect to the set-point-range of SWB. Indeed, since SWB is envisaged as the direct output of the cognitive buffers (Fig. 3), personality is proposed to generate an equivalent set-point-range for each of the control, self-esteem, and optimism buffers.

It would also be expected that high internal control would be related to behaviors consistent with extraversion, since both are being proposed as links to the maintenance of SWB. This has been supported by Abbey and Andrews (1985) who found that high internal locus of control related positively to social performance.

C. Control and the Other Buffers

If it is assumed that the three identified buffers work together as a system, then it would be expected they would show a strong positive relationship to one another. This pattern has generally been found among people under no apparent systematic threat in relation to locus of control and self-esteem (Kopp & Ruzicka, 1993; Ralph et al., 1995).

Within samples which may be expected to be suffering challenge from an extrinsic threat, the expected situation is less clear. The issue revolves around the question of whether the three buffering systems buffer one another? The evidence is as follows.

Positive significant relationships:

- Locus of control and self-esteem: people with an intellectual disability (Mattika, 1996), people who are unemployed (Cvetanovski & Jex, 1994), and at-risk adolescents (Enger et al., 1994).
- Locus of control, self-esteem, and optimism (Sanna, 1996; Scheier & Carver, 1985; Shepperd et al., 1996).

Non-significant relationships:

- Locus of control and self-esteem: children with emotional behavior problems (Rawson, 1992).

It can be concluded that these data are generally supportive of the proposition that the buffers are functionally linked with one another.

D. Self-Esteem

The construct of self-esteem must be one of the most researched in psychology. Even by 1970 over 2000 articles had been published on the topic (Rosenberg, 1979) and its popularity among researchers currently remains high. Because of this extraordinary degree of attention, the construct has been dissected and examined in elaborate detail, with substantial argument being devoted to the distinction between self-concept and self-esteem (e.g., Hattie, 1992) and the character of putative subdomains (e.g., James, 1892; Luk & Bond, 1992). However, such distinctions are very marginally relevant to this review. Here, we will consider self-concept and self-esteem as synonyms, as also suggested by Josephs et al. (1992) and Marsh (1994), and we will regard the construct as a single factor, consistent with the most commonly used scale (Rosenberg, 1968).

It is generally agreed that self-esteem is a cognition (Sherwood, 1965) employed to evaluate our overall worthiness by comparing our perceived self against our ideal self (Endo, 1992). Included in this self-evaluation is personal dignity and merit (Chrzanowski, 1981), social confidence and ability (Fleming & Courtney, 1984), capability and success (Coopersmith, 1981), and personal respect (Rosenberg, 1968). While such self-evaluations could be made in relation to any number of self-situations, in fact they are dominated by social interaction with family and friends (Josephs et al., 1992; Medora et al., 1993; Sherwood, 1965) much along the lines of Festinger's (1954) social comparison theory. It should also be noted that self-esteem has particular relevance to the area of intellectual disability since it has been linked to adaptive personality characteristics (Glick, 1999) and the motivation to develop effective coping strategies (Switzky, 1997) that are so crucial to the maintenance of SWB.

Several previous authors have overtly considered self-esteem to be a determinant of SWB (e.g., Pugliesi, 1988) while many more infer the presumed direction of causation. Certainly its link to SWB is legendary, with most authors reporting correlations that are so high (e.g., Boschen, 1996 [0.77]; Coyle et al., 1994 [0.62]; Ralph et al., 1995 [0.78]) that Diener and Diener (1995) were moved to report a study establishing that the constructs were discriminable from one another. The link between SWB and self-esteem has also been reported for people with an intellectual disability (Mattika, 1996), which reinforces the importance of self-esteem maintenance since such people may frequently encounter negative life experiences that threaten their self-esteem and, therefore, their SWB (Weisz, 1981; Zigler, 1971).

In terms of its description as a homeostatic device, Kitayama, Markus, Matsumoto, and Norasakkunkit (1997) have noted the 'numerous studies' that demonstrate a robust and pervasive tendency to maintain and enhance self-esteem. This maintenance, according to Verkuyten (1993) is derived through the interaction of three processes: social comparison (Festinger, 1954); symbolic interaction, in which people come to view themselves as significant others see them (Cooley, 1902); and self-attribution, in which people gain a sense of self from their own actions (Gecas & Schwalbe, 1983). Thus, self-esteem can be viewed as a robust device drawing on many sources for its maintenance, especially social interaction.

The centrality of self-esteem as a homeostatic device has been reinforced through the finding that people with high self-esteem show SWB resilience in the face of negative life events (e.g., DuBois et al., 1998; Long & Spears, 1998). Moreover, Brown and Mankowski (1993) have provided further understanding of the cognitive processes involved. They argue that people with low self-esteem react to events in an even-handed fashion. That is, positive events produce positive reactions and negative events produce negative reactions. This is not so, however, for people with high self-esteem.

Such people embrace positive events but reject, limit, or offset negative events. As a consequence their reactions to negative events are less severe.

Given the aforementioned connections and consequences of self-esteem, it is not difficult to imagine that high self-esteem is self-perpetuating through the kinds of behavior such people are motivated to perform. Consider, for example, the following paraphrased from Coopersmith (1967, pp. 70–71):

> "people with high self-esteem approach tasks and persons with the expectation that they will be well received and successful, they follow their own judgement and consider novel ideas, they hold a conviction they are correct and the courage to express those convictions, they have high social independence and creativity, are assertive and likely to take 'vigorous social actions'. They are more likely to be participants then listeners in group discussions, report less difficulty in forming friendships, have a lack of self-consciousness, and a lack of preoccupation with personal problems."

The tight link between self-esteem and SWB mentioned earlier seems easy to understand in the light of such attributes.

E. Self-Esteem and Motivation

Since high self-esteem is associated with so many desirable behavioral attributes, as well as with high SWB, it could be imagined that people with low self-esteem might be motivated to achieve higher levels. This has been formulated as Self-Enhancement Theory (Shrauger, 1975). However, there is little evidence to support this proposition. On the contrary, people with low self-esteem have lower overall motivation to engage life (e.g., Baumeister et al., 1989; Klein, 1995; Neugarten et al., 1961) and employ cognitive strategies that allow them to feel comfortable with a relatively disengaged lifestyle.

This idea was formalized as Self-Consistency Theory (Lecky, 1945) and is consistent with self-esteem having a high level of determination from personality, and to employ buffering strategies consistent with the self-esteem set-point-range. From this perspective, people with high self-esteem exhibit more self-enhancing biases because such biases strengthen the self-image. Such biases, on the other hand, would be threatening to the self-image of people with less positive self-views. Thus, as argued by Brown, Bayer, and Brown (1988), both high and low self-esteem people engage in the process of self-enhancement, but they do so in different ways. People with high self-esteem engage in direct forms of self-enhancement. The self is linked to positive identities and outcomes, and such people over-evaluate their own product rather than devaluing the out-group product. People with low self-esteem, on the other hand, engage in indirect forms of self-enhancement. The self is only indirectly linked to positive identities and outcomes by virtue of one's association with others. These people show little evaluation of their own product but derogate the out-group product (e.g., Hogg & Sunderland, 1991).

In summary, both high and low self-esteem is associated with motivation to engage in particular behaviors and cognitive strategies. The precise behaviors, however, differ between the two groups and, most importantly, are directed to maintain the status quo. In other words, self-esteem has a strong personality component (Campbell et al., 1976; Hattie, 1992) which makes it quite stable over time (e.g., Block & Robins, 1993; O'Malley & Bachman, 1979).

However, self-esteem does exhibit short-term variation due to either intentional intervention (e.g., Omizo et al., 1992) or life events, and several authors have suggested self-esteem lability as a predictive index for depression (e.g., Butler et al., 1994; Roberts & Gotlib, 1997). This is interesting and consistent with the homeostatic model. Low self-esteem would be predicted to correlate with low values for the other two buffers (see section 6.1.2), reflecting a weak buffering system that is susceptible to homeostatic defeat by negative live events. Thus, the level of self-esteem should be highly and negatively correlated with depressive symptoms; this has been found to be the case (e.g., Lau et al., 1998; Penland et al., 2000; Rawson, 1992).

Low self-esteem may also, of course, reflect homeostatic defeat due to the chronic imposition of strongly negative life circumstances Such a reduction has been reported, for example, among mothers who are intellectually disabled, due to their chronic exposure to circumstances involving low levels of perceived control (Tymchuk, 1991). In such a condition, where the level of self-esteem reflects extrinsic circumstances rather than personality, the Self-Enhancement Theory, previously dismissed as being applicable to normative samples, may come into its own. That is, it predicts a personality-derived motivation to restore self-esteem to the appropriate set-point-range.

Some evidence in support of such an idea has been provided by Engel (1959), who studied the self esteem of adolescents over a two-year period. It was found that those with a high initial self-esteem, who were in the top 20%, had a significantly more stable self-esteem than those who initially presented in the bottom 20%. If it is assumed that the lower, but not the higher 20%, included some adolescents with an extrinsically-driven level of self-esteem, these findings are consistent with the operation of Self-Enhancement Theory for such individuals.

In summary, self-esteem is linked to the other components depicted in Fig. 3 in a manner consistent with the model. It is strongly linked to personality and to the other cognitive buffers, and appears to be a powerful determinant of SWB. It also has a robust tendency for self-maintenance that is linked to motivation in such a manner as to perpetuate the set-point-range levels of self-esteem for the individual.

F. Optimism

Optimism is defined as a perception that the future will be to the perceiver's advantage or for their pleasure (for an elaboration, see Peterson, 2000; Tiger, 1979). General population studies have consistently shown that people view themselves on an upward path of 'life getting better', with the past remembered as less good than the present, and the future anticipated as being better still (Bortner & Hultsch, 1970; Cantril, 1965; Gallup, 1998), even though the strength of this effect may diminish in elderly people (Ryff, 1991; Shmotkin, 1991). The effect may also apply to domain-level satisfactions. For example, Vaillant and Vaillant (1993) demonstrated a present > past bias in marital satisfaction.

The most substantial empirical demonstration of optimism as a positive cognitive bias has been provided by Glatzer (1991) who reported the results of a large, general population, longitudinal study conducted in West Germany between 1978 and 1984. On each of three occasions people were asked to rate their life satisfaction as they remembered it to be five years ago, in the present, and as they anticipated it would be five years hence. The mean scores, in %SM units, were as follows: past (73, 71, 74), present (78, 77, 77), and future (80, 75, 76). These data do not confirm the future bias, perhaps due to the prevailing uncertainty in the country at that time. The present > past bias is clearly evident, however, and is consistent with the idea that the optimism buffer helps to maintain SWB through a downward comparison with the past.

Measures of optimism, usually made through the Life Orientation Test (Scheier & Carver, 1985), behave in very similar ways to the other two buffers, as previously described. In the first place, optimism shows a high and robust relationship with internal control and self-esteem (see Section VII). It also shows a strong link with personality, as argued by Tiger (1979) and Peterson (2000) in their major reviews of this topic. Moreover, as expected, it is predictive of life satisfaction (e.g., Fitzgerald et al., 1993) and relates inversely to depression (e.g., Pyszczynski et al., 1987; Scheier & Carver, 1985).

The buffering aspect of optimism lies within the global expectation that things are going to get better with time. Thus, the impact of negative events on SWB is reduced by the prospect that the difficulties that are being experienced will not last. Thus, O'Brien et al. (1995) found optimists to both underestimate their susceptibility to health problems and to report lower levels of stress and physical symptoms. Interestingly, however, their frequency of preventative health behaviors was not different from non-optimists. Thus, even though they under-report negatively valanced events, due to the effectiveness of their buffering system, this did not prevent them from processing and acting on relevant health information in an appropriate and adaptive manner. It must also be acknowledged, however, that optimism may be a risk factor for failure in some situations when it combines with a lack of motivation (e.g., Klaczynski & Fauth, 1996).

In summary, the buffers appear to display the necessary characteristics to justify their role as depicted in Fig. 3. Each one has strong links consistent with SWB being a product of both the buffers and personality, as has been previously described. In addition, each buffer shows a strong link to personality, consistent with the proposition that the interaction between extraversion and neuroticism provides an affective balance that maintains the operation of these buffers within their set-point-range. Finally, the three buffers strongly influence one another, consistent with them constituting a single buffer system for the purpose of SWB output. While it has also been argued that these buffers, through the influence of personality, can be linked to motivation, the most central source of motivation is likely to be the cognitive appraisal of needs.

VIII. MET AND UNMET NEEDS

A seemingly obvious determinant of SWB involves met and unmet needs. This connection has been made by many authors (e.g., Avia, 1997), who propose that well-being arises when events contribute to the meeting of needs and the realization of goals. However, in the proposed scheme of Fig. 3, well-being is depicted as having only an indirect relationship to met needs. In this model, met needs act to enhance the positive buffers, which then yield an elevated sense of SWB. In order to explain this indirect scheme, the theories proposing a direct link between needs and SWB will be examined first.

It is generally accepted that the main purpose of needs is to provide motivation, and this idea has been commonly described within the quality-of-life literature as 'Person-Environment Fit' (e.g., Andrews & Withey, 1976; Edwards & Rothbard, 1999; French et al., 1974). Within such schemes, satisfaction stems from the degree of congruence between the environment, as the person perceives it, and the person's needs or aspirations. Such theories link to the idea that satisfaction is a product of the congruence between multiple potential needs within a person's life, an idea that has its most elegant form as the Multiple Discrepancies Theory (Michalos, 1985). This proposes that net satisfaction is a positive linear function of the perceived differences between what one has versus: (1) what one wants, (2) what others have, (3) the best one has had in the past, (4) what one expected to have in the past, (5) what one expects to have in the future, (6) what one deserves, and (7) what one needs.

The resultant net satisfaction, emanating from the meeting of such multiple needs, has been tied to motivation through the assumption that the desire for satisfaction motivates people to act (Mallard et al., 1997). These authors state: "This applies to satisfaction with income, health, education, and other life facets, as well as with satisfaction with life as a whole" (p. 260).

While it seems eminently reasonable to propose that unmet needs provide the basis for motivation (also see Ryan & Deci, 2000), the idea that they are directly linked to SWB levels is problematic. Assume, for example, that needs exist in some approximate hierarchical form, such as proposed by Maslow (1954). Then it is assumed that, as most basic needs are met, higher-level needs arise which, in Maslow's hierarchy, culminate in needs of self-actualization.

In such a scheme, because needs can be consciously recognized and met, SWB would show marked fluctuations as unmet needs arise, and are then met. But this does not occur. SWB shows a remarkable level of stability. In order to account for such stability, it must be assumed either that some needs cannot be met or that met needs are seamlessly replaced by unmet needs, so as to maintain an average SWB level of 75 %SM.

Both of these ideas seem implausible. First, it is difficult to imagine how such a scheme could work to manage SWB with the required precision. Second, since the majority of people in Western society do not experience chronic unmet needs at the lower levels of Maslow's hierarchy (1954), and have their relationship needs reasonably well met, the assumption of 'unmet' needs, required to fulfill the average 25 %SM deficit from complete life satisfaction, must be maintained via unmet 'self-actualization' needs. There is no evidence of which we are aware to support such an idea.

There is an alternative, which is depicted in Fig. 3. In this scheme, SWB is under the direct control of personality and the buffers, which together act to maintain SWB within its normal range. The varying needs in this model, act directly on the buffers. As a consequence, the buffers have the role of absorbing the impact of unmet needs and maintaining a constant level of SWB. In this scheme, chronic met needs will normally have little influence on SWB levels. While they may make the buffers more resilient to negative extrinsic influences, the level of SWB will remain determined by the dispositional set-point-range.

However, the presence of a strong, chronic, unmet need may affect the levels of SWB. This would act to compromise the buffers, and thereby to reduce SWB. For example, a person who is chronically very hungry or insecure is likely to have a level of SWB that lies below the normal range.

Two distinct systems that interact in the control of SWB are being described. The motivational system, which has as its prime purpose the initiation of behavior to meet needs, interacts with the SWB homeostatic system, which has as its prime purpose the maintenance of SWB.

To summarize, it is proposed that, in the absence of strong unmet needs, the SWB homeostatic system will deliver a level of SWB consistent with its set-point-range. The presence of strong unmet needs can defeat this system and, therefore, cause SWB to fall below its normal range. However, the meeting of needs, as a long-term state, will not cause SWB to rise above its set-point-range except for brief periods prior to adaptation (see Section IX).

What, then, is the nature of the interaction between these two systems? Fig. 3 indicates that the motivational system has a direct link with the buffers. That is, met and unmet needs are interpreted by the buffers in terms of their own concern with perceived control, self-esteem, or optimism. Then, the differential strength of the three buffers combine to produce different sensations of the SWB experience.

In order to demonstrate how this might work, the following taxonomy of SWB is offered, derived from Orton et al. (1988) and Avia (1997), with the relevant buffer indicated in parentheses.

> Empathy: understanding (perceived control over) the experiences of another person.
> Gloating: a bad event (loss of control) has happened to a bad person, reinforcing just-world beliefs (perceived control).
> Hope: the anticipation of a desirable event (optimism).
> Relief: disconfirmation of the occurrence of an unmet need (control).
> Pride and Admiration: approving praiseworthy action reflecting on oneself (self-esteem).
> Gratitude: the re-establishment of control, self-esteem, or optimism.

Two other positive emotions listed by these authors are 'Joy' and 'Love,' both of which appear to involve all buffers as a global response. Thus, with these exceptions, the conscious awareness of positive emotions based on met needs can be seen to involve one or more of the buffers. This is consistent with our proposition that SWB is a direct output of the buffers, not met needs per se.

A. Met Needs and the Buffers

Figure 3 indicates a link between met needs and the buffers. This is intended to imply that met needs strengthen the cognitive buffers. For example, a strong intimate relationship, constituting a powerful met need, is likely to engender a sense of perceived control, self-esteem, and optimism.

Indirect evidence for this proposition emerged from a review of personal wealth and SWB (Cummins, 2000a). It was found that while, as expected, very low income increased the probability of homeostatic defeat and, therefore, low SWB, a very high income induced levels of SWB to approximately 80 %SM on a group basis. Such levels were shown to be significantly higher than the population average.

The explanation offered rested on differential access to general resources, not only to meet needs but also to avoid or attenuate negative events. In essence, people who are very poor are highly vulnerable to their environment. They are required to perform tasks, such as child-minding, which they may not wish to perform and are unable to effectively counteract the influence of major negative events, such as the theft of property. People who are very rich, on the other hand, are able to use their money to acquire resources that allow them to be minimally affected by such concerns. They can employ a child-minder and afford insurance against property loss. Thus, while wealth cannot induce SWB above the set-point-range, it can allow rich people to approximate their SWB potential.

Additional evidence for this idea has been provided by Wolinski et al. (1985). Over the course of a one-year longitudinal study they found that people with high or low levels of SWB, at the time of initial measurement, scored lower and higher, respectively, 5 or 12 months later. Such a result would be expected as a consequence of regression to the mean. Interestingly, however, they also found that socio-economic status over-rode this effect, in that there was a direct relationship between socio-economic status and SWB improvement over the course of the study. The authors' conclusion is consistent with that emerging from the aforementioned review. They state that their results "suggest a vicious cycle wherein lower socio-economic status (SES) elderly people will increasingly face declining SWB, while their higher SES counterparts will somehow be able to avoid and/or compensate for the circumstances and problems that would otherwise result in reducing their subjective well-being" (p. 102).

In summary, unmet needs are seen as an important motivational component within the SWB homeostatic system, having their origin in the desire for satisfaction. However, meeting needs is not regarded as yielding SWB, but rather as an influence on the cognitive buffers. The perception of needs is also strongly influenced by personality (Fig. 3), as argued previously, and influenced by adaptation to extrinsic circumstances.

IX. ADAPTATION

The most basic process in the homeostatic model is adaptation, suggested by Andrews and Withey (1976) to be essential to any full explanation of SWB. This is a psychological process that allows people, over some period of time, to experience a reduced reaction to some changed life circumstance that comes to represent their extrinsic experience. For example, when people move from institutions and back into their community, the contrast between their new and past living environment will initially seem very great. However, the relocated people will gradually become used to their new home and, as this occurs, their new circumstances will cease to be a major source of contrast.

The most popular explanation of how such adaptation occurs in response to life events involves the Adaptation Level Theory (Helson, 1964). Excellent descriptions of this process have been supplied by Brickman and Campbell (1971), Brickman et al. (1978), and Zautra and Goodhart (1979) (which should be consulted for a detailed account). A brief description is as follows:

> The basic principle of the Adaptation Level Theory is that people's judgements of their current level of stimulation (positive or negative) depends upon whether this is higher or lower than the level to which they are accustomed. If it is higher, for example, then the person immediately experiences change. However, two processes then act to make the future experience of this new level of stimulation seem less remarkable. The first is an upward shift in adaptation level because the novel stimulation has been added to the 'accustomed' level of stimulation. The second is habituation, which describes the idea that events are judged by the extent to which they deviate from the adaptation level.

Brickman et al., (1978) is the most widely cited study to exemplify the operation of these processes. The popularity of this citation continues unabated despite the methodological limitations documented by Headey and Wearing (1989). Brickman et al. (1978) compared the reported happiness of major lottery winners, people who had been rendered paraplegic, and a general non-event control group. The data from the former two groups were collected some 1 to 18 months following the event and, remarkably, when the three groups were compared only minor differences in SWB were apparent. The explanation, in terms of the Adaptation Level Theory is as follows:

The lottery winners' initial euphoria and changed lifestyle caused a massive upward shift in adaptation level. As a consequence, the new pleasures lost their capacity to excite, and the ordinary events of their previous lives that had been sources of pleasure were now unable to do so because they fell below the new adaptation level. In contrast, the reduced level of positive stimulation experienced by people who had acquired paraplegia caused their adaptation level to fall. As a consequence, these people increasingly experienced pleasure from minor positive events that would have previously gone unnoticed. Thus, due to the changed adaptation levels of these groups, their levels of happiness had returned close to the levels they had experienced prior to their life event.

Authors have offered several extensions to this theme in terms of what, precisely, adapts. Thus, Zautra and Goodhart (1979) incorporate comparisons made with others, while Headey and Wearing (1986) incorporate role performance. There are undoubtedly many other psychological processes that could be nominated as being susceptible to adaptation, but it is interesting to note that the empirical evidence for the operation of adaptation level in relation to SWB is, in fact, quite modest. Some studies even appear to report data inconsistent with predictions based on the Adaptation Level Theory.

The earliest such data were reported by Andrews and Withey (1976) who asked people to rate their SQOL five years ago, in the present, and five years hence. They found the past and future estimations to be virtually independent, but that the present estimation correlated much more strongly with the future (0.44) then with the past (0.25) estimations—a three-fold difference in shared variance.

This could be interpreted as evidence against the Adaptation Level Theory. That is, assuming that current adaptation level had incorporated past levels of SWB, this should make past and present estimates co-vary. Future estimates, on the other hand, could not influence the current adaptation level, and so it would be expected to have a lower level of shared variance.

Such a proposition, however, fails to take account of the optimism buffer which predicts the opposite pattern. That is, present SWB and levels of optimism are normally highly correlated (see Section VII). Therefore, since future estimates of SWB and optimism must be considered virtually synonymous, present and future estimates of SWB should be strongly correlated. So, the fact that Andrews and Withey (1976) found the pattern they did, more likely reflects the influence of optimism than adaptation level.

A second study—Zautra and Reich (1980)—provided data seemingly against the adaptation level. They reported that people who experienced a high incidence of self-originated positive events actually rated the pleasantness of mundane events higher than people with low incidence. The authors interpreted this as evidence against the Adaptation Level Theory since the experience of positive self-generated life events appeared to enhance the pleasure gained from mundane events. However, there are problems with such an interpretation. Perhaps most important is the understanding, argued in Section IV, that people with a high set-point-range for SWB are predicted to experience more positive events and also to rate the events in their lives as more pleasurable. In this context, the findings by Zautra and Reich (1980) can be interpreted as confirmation of the high personality contribution to SWB.

Other evidence apparently against the Adaptation Level Theory is the finding by Hunskaar and Vinsnes (1991) that the quality of life of women with incontinence was not related to the duration of their condition. However, two matters make such data insubstantial for this purpose. First, the Sickness Impact Profile (Bergner et al., 1981), which they used as a measure of outcome, comprises mainly functional status and objective quality of life indices. It is certainly not a measure of SWB. Second, some aversive circumstances do not readily permit adaptation, and the social and practical considerations imposed by incontinence may well fall into this category.

While this cannot be a complete list of relevant studies, those mentioned in the preceding text are the only ones known to the authors that could be cited against the theory. On the other hand, the only known study in support of the theory, in addition to the Brickman et al. (1978) report which has already been cited, is that of Rigby et al. (1990) who studied people who were both disabled and living in an institution. In support of the Adaptation Level Theory, they found less negative affect among the longer-stay residents. However, they found no such difference in positive affect.

It seems curious that so little research attention has been directed to the testing of the Adaptation Level Theory in the context of SWB. Perhaps it is the case that authors simply assume it has been validated from its wide acceptance in the literature. However, this appears to be a premature supposition, at least from the evidence we have been able to gather. In fact, it appears this area deserves far more attention, not only to confirm or disconfirm the theory, but also to answer important questions concerning the type of experience that does or does not yield to adaptation. Moreover, the whole question of the time taken for successful adaptation is a critical practical and theoretical issue (see later text).

It needs to be acknowledged, however, that this is also a difficult area to research for a number of reasons. One is that evidence for adaptation cannot be reliably sought from the presentation of nonsignificant data. For example, the study by Borgen et al. (1996) followed-up high school graduates for two years and found that neither employment-unemployment or study continuation differentially influenced either self-esteem or depression. However, several factors other than the success of adaptation could have caused this result, including the fact that the authors used a relatively insensitive form of analysis.

Finally, given the homeostatic model that has been described, it is going to be difficult to disentangle adaptation to extrinsic events from other forms of adaptation occurring elsewhere in the model, such as at the level of needs. But for the purpose of this paper it is clear that adaptation to altered circumstances of living does occur through one means or another, and that such processes are involved in maintaining the set-point-range of SWB, as has been described.

Just how long the system takes to adapt to changed circumstances will undoubtedly depend on such parameters as the perceived magnitude of the event and the resilience of the system. Some indications of this time-span can be derived from the study by Suh et al. (1996) of college students. This combined longitudinal and cross-sectional study found that only events within the previous six months exerted an influence on SWB. This appears a reasonable starting point for such estimations.

In summary, while data confirming the validity of the Adaptation Level Theory in relation to SWB are currently unimpressive, the theory does have a strong level of acceptance within the literature. It also seems logical to apply this theory, which originated in the context of perception, to the SWB area, as argued by Brickman et al., 1978. Finally, no telling arguments or data have been provided that reasonably question the validity of this idea. Therefore, for these reasons the Adaptation Level Theory has been incorporated into the homeostatic model.

X. HOMEOSTATIC MAINTENANCE AND FAILURE

The maintenance of SWB within its set-point-range requires some form of feedback loop. While the nature of such a device is speculative at this stage, a recent suggestion by Carver (2000) provides one explanation for how the set-point-range might be maintained.

Carver's idea involves the assumption that action is goal-directed and managed by feedback loops. Some of the loops are goal seekers, others are 'anti-goal' avoiders. These loops make comparisons between current conditions and the goal (or reference point) and make adjustments as necessary. As a consequence, in the absence of distractions or other forces, people tend to do what they intend to do (goal-seeking and -matching) and avoid doing the things they regard as unpleasant (anti-goal avoiding). Carver (2000) states:

> "The affect portion of the theory uses much the same logic but with the incorporation of time as a parameter. It proposes a loop that monitors the rate at which the behavioral systems (goal-seeking and anti-goal avoiding) are doing what they are trying to do ... The loop takes sensed velocity and compares it to a velocity goal. If the sensed velocity is less than the reference point, the result is a negative affect; if it exceeds the reference point, the result is positive affect" (p. 339).

In the context of the homeostatic model, it could be supposed that SWB lying either above or below the set-point-range constitutes a deviation from the velocity goal. Such deviations will then lead to internal adjustments that will eventually restore SWB to a level within its set-point-range. Thus, in terms of the goal-seeking loop, which Carver (2000) presumes to be the affect loop, levels of SWB lying above the set-point-range should lead to 'coasting'. That is, withdrawal of effort, basking, or taking it easy. Levels of SWB lying below the set-point-range should lead the goal-seeking loop to try harder. Thus, this system acts to prevent the maintenance of SWB levels outside the set-point-range.

While this proposition is speculative at this stage, it does represent an attempt to explain the nature of the feedback loops underpinning the homeostatic set-point-range. Such considerations, however, and the bulk of the discussion so far, have concentrated on the chronic maintenance of SWB within its set-point-range. Consideration will now be given to variations of SWB that lie outside this range.

A. Joy

The buffers are not normally delivering SWB to its maximum (100 %SM). They are constrained by their own set-point which has, as its cognitive manifestation, the understanding that we do not have absolute control, that we are not perfect, and that the future will not be uniformly positive. However, higher than normal SWB can be induced in the short-term by meeting a need (e.g., a satisfying meal) or experiencing a highly positive life event. Such situations represent homeostatic failure at the level of the cognitive buffers.

In support of this idea, Mikulincer and Peer-Golden (1991) found that short-term happiness reflected situational validation of the ideal self ('the person you would like ideally to be'). They found that happiness in a given event increased with the congruence between the ideal self and the perceived self in that event. Therefore, we hypothesize that other forms of situational validation, involving ideals based on control or optimism, can also yield above-range levels of SWB. Such deviations however, will be short-lived due to the influence of adaptation.

B. Depression

If depression is conceptualized as the loss of SWB homeostasis, then the relationship between dysthymia and SWB should approximate the relationship between SWB and extrinsic factors as shown in Fig. 2. That is, provided that some negative influence lacks the power to defeat homeostasis, the symptoms of depression should be virtually absent. As Kammann and Flett (1983) commented: "an absence of depression can occur with many different levels of positive well-being" (p. 261).

This changes, however, as the negative influence starts to induce dysthymia by defeating homeostasis and forcing SWB to lower levels. Under such conditions, the lower values for SWB and the symptoms of depression start to co-vary in the manner depicted by Fig. 2. Thus, the model predicts a curvilinear relationship between extrinsic conditions and depression, precisely as has been reported in relation to depression and martial satisfaction (Fincham & Bradbury, 1993), life satisfaction (Coyle et al., 1994; Lewinsohn et al., 1991), and positive affect (Kammann & Flett, 1983).

Further predictions from the model are as follows. First, under conditions of homeostatic defeat, the symptoms of depression (i.e., scores on depression indices) are coincident with low values within the buffer systems. This pattern of relationships has been verified in relation to self-esteem, both within a general population sample (Fincham & Bradbury, 1993) and for people with an intellectual disability (Benson & Ivins, 1992). Thus, as the buffer systems fail to successfully absorb the impact of negative events, their own values decrease and the consequential fall in SWB is mirrored by a rise in the indices of depression.

The second prediction is that the level of the set-point-range should mirror the extent to which the homeostatic system is robust to negative life events. A relatively high setting, determined by personality, should indicate a high level of resilience, while a low setting predicts a fragile system that is prone to failure and, therefore, to depression. This prediction has already been discussed in Section VII. Further support comes from Lewinsohn et al. (1991) who found low levels of life satisfaction to be a significant risk factor for future depression.

The third prediction is that people with a high level of neuroticism would be predisposed to depression. This is consistent with the logic that their personality structure would not only give them a low SWB set-point-range but would also predispose them to reward insensitivity and relative inability to counteract the negative influence of stressful situations (Flynn & Cappeliez, 1993). Just such a finding has been reported by Roberts and Kendler (1999) in a large study of twins. Moreover, high neuroticism is likely to produce a 'depressogenic' attributional style, in which negative life events are very likely to be experienced as stressful, since they are more likely than normal to exceed the threshold of the buffers. So, in this sense, such people 'generate' negative life events (see Simons et al., 1993) with the consequence that their lives are characterized by a predictably high frequency of such events.

In summary, both joy and depression can be regarded as consequences of homeostatic failure. However, whereas joy is inevitably an acute state, defeated by homeostatic processes, depression can be chronic, representing the failure of homeostasis in the face of powerful and persistent negative experiences. This depiction of depression, as representing the loss of SWB through homeostatic failure, is novel.

XI. CONCLUSIONS

The idea that it is normal and adaptive to view one's life positively is revolutionary. As has been pointed out by other authors in this area (e.g., Peterson, 2000), such an idea fundamentally challenges the ideas of many influential psychologists and psychiatrists from the last century as to what constitutes desirable psychological functioning. Most essentially, the idea that the accurate perception of reality equates to optimal psychological functioning is clearly wrong. People who see their lives accurately are generally depressed. Thus, since moderately high levels of SWB are normal, there must be some robust psychological machinery to ensure such levels are maintained.

This chapter has attempted to describe a model that could account for such maintenance. It draws together the idea of a homeostatic system that manages SWB through an interlocking system of psychological devices. In this system, personality provides a steady affective background that sets SWB within a narrow range for each individual. This is achieved through the supply of a direct affective component to SWB and by the influence personality exerts on other components of the homeostatic system.

The cognitive buffers are proposed to be under the influence of personality, which acts to provide them with a determined range of operation such that SWB is held within its set-point-range. Personality is also envisaged as having a powerful influence on motivational systems that seek satisfaction and, thus, predispose behavior that is likely to maintain normal levels of

SWB. This is mainly through the link between extraversion and reward sensitivity, but also in relation to the general influence of personality on the level of perceived needs. Finally, at the most fundamental level of the homeostatic system, are the processes of adaptation and habituation, which constitute the first line of defence against the threat of changed extrinsic conditions influencing levels of SWB.

In the construction of this chapter, all accessed and relevant publications have been incorporated into the description. While these appear to overwhelmingly offer support for the model, an unconscious bias to generate such a fit must be considered as a limitation to our judgement. We also acknowledge that only a fraction of available evidence has been cited, given the breadth of the psychological processes under consideration. Therefore, alternative views can be formed on the interpretation of the cited publications with respect to the model, and that other data may cause a re-evaluation of the structure that has been described. We look forward to such developments and offer this homeostatic model only as a first step in understanding how SWB is so effectively maintained.

ACKNOWLEDGMENTS

The authors thank Pamela de Kort and Ann-Marie James for their assistance in the preparation of this manuscript.

REFERENCES

Aaronson, N. K., Ahmedzai, S., & Bergman, B. (1993). The European Organization for Research and Treatment of Cancer QLQ-C30: A quality of life instrument for use in international clinical trials in oncology. *Journal of the National Cancer Institute, 85,* 365.

Abbey, A., & Andrews, F. M. (1985). Modeling the psychological determinants of life quality. *Social Indicators Research, 16,* 1–34.

Ager, A., & Hatton, C. (1999). Discerning the appropriate role and status of 'quality of life' assessment for persons with intellectual disability: A reply to Cummins. *Journal of Applied Research in Intellectual Disabilities, 12,* 335–339.

Andreasen, N. J. C., & Norris, A. S. (1972). Long-term adjustment and adaptation mechanisms in severely burned adults. *The Journal of Nervous and Mental Disease, 154,* 352–362.

Andrews, F. M., & Withey, S. B. (1976). *Social indicators of well-being: American's perceptions of life quality.* New York: Plenum Press.

Argyle, M., & Lu, L. (1990). The happiness of extraverts. *Personality and Individual Differences, 11,* 1011–1017.

Avia, M. D. (1997). Personality and positive emotions. *European Journal of Personality, 11,* 33–56.

Bach, J. R., & Tilton, M. C. (1994). Life satisfaction and well-being measures in ventilator assisted individuals with traumatic tetraplegia. *Archives of Physical Medicine and Rehabilitation, 75,* 626–632.

Baumeister, R. F., Tice, D. M., & Hutton, D. G. (1989). Self-presentational motivations and personality differences in self-esteem. *Journal of Personality, 57*(3), 547–579.

Benson, B. A., & Ivins, J. (1992). Anger, depression and self-concept in adults with mental retardation. *Journal of Intellectual Disability Research, 36*, 169–175.

Bergeman, C. S., Plomin, R., Pedersen, N. L., & McClearn, G. E. (1991). Genetic mediation of the relationship between social support and psychological well-being. *Psychology & Aging, 6*, 640–646.

Bergner, M., Bobbitt, R. A., Carter, W. B., & Gilson, B. S. (1981). The sickness impact profile: Development and final revision of a health status measure. *Medical Care, 19*, 787–805.

Block, J., & Robins, R. W. (1993). A longitudinal study of consistency and change in self-esteem from early adolescence to early adulthood. *Child Development, 64*, 909–923.

Bloom, J. R., Fobair, P., Spiegel, D., Cox, R. S., Varghese, A., & Hoppe, R. (1991). Social supports and the social well-being of cancer survivors. *Advances in Medical Sociology, 2*, 95–114.

Borgen, W. A., Amundson, N. E., & Tench, E. (1996). Psychological well-being throughout the transition from adolescence to adulthood. *Career Development Quarterly, 45*, 189–199.

Bortner, R. W., & Hultsch, D. F. (1970). A multivariate analysis of correlates of life satisfaction in adulthood. *Journal of Gerontology, 25*, 41–47.

Boschen, K. A. (1996). Correlates of life satisfaction, residential satisfaction, and locus of control among adults with spinal cord injuries. *Rehabilitation Counseling Bulletin, 39*, 230–243.

Bowling, A. (1996). Associations with changes in life satisfaction among three samples of elderly people living at home. *International Journal of Geriatric Psychiatry, 11*, 1077–1087.

Bradburn, N. M. (1969). *The structure of psychological well-being.* Chicago: University of Chicago Press.

Brickman, P., & Campbell, D. T. (1971). Hedonic relativism and planning the good society. In M. H. Appley (Ed.), *Adaptation-level theory: A symposium* (pp. 287–302). New York: Academic Press.

Brickman, P., Coates, D., & Janoff-Bulman, R. (1978). Lottery winners and accident victims: Is happiness relative? *Journal of Personality and Social Psychology, 36*, 917–927.

Brief, A. P., Butcher, A. H., George, J. M., & Link, K. E. (1993). Integrating bottom-up and top-down theories of subjective well-being: The case of health. *Journal of Personality and Social Psychology, 64*, 646–653.

Brown, R. I., Bayer, M. B., & Brown, P. M. (1988). Quality of life: A challenge for rehabilitation agencies. *Australian and New Zealand Journal of Developmental Disabilities, 14*, 189–199.

Brown, J. D., & Mankowski, T. A. (1993). Self-esteem, mood, and self-evaluation: Changes in mood and the way you see you. *Journal of Personality and Social Psychology, 64*, 421–430.

Brown, R. I., & Timmons, V. (1994). Quality of life—Adults and adolescents with disabilities. *Exceptionality Education Canada, 4*, 1–11.

Brown, I. (1996). Lessons from a quality of life project in Canada. *Paper presented at the 10th Conference of the International Association for the Scientific Studies of Intellectual Disabilities.* Helinski, Finland.

Butler, A. C., Hokanson, J. E., & Flynn, H. A. (1994). A comparison of self-esteem lability and low trait self-esteem as vulnerability factors for depression. *Journal of Personality and Social Psychology, 66*, 166–177.

Campbell, A., Converse, P. E., & Rodgers, W. L. (1976). *The Quality of American life: Perceptions, evaluations, and satisfactions.* New York: Russell Sage Foundation.

Cantril, H. (1965). *The pattern of human concerns.* New Jersey: Rutgers University Press.

Carver, C. S. (2000). On the continuous calibration of happiness. *American Journal of Mental Retardation, 105*, 336–341.

Chrzanowski, G. (1981). The genesis and nature of self-esteem. *American Journal of Psychotherapy, 35,* 38–46.
Cooley, C. H. (1902). *Human nature and the social order.* New Brunswick: Transaction Books.
Coopersmith, S. (1967). Some expressions of self-esteem. In W. H. Freeman (Ed.), *The antecedents of self-esteem.* W. H. Freeman: San Francisco.
Coopersmith, S. (1981). *Manual for the Coopersmith Self-Esteem Inventory (SEI).* Palo Alto, CA: Consulting Psychologists Press.
Costa, P. T. Jr., & McCrae, R. R. (1989). Personality as a lifelong determinant of welbeing. In L. Z. Malatesta & C. E. Izzard (Eds.), *Emotion in adult development* (pp. 141–157). Beverly Hills, CA: Sage.
Coyle, C. P., Lesnik-Emas, S., & Kinney, W. B. (1994). Predicting life satisfaction among adults with spinal cord injuries. *Rehabilitation Psychology, 39,* 95–112.
Cummins, R. A. (1995). On the trail of the gold standard for life satisfaction. *Social Indicators Research, 35,* 179–200.
Cummins, R. A. (1996). The domains of life satisfaction: An attempt to order chaos. *Social Indicators Research, 38,* 303–332.
Cummins, R. A. (1997a). *Comprehensive Quality of Life Scale—Adult.* Manual: Fifth Edition. Melbourne: School of Psychology, Deakin University.
Cummins, R. A. (1997b). *Comprehensive Quality of Life Scale—Intellectual/cognitive disability.* Manual: Fifth Edition. Melbourne: School of Psychology, Deakin University.
Cummins, R. A. (1997c). Assessing quality of life for people with disabilities. In R. I. Brown (Ed.), *Quality of life for handicapped people* (2nd ed., pp. 116–150). Cheltenham, England: Stanley Thomas.
Cummins, R. A. (1997d). Self-rated quality of life scales for people with an intellectual disability: A review. *Journal of Applied Research in Intellectual Disability, 10,* 199–216.
Cummins, R. A. (1998). The second approximation to an international standard of life satisfaction. *Social Indicators Research, 43,* 307–334.
Cummins, R. A. (1999). A psychometric evaluation of the comprehensive quality of life scale—fifth Edition. In L. L. Yran, B. Yuen, & C. Low (Eds.), *Urban quality of life: Critical issues and options* (pp. 32–46). Singapore: National University of Singapore.
Cummins, R. A. (2000a). Personal income and subjective well-being: A review. *Journal of Happiness Studies, 1,* 133–158.
Cummins, R. A. (2000b). A homeostatic model for subjective quality of life. *Proceedings, Second Conference of Quality of Life in Cities* (pp. 51–59). Singapore: National University of Singapore.
Cummins, R. A. (2000c). Objective and subjective quality of life: An interactive model. *Social Indicators Research, 52,* 55–72.
Cummins, R. A. (2001a). *Directory of instruments to measure quality of life and cognate areas.* Melbourne: School of Psychology, Deakin University. Sixth Edition.
Cummins, R. A. (2001b). Self-rated quality of life scales for people with an intellectual disability: A reply to Ager and Hatton. *Journal of Applied Research in Intellectual Disabilities, 14,* 1–11.
Cummins, R. A. (2003). Normative life satisfaction: Measurement issues and a homeostatic model. *Social Indicators Research, 64,* 225–256.
Cummins, R. A., & Nistico, H. (2002). Maintaining life satisfaction: The role of positive cognitive bias. *Journal of Happiness Studies, 3,* 37–69.
Cvetanovski, J., & Jex, S. M. (1994). Locus of control of unemployed people and its relationship to psychological and physical well-being. *Work & Stress, 8,* 60–67.
DeNeve, K. M. (1999). Happy as an extraverted clam? The role of personality for subjective well-being *Psychological Science, 8,* 141–144.

De Neve, K., & Cooper, H. (1998). The happy personality: A meta-analysis of 137 personality traits and SWB. *Psychological Bulletin, 124,* 197–229.

Depue, R. A., & Montoe, S. M. (1986). Conceptualization and measurement of human disorder in life stress research: The problem of chronic disturbance. *Psychological Bulletin, 99,* 36–51.

Diener, E. (1984). Subjective well-being. *Psychological Bulletin, 95,* 542–575.

Diener, E., & Diener, M. (1995). Cross-cultural correlates of life satisfaction and self-esteem. *Journal of Personality and Social Psychology, 68,* 653–663.

Diener, E., Emmons, R. A., Larsen, R. J., & Griffin, S. (1985). The satisfaction with life scale. *Journal of Personality Assessment, 49,* 71–75.

Diener, E., & Larsen, R. J. (1984). Temporal stability and cross-situational consistency of affective, behavioral, and cognitive responses. *Journal of Personality and Social Psychology, 47,* 871–883.

Diener, E., Sandvik, E., Pavot, W., & Fujita, F. (1992). Extraversion and subjective well-being in a U.S. national probability sample. *Journal of Research in Personality, 26,* 205–215.

Diener, E., Suh, E. M., Lucas, R. E., & Smith, H. L. (1999). Subjective well-being: Three decades of progress. *Psychological Bulletin, 125,* 276–302.

Doyle, K. O., & Youn, S. (2000). Exploring the traits of happy people. *Social Indicator Research, 52,* 195.

DuBois, D. L., Bull, C. A., Sherman, M. D., & Roberts, M. (1998). Self-esteem and adjustment in early adolescents: A social contextual perspective. *Journal of Youth and Adolescence, 27,* 557–583.

Duckitt, J. H. (1983). Psychological factors related to subjective health perception among elderly women. *Humanitas, Journal of Research in the Human Sciences, 9,* 441–449.

Depue, R. A., & Collins, P. F. (1999). Neurobiology of the structure of personality: Dopamine facilitation of incentive motivation and extraversion. *Behavioral and Brain Sciences, 22,* 491–569.

Edgerton, R. B. (1990). Quality of life from a longitudinal research perspective. In R. L. Schalock (Ed.), *Quality of life: Perspectives and issues* (pp. 149–160). Washington: American Association on Mental Retardation.

Edwards, J. R. (1998). Cybernetic theory of stress, coping, and well-being: Review and extension to work and family. In C. L. Cooper (Ed.), *Theories or organizational stress* (pp. 122–153). New York: Oxford University Press.

Edwards, J. R., & Rothbard, N. P. (1999). Work and family stress and well-being: An examination of person-environment fit in their work and family domains. *Organizational Behavior and Human Decision Processes, 77,* 85–129.

Elliott, T. R., Marmarosh, C., & Pickelman, H. (1994). Negative affectivity, social support, and the prediction of depression and distress. *Journal of Personality, 62,* 299–319.

Endo, Y. (1992). Personalized standard of self-esteem. *Japanese Journal of Educational Psychology, 40,* 157–163.

Engel, M. (1959). The stability of self-concept in adolescence. *Journal of Abnormal Psychology, 58,* 211–215.

Enger, J. M., Howerton, D. L., & Cobbs, C. R. (1994). Internal/external locus of control, self-esteem, and parental verbal interaction of at-risk black male adolescents. *The Journal of Social Psychology, 134,* 269–274.

Felce, D., & Perry, J. (1995). Quality of life: Its definition and measurement. *Research in Developmental Disabilities, 16,* 51–74.

Festinger, L. (1954). A theory of social comparison processes. *Human Relations, 7,* 117–140.

Filipp, S., & Klauer, T. (1991). Subjective well-being in the face of critical life events: The case of successful copers. In F. Strack, M. Argyle, & N. Schwarz (Eds.), *Subjective well-being: An interdisciplinary perspective* (pp. 213–234). New York: Plenum Press.

Fincham, F. D., & Bradbury, T. N. (1993). Marital satisfaction, depression and attributions: A longitudinal analysis. *Journal of Personality and Social Psychology, 64,* 442–453.

Fitzgerald, T. E., Tennen, H., Affleck, G., & Pransky, G. S. (1993). The relative importance of dispositional optimism and control appraisals in quality of life after coronary artery bypass surgery. *Journal of Behavioral Medicine, 16,* 25–43.

Flanagan, J. C. (1978). A research approach to improving our quality of life. *American Psychologist, 33,* 138–147.

Fleming, J. S., & Courtney, B. E. (1984). The dimensionality of self-esteem: II. Hierarchical facet model for revised measurement scales. *Journal of Personality and Social Psychology, 46,* 404–421.

Flynn, R. J., & Cappeliez, P. (1993). An integrative cognitive-environmental view of depression. In P. Cappeliez & R. J. Flynn (Eds.), *Depression and the social environment* (pp. 1–11). Montreal: McGill-Queens University Press.

Fogarty, G. J., Machin, M. A., Albion, M. J., Sutherland, L. F., Lalor, G. I., & Revitt, S. (1999). Predicting occupational strain and job satisfaction: The role of stress, coping, personality and affectivity variables. *Journal of Vocational Behavior, 54,* 429–452.

Francis, L. J. (1999). Happiness is a thing called stable extraversion: A further examination of the relationship between the Oxford Happiness Inventory and Eysenck's dimensional model of personality and gender. *Personality and Individual Differences, 26,* 5–11.

French, J. R. P. Jr., Rodgers, W., & Cobb, S. (1974). Adjustment as person-environment fit. In G. V. Coelho, B. A. Hamburg, & J. E. Adams (Eds.), *Coping and adaptation* (pp. 316–333). New York: Basic Books.

Fyrand, L., Wichstom, L., Moum, T., Glennas, A., & Kvien, T. K. (1997). The impact of personality and social support on mental health for female patients with rheumatoid arthritis. *Social Indicators Research, 40,* 285–298.

Gallup, (1998). Have and have-nots. Perceptions of fairness and opportunity 1998. *Princeton: Gallop Poll Social Audit,* The Gallop Organization.

Gecas, V., & Schwalbe, M. L. (1983). Beyond the looking-glass self: Social structure and efficacy based self-esteem. *Social Psychology Quarterly, 46,* 77–88.

Glatzer, W. (1991). Quality of life in advanced industrialized countries: The case of West Germany. In F. Strack, M. Argyle, & N. Schwarz (Eds.), *Subjective well-being: An interdisciplinary perspective* (pp. 261–279). New York: Plenum Press.

Glick, M. (1999). Developmental and experiential variables in the self-images of people with mild mental retardation. In E. Zigler & D. Bennett-Gates (Eds.), *Personality development in individuals with mental retardation* (pp. 135–156). Cambridge University Press.

Gray, J. A. (1970). The psychophysiological basis of introversion-extraversion. *Behavior Research and Therapy, 8,* 249–266.

Groot, W., & VandenBrink, M. (2000). Life satisfaction and preference drift. *Social Indicators Research, 50,* 315–329.

Hagerty, M. R., Cummins, R. A., Ferriss, A. L., Land, K., Michalos, A. C., Peterson, M., Sharpe, A., Sirgy, J., & Vogel, J. (2001). Quality of life indexes for national policy: Review and agenda for research. *Social Indicators Research, 55,* 1–91.

Hattie, J. (1992). *Self-concept.* Hillsdale, NJ: Lawrence Erlbaum Associates Publishers.

Headey, B., Holmstrom, E., & Wearing, A. (1985). Models of well-being and ill-being. *Social Indicators Research, 17,* 211–234.

Headey, B., & Wearing, A. (1986). *The sense of relative superiority-central to well-being.* University of Melbourne (unpublished).

Headey, B., & Wearing, A. (1989). Personality, life events, and subjective well-being: Toward a dynamic equilibrium model. *Journal of Personality and Social Psychology, 57*, 731–739.

Headey, B., & Wearing, A. (1992). *Understanding happiness: A theory of subjective well-being.* Melbourne: Longman Cheshire.

Helson, H. (1964). *Adaptation-level theory.* New York: Harper & Row.

Hogg, M. A., & Sunderland, J. (1991). Self-esteem and intergroup discrimination in the minimal group paradigm. *British Journal of Social Psychology, 30*, 51–62.

Huelsman, T. J., Nemanick, R. C., Jr., & Munz, D. C. (1998). Scales to measure four dimensions of dispositional mood: Positive energy, tiredness, negative activation, and relaxation. *Educational and Psychological Measurement, 58*, 804–819.

Hunskaar, S., & Vinsnes, A. (1991). The quality of life in women with urinary incontinence as measured by the sickness impact profile. *Journal of the American Geriatrics Society, 39*, 378–382.

Hunt, S. M., Singer, K., & Cobb, S. (1967). Components of depression. *Archives of General Psychiatry, 16*, 441–447.

Izard, C. E. (1993). Four systems for emotion activation: Cognitive and noncognitive processes. *Psychological Review, 100*, 68–90.

Jacob, J. C., & Brinkerhoff, M. B. (1999). Mindfulness and subjective well-being in the sustainability movement: A further elaboration of multiple discrepancies theory. *Social Indicators Research, 46*, 341–368.

James, W. (1892). *Psychology.* New York: Henry Holt.

Jang, K. L., Livesley, W. J., & Vernon, P. A. (1996). Heritability of the big five personality dimensions and their facets—a twin study. *Journal of Personality, 64*, 577–591.

Josephs, R. A., Markus, H. R., & Tafarodi, R. W. (1992). Gender and self-esteem. *Journal of Personality and Social Psychology, 63*, 391–402.

Kammann, R., & Flett, R. (1983). Affectometer 2: A scale to measure current level of general happiness. *Australian Journal of Psychology, 35*, 259–265.

Kaplan De-Nour, (1981). Prediction of adjustment to chronic hemodialysis. In N. B. Levy (Ed.), *Psychonephrology: Psychological factors in hemodialysis and transplantation* (Vol. 1, pp. 117–132). New York: Plenum.

Kitayama, S., Markus, H. R., Matsumoto, H., & Norasakkunkit, V. (1997). Individual and collective processes in the construction of the self: Self-enhancement in the United States and self-criticism in Japan. *Journal of Personality and Social Psychology, 72*, 1245–1267.

Klaczynski, P. A., & Fauth, J. M. (1996). Intellectual ability, rationality, and intuitiveness as predictors of warranted and unwarranted optimism for future life events. *Journal of Youth and Adolescence, 25*, 755–773.

Klein, H. A. (1995). Self-perception in late adolescence: An interactive perspective. *Adolescence, 30*, 579–592.

Kopp, R. G., & Ruzicka, M. F. (1993). Women's multiple roles and psychological well-being. *Psychological Reports, 72*, 1351–1354.

Landua, D. (1992). An attempt to classify satisfaction changes: Methodological and content aspects of a longitudinal problem. *Social Indicators Research, 26*, 221–241.

Lau, A., Chi, I., & McKenna, K. (1998). Self-perceived quality of life of Chinese elderly people in Hong Kong. *Occupational Therapy International, 5*, 118–139.

Lecky, P. (1945). *Self-consistency: A theory of personality.* New York: Island Press.

Lefcourt, H. M. (1976). *Locus of control: Current trends in theory and research.* Hillsdale, New Jersey: Lawrence Erlbaum.

Lewinsohn, P. M., Redner, J. E., & Seeley, J. R. (1991). The relationship between life satisfaction and psychosocial variables: New perspectives. In F. Strack, M. Argyle, & N. Schwarz (Eds.), *Subjective well-being: An interdisciplinary perspective* (pp. 141–169). Oxford: Pergamon Press.

Long, K. M., & Spears, R. (1998). Opposing effects of personal and collective self-esteem on interpersonal and intergroup comparisons. *European Journal of Social Psychology, 28*, 913–930.

Lu, L., & Shih, J. B. (1997). Sources of happines: A qualitative approach. *The Journal of Social Psychology, 137*, 181–187.

Lucas, R. E., Diener, E., Grob, A., Suh, E. M., & Shao, L. (2000). Cross-cultural evidence for the fundamental features of extraversion. *Journal of Personality and Social Psychology, 79*, 452.

Luk, C. H., & Bond, M. H. (1992). Explaining Chinese self-esteem in terms of the self-concept. *Psychologia, 35*, 147–154.

Macaskill, G. T., Hopper, J. L., White, V., & Hill, D. J. (1994). Genertic and environmental variation in Eysenck Personality Questionnaire scales measured on Australian adolescent twins. *Behavior Genetics, 24*, 481–491.

Mallard, A. G. C., Lance, C. E., & Michalos, A. C. (1997). Culture as a moderator of overall life satisfaction—Life facet of satisfaction relationships. *Social Indicators Research, 40*, 259–284.

Marsh, H. W. (1994). The importance of being important: Theoretical models of relations between specific and global components of physical self-concept. *Journal of Sport and Exercise Psychology, 16*, 306–325.

Maslow, A. H. (1954). *Motivation and Personality.* New York: Harpers.

McCrae, R. R., & Costa, P. T. (1995). Positive and negative valence within the five-factor model. *Journal of Research in Personality, 29*, 443–460.

Medora, N. P., Goldstein, A., & von der Hellen, C. (1993). Variables related to romanticism and self-esteem in pregnant teenagers. *Adolescence, 28*, 159–170.

Mellor, D., Cummins, R. A., & Loquet, C. (1999). The gold standard for life satisfaction: Confirmation and elaboration using an imaginary scale and qualitative interview. *International Journal of Social Research Methodology Theory and Practice, 2*, 263–278.

Michalos, A. C. (1985). Multiple discrepancies theory (MTD). *Social Indicators Research, 16*, 347–413.

Mikulincer, M., & Peer-Goldin, I. (1991). Self-congruence and the experience of happiness. *British Journal of Social Psychology, 30*, 21–35.

Mullis, R. J. (1992). Measures of economic well-being as predictors of psychological well-being. *Social Indicators Research, 26*, 119–135.

Nemanick, R. C. Jr., & Munz, D. C. (1997). Extraversion and neuroticis, trait mood, and state affect: A hierarchical relationship? *Journal of Social Behaviour and Personality, 12*(4), 1079–1092.

Neugarten, B. L., Havighurst, R. J., & Tobin, S. S. (1961). The measurement of life satisfaction. *Journal of Gerontology, 16*, 134–143.

Nieboer, A. P. (1997). *Life events and well-being: A prospective study on changes in well-being of elderly people due to a serious illness event or death of the spouse.* Amsterdam: Thesis Publishers.

O'Brien, W. H., VanEgeren, L., & Mumby, P. B. (1995). Predicting health behaviors using measures of optimism and perceived risk. *Health Values, 19*, 21–28.

O'Malley, P. M., & Backman, J. G. (1979). Self-esteem and education: Sex and cohort comparisons among high school students. *Journal of Personality and Social Psychology, 37*, 1153–1159.

Omizo, M. M., Omizo, S. A., & D'Andrea, M. J. (1992). Promoting wellness among elementary school children. *Journal of Counseling and Development, 71*, 194–198.

Ormel, J. (1983). Neuroticism and well-being inventories. Measuring traits or states? *Psychological Medicine, 13*, 165–176.

Ormel, J., & Schaufeli, W. B. (1991). Stability and change in psychological distress and their relationship with self-esteem and locus of control: A dynamic equilibrium model. *Journal of Personality and Social Psychology, 60*, 288–299.

Pallant, J., & Cummins, R. A. (2002). *The comparative psychometric performance of two scales designed to measure subjective quality of life.* (submitted).

Penland, E. A., Masten, W. G., Zelhart, P., Fournet, G. P., & Callahan, T. A. (2000). Possible selves, depression and coping skills in university students. *Personality and Individual Differences, 29*, 963–969.

Peterson, C. (2000). The future of optimism. *American Psychologist, 55*, 44–56.

Phares, E. J. (1978). Locus of control. In H. London & J. E. Exner (Eds.), *Dimensions of personality* (pp. 263–303). New York: John Wiley & Sons.

Pugliesi, K. (1988). Employment characteristics, social support and the well-being of women. *Women and Health, 14*, 35–58.

Ralph, A., Merralls, L., Hart, L., Porter, J. S., & Tan Su-Neo, A. (1995). Peer interactions, self-concept, locus of control, and avoidance of social situations of early adolescents. *Australian Journal of Psychology, 47*, 110–118.

Rawson, H. E. (1992). The interrelationship of measures of manifest anxiety, self-esteem, locus of control and depression in children with behaviour problems. *Journal of Psychoeducational Assessment, 10*, 319–329.

Rigby, K., McCarron, L., & Rigby, J. (1990). *Quality of life in a nursing home: A report on the perceptions of residents and staff at Julia Farr Centre.* Adelaide: South Australian Institute of Technology.

Roberts, B. W., & DelVecchio, W. F. (2000). The rank-order consistency of personality traits from childhood to old age: A quantitative review of longitudinal studies. *Psychological Bulletin, 126*, 3–25.

Roberts, J. E., & Gotlib, I. H. (1997). Temporal variability in global self-esteem and specific self-evaluation as prospective predictors of emotional distress: Specificity in predictors and outcome. *Journal of Abnormal Psychology, 106*(4), 521–529.

Roberts, S. B., & Kendler, S. (1999). Neuroticism and self-esteem as indices of the vulnerability to major depression in women. *Psychological Medicine, 29*, 1101–1109.

Romney, D. M., Brown, R. I., & Fry, P. S. (1994). Improving the quality of life: prescriptions for change. *Social Indicators Research, 33*, 237–272.

Rosenberg, G. S. (1968). Age, poverty, and isolation from friends in the urban working class. *Journal of Gerontology, 23*, 533–538.

Rosenberg, M. (1979). *Conceiving the self.* New York: Basic Books.

Rotter, J. B. (1966). Generalized expectancies for internal versus external control of reinforcement. *Psychological Monographs, 80* (Whole No. 609).

Russell, J. A., & Carroll, J. M. (1999). On the bipolarity of positive and negative affect. *Psychological Bulletin, 125*, 3–30.

Ryan, R. M., & Deci, E. L. (2000). Self-determination theory and the facilitation of intrinsic motivation, social development, and well-being. *American Psychologist, 55*, 68–79.

Ryff, C. D. (1991). Possible selves in adulthood and old age: A tale of shifting horizons. *Psychology and Aging, 6*, 286–295.

Sandvik, L., Erikssen, J., Thaulow, E., Erikssen, G., Mundal, R., & Rodahl, K. (1993). Physical fitness as a predictor of mortality among healthy, middle-aged Norwegian men. *New England Journal of Medicine, 328*, 533–537.

Sanna, L. J. (1996). Defensive pessimism, optimism and simulating alternatives: Some ups and downs of prefactual and counterfactual thinking. *Journal of Personality and Social Psychology, 71*(5), 1020–1036.
Saudino, K. J., Gagne, J. R., Grant, J., Ibatoulina, A., Marytuina, T., Ravich-Scherbo, I., & Whitfield, G. K. (1999). Genetic and environmental influences on personality in adult Russian twins. *International Journal of Behavior Development, 23,* 375–389.
Schalock, R. L., Bonham, G. S., & Marcharnd, C. B. (2000). Consumer based quality of life assessment: A path model of perceived satisfaction. *Evaluation and Program Planning, 23,* 75–85.
Scheier, M. F., & Carver, C. S. (1985). Optimism, coping, and health: Assessment and implications of generalized outcome expectancies. *Health Psychology, 4,* 219–247.
Shmotkin, D. (1991). The structure of the Life Satisfaction Index A in elderly Israeli adults. *International Journal of Aging and Human Development, 32,* 131–150.
Shepperd, J. A., Ouellette, J. A., & Fernandez, J. K. (1996). Abandoning unrealistic optimism: Performance estimates and the temporal proximity of self-relevant feedback. *Journal of personality and Social Psychology, 70,* 844–855.
Sherwood, J. J. (1965). Self identity and referent others. *Sociometry, 28,* 66–81.
Shrauger, J. S. (1975). Responses to evaluations as a function of initial self-perceptions. *Psychological Bulletin, 82,* 581–596.
Simons, A. D., Angell, K. L., Monroe, S. M., & Thase, M. E. (1993). Cognition and life stress in depression: Cognitive factors and the definition, rating, and generation of negative life events. *Journal of Abnormal Psychology, 102,* 584–591.
Sloper, P., Knussen, C., Turner, S., & Cunningham, C. (1991). Factors related to stress and satisfaction with life in families of children with Down's Syndrome. *Journal of Child Psychology and Psychiatry, 32,* 655–676.
Suh, E., & Diener, E. (1996). Events and subjective well-being: Only recent events matter. *Journal of Personality and Social Psychology, 70,* 1091–1102.
Suh, E., Diener, E., & Fujita, F. (1996). Events and subjective well-being: Only recent events matter. *Journal of Personality and Social Psychology, 70,* 1091–1102.
Switzky, H. N. (1997). Individual differences in personality and motivational systems in persons with mental retardation. In W. E. MacLean (Ed.), *Ellis' handbook of mental deficiency, psychological theory and research* (3rd ed., pp. 343–377). Hillsdale, NJ: Erlbaum.
Switzky, H. N. (1999). Intrinsic motivation and motivational self-system processes in persons with mental retardation: A theory of motivational orientation. In E. Zigler & D. Bennet-Gates (Eds.), *Personality development in individuals with mental retardation* (pp. 70–106). Cambridge: Cambridge University Press.
Switzky, H. N. (2003). A cognitive-motivational perspective on mental retardation. In H. N. Switzky & S. Greenspan (Eds.), *What is mental retardation? Ideas for an evolving disability.* Washington, DC: American Association on Mental Retardation.
Tiger, L. (1979). *Optimism: The biology of hope.* New York: Simon and Schuster.
Tonkens, E., & Weijers, I. (1999). Autonomy, solidarity, and self-realization: Policy view of dutch service providers. *Mental Retardation, 37,* 468–476.
Tymchuk, A. J. (1991). Self-concepts of mothers who show mental retardation. *Psychological Reports, 68,* 503–510.
Vaillant, C. O., & Vaillant, G. E. (1993). Is the U-curve of marital satisfaction an illusion? A 40-year study of marriage. *Journal of Marriage and the Family, 55,* 230–239.
Verkuyten, M. (1993). Self-esteem among ethnic minorities and three principles of self-esteem formation: Turkish children in the Netherlands. *International Journal of Psychology, 28,* 307–321.

Wakefield, J. A. (1989). Personality, health and cigarette smoking. *Personality and Individual Differences, 10,* 541–546.

Watson, D., & Tellegen, A. (1985). Toward a consensual structure of mood. *Psychological Bulletin, 98,* 219–235.

Watson, D., Clark, L. A., & Tellegen, A. (1988). Development and validation of brief measures of positive and negative affect: The PANAS scales. *Journal of Personality and Social Psychology, 54,* 1063–1070.

Watson, D., & Pennebaker, J. W. (1989). Health complaints, stress, and distress: Exploring the central role of negative affectivity. *Psychological Review, 96,* 234–254.

Watson, D., & Clark, L. A. (1992). On traits and temperament: General and specific factors of emotional experience and their relation to the five-factor model. *Journal of Personality, 60,* 441–476.

Watson, D., Clark, L. A., Weber, K., Assenheimer, J. S., Strauss, M. E., & McCormick, R. A. (1995). Testing a tripartite model: I. Evaluating the convergent and discriminant validity of anxiety and depression symptom scales. *Journal of Abnormal Psychology, 104,* 3–14.

Weisz, J. (1981). Learned helplessness in black and white children identified by their schools as retarded and nonretarded: Performance deterioration in response to failure. *Developmental Psychology, 17,* 499–508.

Wilson, K., & Gullone, E. (1999). The relationship between personality and affect over the life span. *Personality and Individual Differences, 27,* 1141–1156.

Wolinsky, F. D., Coe, R. M., Miller, D. K., & Prendergast, J. M. (1985). Correlates of change in subjective well-being among the elderly. *Journal of Community Health, 10,* 93–107.

Zautra, A., & Goodhart, D. (1979). Quality of life indicators: A review of the literature. *Community Mental Health Review, 4,* 1–10.

Zautra, A., & Reich, J. (1980). Positive life events and reports of well-being: Some useful distinctions. *American Journal of Community Psychology, 8,* 657–670.

Zigler, E. (1971). The retarded child as a whole person. In H. E. Adams & W. K. Boardman (Eds.), *Advances in experimental clinical psychology.* New York: Pergamon.

Quality of Life from a Motivational Perspective

ROBERT L. SCHALOCK

BOB SCHALOCK & ASSOCIATES
HASTINGS COLLEGE

This chapter proposes that the core domains of a quality life can be viewed as motivational states that initiate and direct behavior. To that end, this chapter is based on three assumptions:

- The end-states represented by each of the eight identified core quality-of-life domains represent desired human conditions associated with personal well-being and, therefore, result in incentives that underlie the motivational process.
- The person-centered nature of the concept of quality of life and its application results in an increase in one's internal locus of control, self-regulation, autonomy, self-determination, personal control, and expectancy of success.
- The ecological nature of quality-of-life enhancement techniques based on motivational strategies augment the positive effects of mediated learning experiences, thereby increasing one's intrinsic motivation.

This chapter is divided into five sections: (1) our current understanding of the concept of quality of life; (2) the current focus in personality and motivation research on effectance and intrinsic motivation; (3) the motivational aspects of the core quality-of-life domains; (4) quality-of-life and motivational strategies; and (5) implications of viewing quality of life from a motivational perspective.

I. OUR CURRENT UNDERSTANDING OF THE CONCEPT OF QUALITY OF LIFE

Over the last 15 years, there has been considerable work on the conceptualization, measurement, and application of the quality-of-life construct. Throughout this work, a consensus is emerging regarding its meaning and core domains.

A. Meaning

Throughout the world, the concept of quality of life is being used as a:

- *Sensitizing notion* that gives one a sense of reference and guidance from the individual's perspective, focusing on the person and the individual's environment. As a sensitizing notion, "quality" makes us think of the excellence or "exquisite standard" associated with human characteristics and positive values, such as happiness, success, wealth, health, and satisfaction; whereas "of life" indicates that the concept concerns the very essence or essential aspects of human existence (Lindstrom, 1992; Schalock, 2000; Schalock et al., 2002).
- *Social construct* that is being used as an overriding principle to evaluate person-referenced outcomes and to improve and enhance a person's perceived quality of life. In that regard, the concept is impacting program development, service delivery, management strategies, and evaluation activities in the areas of education, disabilities, mental health, and aging (Schalock, 2001; Schalock & Verdugo, 2002).
- *Unifying theme* that is providing a systematic framework for understanding and applying the quality-of-life concept in education, health, and rehabilitation programs. This systematic framework includes conceptualizing, measuring, and applying the concept from a systems perspective: microsystem—the immediate social setting, including the person, family, and/or advocates; mesosystem—the neighborhood, community, or organization providing education and habilitation services and supports; and macrosystem—the overarching patterns of culture, society, larger populations, and country or sociopolitical influences (Keith & Schalock, 2000; Schalock & Verdugo, 2002).

B. Core Domains

Rather than attempting a simple definition of quality-of-life, the current emphasis in quality-of-life research, application, and evaluation is to realize that quality of life is a multidimensional construct, with both subjective and objective components. The acceptance of the multidimensionality of a

TABLE I
Core Quality of Life Domains and Their Definitions

Emotional Well-Being: the condition of being content (satisfied, happy), having a positive self-concept, and/or being relatively free of stress.

Interpersonal Relations: the experiencing of social interactions and relationships (with family, friends, peers) and/or receiving supports (emotional, physical, financial, feedback) from family, friends, peers, or agencies.

Material Well-Being: the presence of adequate financial status, employment, and adequate housing.

Personal Development: the level of education received, personal competence expressed, and/or performance exhibited (includes creativity and personal expression).

Physical Well-Being: the level of health experienced (physical functioning, disease symptoms, pain, fitness, energy, nutrition); the performance of activities of daily living (walking, dressing, self-feeding) and leisure activities; and/or receipt of health care.

Self-Determination: the expression of autonomy and personal control, the pursuit of personal goals and values, and the opportunity to make choices.

Social Inclusion: the integration into and participation in one's community, the expression of valued social roles, and the receipt of social supports from the community.

Rights: the expression of human rights (respect, dignity, equality) and the guarantee of legal rights (citizenship, access, due process).

---

quality life has led to considerable work in identifying and validating eight individual-level core quality-of-life domains: (1) emotional well-being, (2) interpersonal relation, (3) material well-being, (4) personal development, (5) physical well-being, (6) self-determination, (7) social inclusion, and (8) rights (Schalock & Verdugo, 2002; Schalock et al., 2002). Each of these domains is defined in Table I.

II. THE FOCUS ON EFFECTANCE AND INTRINSIC MOTIVATION

This chapter is written within the context of the emerging work in the area of personality and motivation processes in persons with mental retardation. Although this work suggests a complex interplay among personality, motivation, and cognitive processes, two critical motivational concepts have emerged: effectance (or mastery) motivation, in which it is assumed that everyone has an intrinsic need to feel competent (White, 1959); and self efficacy beliefs, where one is capable of organizing and implementing actions necessary to attain designated levels of performance (Bandura, 1997). Our appreciation of these two concepts has resulted in a better understanding of the concepts of self-regulation, autonomy and self-determination, mediational learning experiences, and personality traits in persons with mental retardation.

In this volume and elsewhere, the reader will find excellent summaries in the area of personality and motivational processes in persons with mental retardation (for example, Lecavalier & Tasse, 2002; Reiss & Havercamp, 1998; Switzky, 1997, 1999; Zigler & Bennett-Gates, 1999; Zigler et al., 2002). Of direct relevance to this chapter is the concept of effectance (or mastery) motivation, which suggests that everyone has an intrinsic need to feel competent, which is associated with internal reinforcement, exploration, play, curiosity, and mastery of the environment (White, 1959). Over the years, research in this area has helped us to better understand the following four concepts that are integral to the next section on "the motivational aspects of the core quality-of-life domains."

1. *Self-regulation*, with the associated principles of: (a) self-efficacy (or beliefs concerning one's capabilities to organize and implement actions necessary to attain designated levels of performance; Bandura, 1997); and (b) goal-setting and goal values as reasons for task engagement (Dweck & Leggett, 1988).
2. *Autonomy and self-determination*, which leads to an internal locus of control (Rotter, 1966), increased intrinsic motivation (Ryan & Deci, 2000), a sense of competence (Deci & Ryan, 1991), and enhanced decision-making (Mithaug, 1996).
3. *Knowledge acquisition strategies* that involve mediational learning experiences (Feuerstein et al., 1991; Tzuriel, 1991) and active problem-solving processes (Sternberg & Berg, 1992; Switzsky, 1997).
4. *Personality traits* in persons with mental retardation suggesting that these individuals have: (a) lower levels of expectancy of success and effectance motivation than those of normal intellect; (b) higher levels of dependency on a supportive adult, with initial wariness when interacting with strange adults; (c) higher levels of outer directedness and looking to others for solutions of difficult or ambiguous problems; and (d) higher levels of extrinsic motivation orientation and learned helplessness (Hodapp & Fidler, 1999; Switzky, 1997, 1999; Zigler et al., 1999).

III. THE MOTIVATIONAL ASPECTS OF THE CORE QUALITY-OF-LIFE DOMAINS

Thus far, this chapter has reviewed our current understanding of the concept of quality of life, focusing on its meaning and core domains, and summarized key personality and motivational concepts (such as self regulation, autonomy and self determination, knowledge acquisition strategies, and personality traits) from the current work on personality and motivational processes in persons with mental retardation. The purpose of this section is to relate each of the eight person-centered core quality-of-life domains to potential motivational states.

The relationships between each of the eight person-centered core quality-of-life domains and potential motivational states are summarized in Table II. The left column lists the eight core person-referenced quality-of-life domains; the right column lists potential literature-based motivation states that can be associated with the respective domain. As discussed later, each of these

TABLE II
CORE QUALITY OF LIFE DOMAINS AND POTENTIAL MOTIVATION STATES

Quality of Life Domain	Potential Motivation State/Reference
Emotional Well-Being	Esteem (M)
	Honor (R)
	Tranquility (R)
	Order (R)
Interpersonal Relations	Relatedness (R & D)
	Social contact (R)
	Family (R)
	Romance (R)
Material Well-Being	Status (R)
	Savings (R)
	Achievement (Mc)
Personal Development	Competence (R & D)
	Goal setting and values (D & L)
	Self-actualization (M)
	Curiosity (R)
Physical Well-Being	Physiological (M)
	Exercise (R)
Self-Determination	Autonomy (R & D)
	Self-actualization (M)
	Intrinsic motivation (D & R)
	Self-efficacy (B)
	Independence (R)
	Power (R)
Social Inclusion	Love and belonging (M)
	Idealism (R)
	Acceptance (R)
Rights	Safety (M)

Key to initials in parentheses: B (Bandura, 1997); D & L (Dweck & Leggett, 1988); D & R (Deci & Ryan, 1991); Mc (McClelland, 1955); M (Maslow, 1954); R (Reiss, 2000); R & D (Ryan & Deci, 2000).

motivational states can lead to domain enhancement and resultant satisfaction. As also shown in Table II, each potential motivational state is followed in parenthesis by an author's initials, with the specific author(s) referenced in the table footnote. The clear relationship between core quality-of-life domains and potential motivational states allows one to view quality of life as a motivational construct. The implications of this fourth perspective are discussed in the following two sections.

IV. QUALITY OF LIFE AND MOTIVATIONAL STRATEGIES

Three premises were stated in the introduction of this chapter: (1) the end-states represented by each of the eight core quality-of-life domains represent desired human conditions associated with personal well-being and, therefore, result in incentives that underlie the motivation process; (2) the person-centered nature of the concept of quality of life and its application results in an increase in one's internal locus of control, self-regulation, autonomy, self-determination, personal control, and expectancy of success; and (3) the ecological nature of quality-of-life enhancement techniques based on motivational strategies augments the positive effects of mediated learning experiences, thereby increasing one's intrinsic motivation. If these premises are correct, which appears to be the case, what strategies might be used to develop skills associated with increased individual motivation? Below are eight motivation-enhancing skills that presumably increase both effectance and instrinsic motivation and can be developed through instruction to promote capacity (skills and knowledge), opportunities to experience control and choice, and the design of supports and accommodations.

- *Choice-making skills.* Examples include choosing between two or more activities or options, deciding when to do an activity, and selecting the person with whom to associate.
- *Problem-solving skills.* Examples include listing relevant action alternatives, identifying consequences of those actions, assessing the probability of each consequence, establishing the relative importance or value of each consequence, and integrating these values and probabilities to identify the most attractive course of action.
- *Decision-making skills.* Most models of decision making incorporate the following steps: listing relevant action alternatives, identifying possible consequences of those actions, assessing the probability of each consequence occurring (if the action were undertaken), establishing the relative importance (value or utility) of each consequence, and integrating

these values and probabilities to identify the most attractive course of action.
- *Goal-setting and attainment skills.* Examples include identification and enunciation of specific goals, the development of objectives and tasks to achieve these goals, and the actions necessary to achieve a desired outcome.
- *Self-management skills.* Examples include self-monitoring, self-evaluation, self-instruction, and self-reinforcement.
- *Self-advocacy and leadership skills.* Examples include being assertive, communicating effectively, negotiating, compromising, using persuasion, being an effective listener, and navigating through systems and bureaucracies.
- *Perceptions of control and efficiency.* These result from choice-making, problem-solving, decision-making, and goal-setting and attainment.
- *Self-awareness and self-knowledge.* These result from one's interpretation of events and experiences such as meaningful activities and meaningful lives (for example, work and home).

V. IMPLICATIONS OF VIEWING QUALITY OF LIFE FROM A MOTIVATIONAL PERSPECTIVE

Increasingly, the quality-of-life literature is approaching the conceptualization, measurement, and application of the concept from a systems perspective that focuses on either the individual (micro), the larger community (meso), or the larger society (macro). Consistent with this approach, this final section suggests three implications of viewing quality of life from a motivational perspective: implications from an individual, program, and policy perspective.

A. Individual Implications

The reader is familiar with the use of a hierarchy to denote the relative value or position of different motivational states. The most familiar example is probably that of Maslow (1954). In addition, reinforcement hierarchies have been used to describe the position of value of a reinforcer for a given person, which is determined by a complex interaction of developmental level, past social learning experience, availability of the reinforcer, and whether or not it has acquired the properties of a higher-order reinforcer (Zigler, 1971, 1999). The use of a hierarchy to describe relative value or position is extended here to include the eight core person-centered quality-of-life domains. Two examples are presented that reflect both the potentially generic nature (the "generalized" quality-of-life hierarchy), and the individualized valence (the "personalized" hierarchy) of these eight domains. The first example is based on work done in Spain (Elorriaga et al., 2000) and a participatory action research project in the state of Maryland (Schalock, Bonham, & Marchand, 2000); the second is based on a case involving a serious burn to a person diagnosed as an individual with "severe/profound mental retardation."

1. THE "GENERALIZED" QUALITY-OF-LIFE HIERARCHY

The core domains of a quality life have been modeled as a triangle (Elorriaga et al., 2000), with a hierarchy built upon the foundation of physical well-being, material well-being, and rights. As shown in Fig. 1, the next level of the hierarchy is personal development and self-determination, followed higher by social inclusion and interpersonal relations. At the top of the hierarchy is emotional well-being. In my work with self-advocates in the U. S. and elsewhere, the motivational aspects of this hierarchy are seen clearly when each of the levels is used to describe what people want:

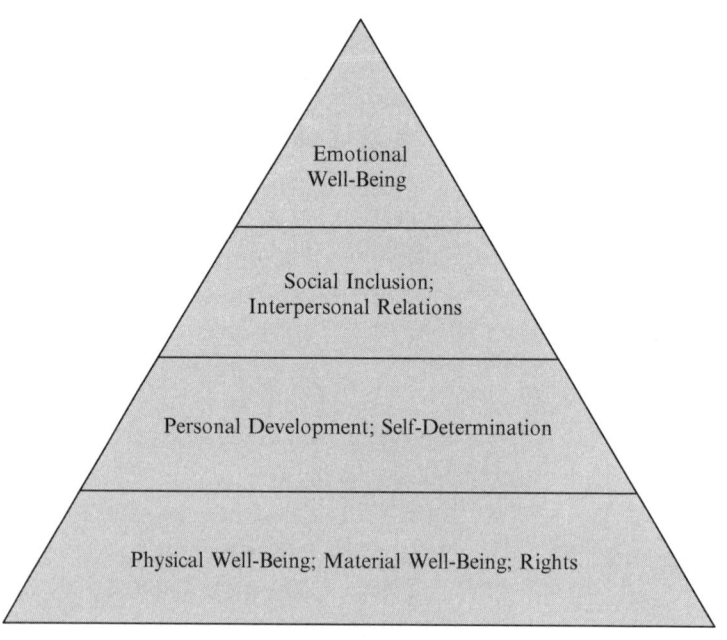

FIG. 1. The quality of life hierarchy.

- To stay healthy and safe (physical well-being, material well-being, and rights);
- To have what and who is important to us in everyday life, and to have people to be with us, things to do, and places to be (personal development and self-determination);
- To have opportunities to meet new people, and to change with whom and where we live (social inclusion and interpersonal relations);
- To have our own dreams and our own journeys (emotional well-being).

The triangle shown in Fig. 1, turned on its side, forms the basis for a path analysis of participatory action research data currently being collected on a group of persons with mental retardation/developmental disabilities receiving services in the state of Maryland (Schalock et al., 2000; Schalock & Bonham, 2003). The project involves self-advocates administering to other self-advocates a 50-item quality-of-life questionnaire based on the eight person-centered core quality-of-life domains listed in Table I. As shown in Fig. 2, physical well-being, material well-being, and rights are shown on the left. They are related, as indicated by the curved arrows among them, but without assuming causality. Physical and material well-being are highly related, as indicated by the path coefficient of 0.69. Rights are significantly related to physical and material well-being, but not as strongly as physical and material well-being are related to each other.

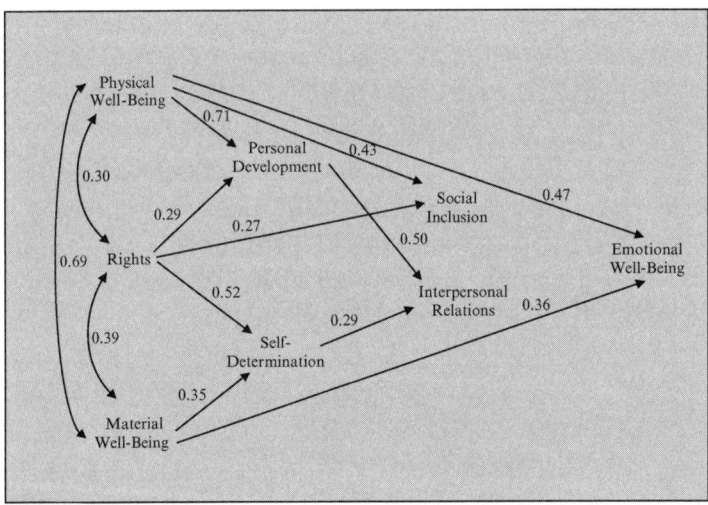

FIG. 2. Path model of quality of life hierarchy.

The foundational life domain of rights affects both domains on the next level of the hierarchy, but rights affect self-determination more than it affects personal development. Physical well-being has a strong impact on personal development, but has no significant impact on self-determination (hence, no arrow is shown between physical well-being and self-determination). Material well-being affects self-determination, but does not affect personal development. Physical and material well-being also have a direct impact on emotional well-being, rather than having all of their impact indirectly through intermediate levels of the hierarchy. The domain of rights also has a direct effect on the domain of social inclusion.

2. A "PERSONALIZED" HIERARCHY

I have recently been involved in a personal injury case that demonstrates that the motivational aspects of the "generalized" hierarchy shown in Fig. 1 can differ depending upon the individual (which is quite consistent with the notion of the subjective nature to both quality-of-life and motivational states). The case involved a 26-year-old male who is diagnosed as an individual with "severe/profound mental retardation." After attending public school until he was 21, John (a fictitious name) was admitted to a community-based, community living facility. Although scoring low on standardized intelligence tests, John demonstrates good sensory-motor skills, minimal receptive language, and some self-help skills (such as self-feeding and partial dressing). Soon after his enrollment in the community living facility, John received serious burns to his lower legs and feet when he sat down in an unattended bathtub. Subsequently, he was admitted to an emergency room and a burn unit. Two days after the burn incident, a naso-gastric tube was inserted since he had refused to eat and drink. The issue that was presented to me was: "What is the impact on John's quality of life, given his earlier history compared to that which has followed the accident (including being placed in a skilled nursing facility due to the need for flushing of the naso-gastric tube twice daily)?"

In observing John for an extended period of time, it was apparent that the "generalized" hierarchy shown in Fig. 1 needed to be revised based on his current needs and potential motivational states. This new configuration of the hierarchy is shown in Fig. 3 and indicates that the foundation levels for John include: rights, personal development, emotional well-being, physical well-being, and social inclusion. Once these levels are addressed, then the quality-of-life domains of material well-being, interpersonal relations, and self-determination will be more involved.

From a motivational perspective, there are at least three major implications from the individual's perspective. First, the relative incentive value of each quality-of-life domain can vary between people and across the

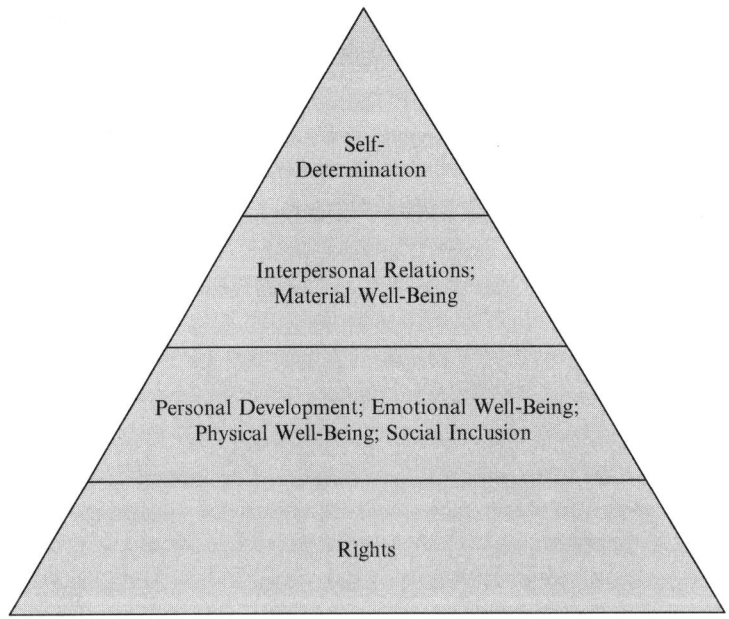

FIG. 3. A personalized quality of life hierarchy.

lifespan. For example, for youth the domains of interpersonal relations, self-determination, and social inclusion may be most important; whereas for people of age, emotional, material, and physical well-being may be relatively more important than the other five domains. Second, the end-states represented by each quality-of-life domain represent desired conditions and thereby result in incentives that underlie the motivational process. The reader may wonder at this point: "What are those end-states?" Increasingly, they appear to be personal well-being as reflected in the concepts of happiness and satisfaction (Crocker, 2000; Cummins, 1996; Diener, 2000; Meyers, 2000; Schalock & Felce, 2004). And third, quality-of-life domains, just as motivational states, are unique to the individual and need to be approached from the perspective of self-determination and personal control. This implication directly affects education and rehabilitation programs.

B. Program Implications

Research guided by a self-determination theory has focused primarily on the social-cultural conditions that facilitate the natural processes of self-motivation and enhanced intrinsic motivation, self-regulation, and well-being. This research has produced two significant results: first, the successful satisfaction of an individual's competence, autonomy, and relatedness motives yield enhanced self-motivation, constructive social development, and personal well-being (Ryan & Deci, 2000); and second, assessed levels of self-determination and quality of life are significantly positively correlated (Wehmeyer & Schwartz, 1998). Given these findings, the logical question to ask is: "What education and rehabilitation programmatic practices might enhance the desired outcomes of enhanced intrinsic motivation, self regulation, and well-being?" Two factors are highlighted in the literature: self-determination and personal control.

1. SELF-DETERMINATION

Self-determined behavior refers to actions that are identified by four essential characteristics (Wehmeyer & Schalock, 2001): (1) the person acts autonomously (according to their own preferences, interests, and/or abilities, and independently which is to be free from undue external influences or interference); (2) the action(s) was self-regulated and includes self-management strategies (for example, self-monitoring, self-instruction, self-evaluation, and self-reinforcement), goal-setting and attainment behaviors, problem-solving behaviors, and observational learning strategies; (3) the person initiated and responded to the event(s) in a psychologically empowered manner reflective of personal efficacy and internal locus of control; and (4) the person acted in a self-realizing and understanding manner that forms through experience with an interpretation of one's environment, and is influenced by evaluations of significant others, reinforcement, and attributions of one's own behavior.

2. PERSONAL CONTROL

According to Stancliffe et al. (2000a), personal control is not the same as self-determination. Specifically, self-determination involves a person controlling those areas of their life that they desire to exercise control; whereas, personal control refers to what happens to them in their lives, when and where it occurs, and with whom it takes place (p. 431). Through a series of studies (Stancliffe et al., 2000a,b) the authors have found that increased personal control is related to:

- Measured self-determination skills (such as choice-making, goal-setting, problem-solving, self-regulation, personal advocacy skills, social and communication skills, and community-living skills).

- Measured self-determination knowledge (such as resources and the system, laws, rights, responsibilities, perceived options, and self awareness).
- Measured self-determination attitudes and beliefs (such as locus of control, self-esteem, self-acceptance, self-confidence/self-efficacy, and value by others).

From a motivational perspective, the components to self-determination and personal control are important for at least two reasons. First, they underscore the critical role that self-determination and personal control should play in the provision of education, habilitation, and social services. In this regard, there is an emerging set of best practices in self-determination that reflect many of these components including (Ficker-Terrill, 2002; Moseley & Nerney, 2000): independent service provision, which minimizes a conflict of interest; flexible individual budgeting; personally directed and controlled planning process; independent support brokerage; autonomous fiscal intermediary services; meaningful activities and lives (work and home); and the provision of a wide array of service and support options.

Second, the components imply a direct relationship between quality of life and self-determination as reflected in the following three findings:

1. One factor contributing to the positive outcomes in the lives of persons with mental retardation and a higher level of assessed quality of life is enhanced self-determination (Wehmeyer & Schwartz, 1998).
2. People who are self-determined make or cause things to happen in their lives; they are causal agents in their lives. However, causal agency implies more than simply making something happen; it implies that the individual who makes or causes things to happen does so to accomplish a specific end. Intuitively, and by definition, these ends or changes are designed to improve or enhance the person's quality of life (Wehmeyer & Schalock, 2001).
3. The degree to which a person is self-determined either influences or is influenced by other core domains of quality of life, and, in combination with these other core domains, influences or impacts global or overall quality-of-life status (Schalock et al., 2000).
4. The person-centered nature of the concept of quality of life and its application results in an increase in one's internal locus of control, enhanced self-regulation, autonomy, self-direction, personal control, and expectancy of success (Schalock & Verdugo, 2002).

C. Policy Implications

A final implication of viewing quality of life from a motivational perspective relates to the increasing emphasis on consumer direction in human services. As discussed by Ficker-Terrill (2002), Kosciulek (2000), and Schalock (2004), if people with disabilities are to experience personal satisfaction, increased motivation, and an enhanced quality of life, they need to play a central role in directing the disability policy development and rehabilitation services delivery that are central to their empowerment. To empower a person is to provide them with the opportunity to make choices and decisions regarding their life. Choice and control are highly valued prerogatives that reflect the autonomy, identity, and independence of an individual, and result in increased motivation and perceived quality of life (Wehmeyer & Schalock, 2001). Given this relationship and the above discussion of the relationship between self-determination and motivation, three principles are emerging in the rehabilitation literature (Kosciulek, 2000):

1. Consumer-directed disability policy and rehabilitation programming should be based on the presumption that consumers with disabilities generally and clearly understand their service needs.
2. Choice and control can be introduced into all service delivery environments.
3. Consumer direction in the provision of services should be available to all.

At least two implications follow from the emergence of consumer empowerment and consumer direction. First, both conditions are logical extensions of the previous discussion of self-determination and personal control, including their impact on service and support provision, quality of life, internal locus of control, and self-efficacy. Second, the consumer movement reflects the ecological nature of quality-of-life enhancement techniques that augment the positive effects of mediated learning experiences and hence increases one's intrinsic motivation.

VI. CONCLUSIONS

In conclusion, writing this chapter has allowed for the appreciated opportunity to extend the concept of quality of life to another dimension—that of a motivational construct. In addition to its use as a sensitizing notion, social construct, and unifying theme, it is quite apparent that the person-centered nature of the quality-of-life concept is consistent with the notion that motivation concerns all aspects of activation and intention: energy, direction, persistence, and equifinality (Ryan & Deci, 2000). As discussed throughout the chapter, the end-states represented by each of the eight core quality-of-life domains represent the perceived personal well-being that serves as an incentive underlying the motivational process. Furthermore, the person-centered nature of the quality-of-life concept and its application result in an increase in one's internal locus of control, self-direction, personal control, autonomy, intrinsic motivation, and expectancy of success.

If the above statements are true, then the current popularity of the concept of quality of life and its application to persons with mental retardation potentially has more impact than once thought. For now, we need to focus not just on the person's perceptions of a quality life and what education and rehabilitation programs can do to enhance that perception, but to realize that from the individual's perspective, the desire for a quality life has motivating and sustaining components as well. Thus, our future research and evaluation challenge is to identify the individual and social-cultural factors that enhance those components and their outcomes.

REFERENCES

Bandura, A. (1997). *Self-efficacy*. New York: W. H. Freeman.
Crocker, A. C. (2000). Introduction: The happiness in all our lives. *American Journal on Mental Retardation, 105*(5), 319–325.
Cummins, R. A. (1996). The domains of life satisfaction: An attempt to order chaos. *Social Indicators Research, 38,* 303–328.
Deci, E. L., & Ryan, R. M. (1991). A motivated approach to self: Integration in personality. In R. Dienstbier (Ed.), *Nebraska symposium on motivation, Vol. 38: Perspectives on motivation* (pp. 237–288). Lincoln: University of Nebraska Press.
Diener, E. (2000). Subjective well-being: The science of happiness and a proposal for a national index. *American Psychologist, 55*(1), 34–43.
Dweck, C. S., & Leggett, E. L. (1988). A social-cognitive approach to motivation and personality. *Psychological Review, 95,* 256–273.
Elorriaga, J., Garcia, L., Martinez, J., & Unamunzaga, E. (2000). Quality of life of people with mental retardation in Spain: One organization's experience. In K. D. Keith & R. L. Schalock (Eds.), *Cross-cultural perspectives on quality of life* (pp. 113–124). Washington, DC: American Association on Mental Retardation.
Feuerstein, R., Klein, P. S., & Tannenbaum, A. J. (Eds.) (1991). *Mediated learning experience (MLE): Theoretical, psychosocial and learning implications.* London: Freund Publishing House Ltd.
Ficker-Terrill, K. (2002). The future. In R. L. Schalock, P. C. Baker, & M. D. Croser (Eds.), *Embarking on a new century: Mental retardation at the end of the 20th century* (pp. 237–245). Washington, DC: American Association on Mental Retardation.
Hodapp, R. M., & Fidler, D. J. (1999). Parenting, etiology, and personality-motivational functioning in children with mental retardation. In E. Zigler & D. Bennett-Gates (Eds.),

Personality development in individuals with mental retardation (pp. 226–248). Cambridge, UK: Cambridge University Press.

Keith, K. D., & Schalock, R. L. (2000). *Cross-cultural perspectives on quality of life*. Washington, DC: American Association on Mental Retardation.

Kosciulek, J. F. (2000). Implications of consumer direction for disability policy development and rehabilitation service delivery. *Journal of Disability Policy Studies, 11*(2), 82–89.

Lecavalier, L., & Tasse, M. (2002). Sensitivity theory of motivation and psychopathology: An exploratory study. *American Journal on Mental Retardation, 107*(2), 105–115.

Lindstrom, B. (1992). Quality of life: A model for evaluating health for all. *Soz Praventivimed, 37*, 301–306.

Maslow, A. H. (1954). *Motivation and personality*. New York: Harper & Row.

McClelland, D. C. (1955). Some social consequences of achievement motivation. In M. R. Jones (Ed.), *Nebraska symposium on motivation* (pp. 50–102). Lincoln: University of Nebraska Press.

Meyers, D. G. (2000). The funds, friends, and faith of happy people. *American Psychologist, 55*(1), 56–67.

Mithaug, D. E. (1996). The optimal prospects principle: A theoretical basis for rethinking instructional practices for self-determination. In D. J. Sands & M. L. Wehmeyer (Eds.), *Self-determination across the life span: Independence and choice for people with disabilities* (pp. 147–165). Baltimore: Paul H. Brookes.

Moseley, C., & Nerney, T. (2000, December/November). Emerging best practices in self-determination. *AAMR News and Notes.* 1–5.

Reiss, S. (2000). A mindful approach to mental retardation. *Journal of Social Issues, 56*(1), 65–80.

Reiss, S., & Havercamp, S. H. (1998). Toward a comprehensive assessment of fundamental motivation: Factor structure of the Reiss profiles. *Psychological Assessment, 10*, 97–106.

Rotter, J. B. (1966). Generalized expectancies for internal vs. external control of reinforcement. *Psychological Monographs, 80* (1, Whole No. 609).

Ryan, R. M., & Deci, E. L. (2000). Self-determination theory and the facilitation of intrinsic motivation, social development, and well-being. *American Psychologist, 55*(1), 68–78.

Schalock, R. L. (2000). Three decades of quality of life. In M. L. Wehmeyer & J. R. Patton (Eds.), *Mental retardation in the 21st century* (pp. 335–358). Austin, TX: Pro-Ed.

Schalock, R. L. (2001). *Outcome-based evaluation: Second edition*. New York: Kluwer Academic/Plenum Publishers.

Schalock, R. L. (2004). The emerging disability paradigm and its implications for policy and practice. *Journal of Disability Policy Studies, 14*(4), 204–215.

Schalock, R. L., & Bonham, G. S. (2003). Measuring outcomes and managing for results. *Evaluation and Program Planning, 24*(3), 229–235.

Schalock, R. L., Bonham, G. S., & Marchand, C. B. (2000). Consumer-based quality of life assessment: A path model of perceived satisfaction. *Evaluation and Program Planning, 23*(1), 77–88.

Schalock, R. L., Brown, I., Brown, R., Cummins, R. A., Felce, D., Matikka, L., Keith, K. D., & Parmenter, T. (2002). Conceptualization, measurement, and application of quality of life for persons with intellectual disabilities: Results of an international panel of experts. *Mental Retardation, 40*(6), 457–470.

Schalock, R. L., & Felce, D. (2004). Quality of life and subjective well-being. In E. Emerson, T. Thompson, T. Parmenter, & C. Hatton (Eds.), *International handbook of methods for research and evaluation in intellectual disabilities* (pp. 261–279). West Sussex, England: John Wiley and Sons.

Schalock, R. L., & Verdugo, M. A. (2002). *Handbook on quality of life for human service practitioners.* Washington, DC: American Association on Mental Retardation.

Stancliffe, R. J., Abery, B. H., & Smith, J. (2000a). Personal control and the ecology of community living settings: Beyond living-unit size and type. *American Journal on Mental Retardation, 105*(6), 431–454.

Stancliffe, R. J., Abery, B. H., Springborg, H., & Elkin, S. (2000b). Substitute decision-making and personal control: Implications for self-determination. *Mental Retardation, 38*(5), 407–421.

Sternberg, R. J., & Berg, C. A. (Eds.) (1992). *Intellectual development.* New York: Cambridge University Press.

Switzky, H. N. (1997). Individual differences in personality and motivational systems in persons with mental retardation. In W. E. MacLean, Jr. (Ed.), *Ellis' handbook of mental eficiency, psychological theory and research,* (3rd ed., pp. 343–377). Mahwah, NJ: Erlbaum.

Switzky, H. N. (1999). Intrinsic motivation and motivational system process in persons with mental retardation: A theory of motivational orientation. In E. Zigler & D. Bennett-Gates (Eds.), *Personality development in individuals with mental retardation* (pp. 70–106). Cambridge, UK: Cambridge University Press.

Tzuriel, D. (1991). Cognitive modifiability, mediated learning experience and affective motivational processes: A transactional approach. In R. Feuerstein, P. S. Klein, & A. J. Tannenbaum (Eds.), *Mediated learning experience (MLE): Theoretical, psychosocial and learning implications* (pp. 95–120). London: Freund Publishing House Ltd.

Wehmeyer, M. L., & Schalock, R. L. (2001). Self-determination and quality of life: Implications for special education services and supports. *Focus on Exceptional Children, 33,* 1–16.

Wehmeyer, M. L., & Schwartz, M. (1998). The relationship between self-determination, quality of life, and life satisfaction for adults with mental retardation. *Education and Training in Mental Retardation and Developmental Disabilities, 33,* 3–12.

White, R. (1959). Motivation reconsidered: The concept of competence. *Psychological Review, 88,* 297–333.

Zigler, E. (1971). The retarded child as a whole person. In H. E. Adams & W. K. Boardman (Eds.), *Advances in experimental clinical psychology* (pp. 34–60). New York: Pergamon Press.

Zigler, E. (1999). The individual with mental retardation as a whole person. In E. Zigler & D. Bennett-Gates (Eds.), *Personality development in individuals with mental retardation* (pp. 1–16). Cambridge, UK: Cambridge University Press.

Zigler, E., & Bennett-Gates, D. (1999). *Personality development in individuals with mental retardation.* Cambridge, UK: Cambridge University Press.

Zigler, E., Bennett-Gates, D., & Hodapp, R. (2000). Assessing personality traits of individuals with mental retardation. In E. Zigler & D. Bennett-Gates (Eds.), *Personality development in individuals with mental retardation* (pp. 206–225). Cambridge, UK: Cambridge University Press.

Zigler, E., Bennett-Gates, D., Hodapp, R., & Henrich, C. C. (2002). Assessing personality traits of individuals with mental retardation. *American Journal on Mental Retardation, 107*(3), 181–193.

Index

A

Ability, 202
  motivation vs., 191–192
Achievement, exceptional students' intrinsic motivation associated with, 198
Achievement motivation
  expectancy-value theory of, 202–203
  goal theory of, 200–201
  study of, 192
Adaptation
  evidence for, 287–288
  in homeostatic model of SWB, 285–288
Adaptation Level Theory, 285–288
Adaptive Learning Environments Model (ALEM), 96
ALEM. *See* Adaptive Learning Environments Model
Amotivation, motivation vs., 2–3
Anxiety, performance goals
  relation to, 70
Aptitude tests, 147
Attachment, as root of loneliness, 228
Attributes, adaptive pattern of, 64
Autonomous behavior. *See* Self-determined behavior
Autonomy, 4, 306
  support, 12–13

B

Behavior
  autonomous vs. controlled, 3–4
  control/regulation of, 52–53
  disruptive, 215
  emotional regulation of, 238
  forethought/planning/activation of, 51
  intentions linked to, 51
  LD/regulation of, 56–57
  of lonely children, 234–235
  mastery goals/regulation of, 65–66
  monitoring/awareness of, 51–52
  motivated, 2–3
  performance goals/regulation of, 70–71
  reaction/reflection of, 53
  regulation of, 34, 50–53
  self-determined, 3–4
  social proof for acceptable, 128
  socially incompetent, 125
Behavioral Activating System, 271–272

C

CFL program. *See* Community for Learning program
Cognition
  activation of prior knowledge in, 37
  control/regulation of, 39–40
  development of, 148, 177–178
  difficulties with, 237
  mastery goals/regulation of, 61–63
  metacognition knowledge activation for, 37–38
  monitoring of, 38–39
  performance goals/regulation of, 67–68
  planning/activation of, 36–38
  reaction/reflection of, 40–41
  regulation of, 34, 36–43
  scaffolding and socially mediated development of, 148–161, 149, 155
  self-esteem as, 276–277
  self-monitoring, 62
  self-regulating, 42

Cognition (*cont.*)
  situational pressure factors/motivational tendencies contribution to, 167, 169–170, 169
  strategies for, 38, 40, 62
  subnormal reading achievement development factors of, 162–177, 167, 168, 169, 171–172, 176, 177
  SWB component of, 257
  task oriented students' strategies of, 156
Communication
  everyday intelligence activation of, 137–138
  in MST, 137–138
  skills of people with MR, 137
Community(ies)
  caring as product of, 99
  from collaboration, 112
  learner-centered learning, 111–112
  school as, 97–98
  social/emotional support from, 94
Community for Learning (CFL) program, 95–96
Companionship
  adult-/peer-mediated approaches to promote, 245
  environment promoting, 244
  social status and, 240–241
Comprehensive Quality of Life Scale (ComQol), 257
  SQOL measured through, 260
ComQol. *See* Comprehensive Quality of Life Scale
Context
  control of, 55–56
  forethought/planning/activation of, 34, 54
  LD/regulation of, 56–57
  mastery goals/regulation of, 65–66
  monitoring of, 54–55
  performance goals/regulation of, 70–71
  reaction/reflection of, 56
  regulation of, 34, 53–57
  self-regulated learning and, 53–57
Control, concept of, 4
Controlled behavior, self-determination behavior *vs.*, 3–4
Coping strategies, 166
  coherence and, 243
  ego-defensive, 158–159, 167, 168
  formation of, 178

  for loneliness, 241–242
  non-task-oriented *vs.* task oriented, 180
  problem-focused, 156
  research, 217
  self-esteem/developing, 277
  social dependence, 160–161
  task-oriented, 156–157
  teachers and loneliness, 244
Creativity, intrinsic motivation linked to, 17
Credulity
  everyday intelligence aspect of, 129
  of persons with developmental disabilities, 126
  social adaptation relevance of, 129–130

D

Development. *See also* Zone of proximal development
  child-adult interactions determinant of, 228–229
  of higher mental functions through social mediation, 148–149
  of maturing competencies, 149–150, 149
  of morality, 141
  of self-regulation, 148
  socially mediated cognition/motivation, 148–161, 149, 155
Development disabilities
  companionship of children with, 240–241
  comprehensibility/manageability/meaningfulness of children with, 243–244
  development tasks of children with, 236
  knowledge acquiring structure of children with, 238
  loneliness of people with, 225–226
  loneliness/social difficulties in, 230–231
  risk factors for, 229
  social competence/loneliness self-reports of students with, 231–232
  social difficulties of people with, 225, 234
  staying alone of children with, 235
Disabilities. *See also* Intellectual disabilities; Learning Disabilities
  defining, 87–88
  functional vulnerability of children with, 241

gullibility/credulity of persons with developmental, 126
loneliness of children with, 242–243
negative trends for students with, 87–88

E

Education. *See also* Special education
living systems framework for, 108–109
Effectance, current focus on, 305–306
Ego-defensive orientation
adaptive focus of, 157
ego-defensive coping and, 158–159
reading skills and, 166–167, 167
Emotions
affective-cognitive approach assumptions of, 235–236
cognitive functioning impact of, 235
cognitive processing role of, 237
community support of, 94
informational effects of, 236–237
MR and problems with, 135
MST role of, 135
regulation of, 238–240, 239–240, 239
self-regulation and, 48, 135
Environments
companionship promoting, 244
exceptional students' motivation and classroom, 215
learning, 94, 114–115
loneliness and social, 233
loneliness contributions of, 228
motivation and classroom, 213–215
Everyday intelligence
as activator of communication, 137–138
as aspect of credulity, 129
intellectual deficits in, 130
of people with MR, 129
raw information processing power/accumulated knowledge of, 129
social incompetence contributions of, 128–130
social/practical intelligence domains of, 128
Exceptional students. *See also* Non-exceptional students
classroom environment/motivation of, 215
expectancies/values of, 202–203
goal orientation of, 201
intrinsic motivation framework of research on, 197
intrinsic motivation of non-exceptional *vs.*, 198–199
intrinsic motivation/achievement associations of, 198
mastery orientation of, 212
motivation of, 197–208
social relationships of, 206–207
External regulation, 7
Extraversion, 267–268, 273
Extrinsic motivation. *See also* External regulation
behavior as becoming self-determined, 6
behaviors of, 4
helplessness and, 170
internalization of, 6–9
internalization/integration caused types of, 7–9
intrinsic motivation *vs.*, 197
for performing intrinsically motivated behavior, 4–5
in SDT, 5–6
social contexts' effects on, 9
strategies to increase, 37
types of, 7–9, 9

F

Facilitated communication (FC), 139–140
FC. *See* Facilitated communication

G

Goal(s). *See also* Goal orientation; Mastery goals; Performance goals
academic alienation, 61
achievement, 204
classes of, 57–58
in classroom setting, 61
mastery avoidance, 60, 63, 66
of mastery/performance, 59, 60
MR and coordination of, 133
in MST, 131–133
performance, 59
purpose, 58
selection of, 132
social, 61, 204

Goal(s) (cont.)
　social competence contribution to
　　academic, 121
　target/purpose, 57–58
　theory, 200–201
　work avoidant, 61
Goal orientation
　achievement, 200
　approach/avoidance forms of, 59,
　　59, 61
　ego and, 60–61
　exceptional vs. non-exceptional
　　students', 201
　general performance, 60
　learning, 104
　mastery, 200, 211
　models of, 58–62, 59
　performance-approach, 200–201
　research on, 61, 71–73
　self-regulated learning and, 57–72, 59
　social, 200
　special education/performance, 209, 210
　of students with LD, 201

I

Identified regulation, 7–8
Inclusion, reducing policy isolation/barriers
　to, 109–110
Instruction. See also Teachers
　in CFL program, 95–96
　forms of, 179
　LCPs and, 89
　learner-centered project-based, 101
　learning interaction with, 148–149
　minimal-sufficiency principle/maximal-
　　operant principle and, 150–151
　models of, 148
　project-based, 55–56
Integrated regulation, 8–9
Integration
　of extrinsic motivation, 6–8
　facilitating, 6
　in organismic theories of behavior, 6
　processes of, 13
　in SDT, 13–14
Intellectual disabilities
　external control/reduction in, 274
　motivation in field of, 271
　perceived control for people
　　with, 274–275
　self-esteem's relevance to, 277
　SWB as outcome measure of people
　　with, 264
Intelligence. See also Everyday intelligence
　academic, 128
Intention, as feature of motivated
　behavior, 2
Interest(s)
　mastery goals related to, 66
　recognizing individual, 94
　self-regulated learning and, 45–46
Internalization
　of extrinsic motivation, 6–9
　processes of, 13
　in SDT, 6, 13–14
　social context and, 13–14
Intrinsic motivation, 6
　behaviors of, 4
　contextual factors effect on, 11
　controlling event undermining, 10–11
　creativity linked to, 17
　current focus on, 305–306
　disruptive behavior and, 215
　exceptional students' achievement
　　associated with, 198
　exceptional vs. non-exceptional
　　students', 198–199
　extrinsic motivation vs., 197
　extrinsic rewards' effects
　　on, 4–5, 10
　increased, 170
　LD vs. non-LD students', 199
　learning and, 14–15
　negative feedback as decreasing, 11–12
　positive feedback as strengthening, 11
　relatedness facilitating, 10
　rewards' effect on, 199
　social context and, 10–13
　social contexts' effects on, 9
　in students with MR, 20–21
　of students with MR/LD, 198
　task orientation indicated by, 154

J

JOLs. See Judgments of learning
Judgments of learning (JOLs), 38–39

INDEX

K

Knowledge
  deficit, 234
  representations/organization of, 238
  specialization of, 193–195

L

LCPs. *See* Learner-centered psychological principles (LCPs)
LD. *See* Learning disabilities
Learner-centered psychological principles (LCPs), 85, 116
  applying, 100–107
  balance addressed in, 109
  conditions for addressing, 106–107
  domains of, 89, 90–91
  as fundamental framework, 88–92
  as fundamental knowledge base, 87–92, 90–91
  instruction and, 89
  learner motivation/achievement enhanced by, 91
  learner-centered defined by, 89
  origin of, 88–89
  personal/social responsibility and, 96–97
  practice of, 93–100
  student perceptions/voice focus of, 97–99
  surveys based on, 91–92
Learners
  developing potential of, 95
  focus on, 109
  knowledge base underlying principles of, 88
  LCPs application to, 89
  natural interests of, 94
Learning. *See also* Learners; Self-regulated learning
  autonomy support/involvement studies on, 15–17
  barriers to, 115–116
  behavioral strategies for, 52–53
  building culture of, 110–112
  caring necessary for establishing culture for, 99–100
  classroom participatory structures' role in, 180
  community of, 111–112
  emotional regulation and, 238
  environments for, 94, 114–115
  instruction interaction with, 148–149
  instructional contexts/practices interventions for, 105–106
  interventions enhancing motivation for, 102–107
  intrinsic motivation/integrated self-regulation and, 14–15
  learner-centered practiced implemented in, 109
  learner-centered research directions for, 113–115
  learner-focused interventions for, 103–104
  learning tasks/instructional materials interventions for, 104–105
  mastery goals influence on, 62
  motivational beliefs related to, 216
  motivation's trajectories and, 173–177, 176, 177–178
  multi-disciplinary, 109
  parents' involvement with, 17
  responsibility for, 107
  self-determination for, 16–17
  social, 245
  socially-mediated sequence of, 150–151
  successful programs for, 93–94
Learning disabilities (LD). *See also* Special education; Subnormal cognitive performance
  behavioral/contextual regulation applications to students with, 56–57
  caring for students with, 99
  computers/loneliness and, 248
  definitions of, 194
  enhancing motivation/achievement for children with, 100–101
  goal orientation of students with, 201
  interventions for, 56–57
  intrinsically motivated students with, 198–199
  LCPs practice and, 93
  learner-focused interventions for students with, 103–104
  learning-centered activities for students with, 100–102
  medication for, 56–57
  metacognitive weaknesses of students with, 41–42
  motivation enhanced of students with, 110, 112–115

Learning disabilities (LD) (*cont.*)
  motivation of students with, 48–50, 115–116
  motivational beliefs/attributions of students with, 48–50
  needs of students with, 85
  SDT-related processes' studies of students with, 18–19
  self-regulated learning for individuals with, 41–43
  self-regulation of individuals with, 42
  self-regulation training for students with, 43
  social reality of students with, 241
  teachers relationship to students with, 207
Learning problems. *See* Learning disabilities
Life satisfaction, domains of, 257
Loneliness
  in adolescents, 232
  affective-cognitive model of, 235–240, 239
  children's understanding of, 227
  components of, 235
  computers and, 248
  construct, 230
  coping/intervention for, 241–247
  defining, 226
  developmental trends of, 232–233
  of developmentally disabled children, 235, 242–243
  emotional/social, 230
  empowerment approaches to, 249
  environmental contributions to, 228
  genetic family factors contribution to, 227–230
  heritable factors in, 227
  interventions for, 245–246
  of people with development disabilities, 225–226
  predictors of, 247–248
  reaction to, 241–242
  regulation module, 246
  repeated experience of, 234–235
  self-reports of social competence and, 231–232
  social difficulties/developmental disabilities and, 230–231
  social environments and, 233
  social status/companionship and, 240–241
  sources of, 229
  technology and, 247–249

M

Mastery goals, 59
  adaptive attributions for performance and, 64
  adaptive help-seeking associated with, 66
  approach/avoidance forms of, 65
  behavioral/contextual regulation of, 65–66
  cognitive regulation and, 62–63
  influence of, 65
  interest related to, 66
  motivational beliefs linked to, 63
  motivational regulation and, 63–65
  research on, 63–65
  self-regulated learning influence by, 62–66
Memory
  cognitive research on, 44–45
  emotional information affect on, 238
Mental retardation (MR). *See also* Special education; Subnormal cognitive performance
  adults with, 22
  communicative skills of people with, 137
  educational research on, 113
  emerging view of, 1–2
  emotional/attention problems of people with, 135
  everyday intelligence of people with, 129
  family climate/presence of children with, 229–230
  FC for, 139–140
  goal coordination of people with, 133
  goal selection of people with, 132–133
  high-pressure social situations for people with, 134
  intrinsic motivation in students with, 20–21, 198
  knowledge deficit of children with, 234
  loneliness of children with, 230–231, 246
  maladaptive behaviors of people with, 132–133
  mastery goals and, 63
  metacognitive/strategic difficulties of children with, 42
  morality of people with, 136–137
  motivation of students with, 48–50
  motivational orientations of students with, 20–21
  novel challenges for people with, 122
  performance deficit of children with, 234

INDEX 327

personality/motivational processes in people with, 305–306
physical competence and, 138–139
relationships and, 127
SDT's possible implications for field of, 19–24
self-determination interventions for individuals with, 21–24
self-determination promotion for, 2
self-regulation of individuals with, 42
self-regulation training for students with, 43
social competence for, 225
social incompetence of people with, 121, 140
social skills of students with, 206
symptoms of, 146
terms in domain of, 195
as thinking disorder, 122
traditional view *vs.* emerging view of, 19–20
Morality, 136–137
 development of, 141
Motivated behavior, intention as feature of, 2
Motivation. *See also* Achievement motivation; Extrinsic motivation; Intrinsic motivation; Motivational orientations; Social motivation
 ability *vs.*, 191–192
 achievement, 58
 amotivation *vs.*, 2–3
 autonomous *vs.* controlled, 3–4
 barriers to integration of special education research and, 193–196
 changing personal conceptions of, 94–96
 classroom environment and student, 213–215
 control/regulation of, 46–48
 development of, 148, 177–178
 of early adolescents in special education classes, 208–215, 210–211
 effectance/intrinsic motivation focus in research on, 305–306
 engagement correlations with, 212
 environments of, 213–214, 216
 exceptional students', 197–208
 factors of, 126, 127
 importance of integrating special education research with, 196–197
 intellectual disabilities in field of, 271
 interactionist model for orientations of, 148
 interventions for, 46, 102–107
 LCPs enhanced, 91, 116
 longitudinal studies on formation of reading competencies and, 164–177, 167, 168, 169, 171–172, 176, 177
 for low performing groups, 94
 mastery goals and, 63–65
 measurement of, 195–196
 models of, 126, 126, 131
 monitoring of, 46
 MST definition of, 131
 needs as providing, 281–282, 284–285
 performance goals/regulation of, 68–70
 personality/needs and, 271–273
 personality's genetic link to, 271
 planning/activation of, 34, 44–46
 problems with, 48–49
 quality-of-life as construct of, 316–317
 quality-of-life domains related to potential states of, 307–308, 307
 quality-of-life/strategies of, 308
 reaction/reflection of, 48
 reading skill developmental interaction with, 165–170, 167, 168, 169
 reading/writing difficulties and vulnerability development of, 170–173
 regulation of, 43–50
 research integration in special education field, 192
 research on exceptional students', 193
 scaffolding and socially mediated development of, 148–161, 149, 155
 school learning-related outcomes of, 121
 self-determination relationship with, 316
 self-determined forms of, 15
 self-esteem and, 278–280
 skills enhancing, 308–309
 social competence and, 140–141
 social functioning role of, 122
 social incompetence contribution of, 126, 131–137
 specialization in field of, 193
 spelling skills role of, 169, 169
 strategies for, 46–47, 52, 65

Motivation (cont.)
  for students with LD research, 112–115
  of students with LD/MR, 48–50, 110
  subnormal reading achievement development factors of, 162–177, 167, 168, 169, 171–172, 176, 177
  support perceptions related to, 205
  SWB challenges causing, 225
  task-related interaction and, 214
  teacher-student relationships' role in, 207
  terminology in field of, 193–194
  theories of, 194–195, 207–208
  tracing trajectories of learning and, 173–177, 176, 177–178
Motivational orientations, 166. *See also* Ego-defensive orientation; Social dependence orientation; Task orientation
  as coping strategies/emotional responses sets, 153–154
  personality and, 271–273
  qualitative features/socio-cognitive origins of, 155
  three-part model for, 153–161, 155
  types of, 153–154
Motivational systems theory (MST)
  affect in, 135–136
  communication in, 137–138
  emotions role in, 135
  goals in, 131–133
  motivation defined in, 131
  PABs in, 131, 133–134
MR. *See* Mental retardation
MST. *See* Motivational systems theory
Multiple Discrepancies Theory, 257, 282

N

Needs
  in homeostasis model, 255–256
  personality influencing, 284–285
  as providing motivation, 281–282
  SWB and met/unmet, 265, 281–285
Neuroticism, 267–268, 273
Non-exceptional students. *See also* Exceptional students
  expectancies/values of, 202–203
  goal orientation of, 201
  intrinsic motivation of exceptional *vs.*, 198–199
  motivation of, 197–208

O

Optimism
  as maintaining SWB, 280–281, 286
  measures of, 280
  as positive cognitive basis, 280

P

PABs. *See* Personal agency beliefs
Performance goals, 194
  anxiety relation to, 70
  behavioral/contextual regulation and, 70–71
  cognitive regulation and, 67–68
  efficacy beliefs and, 68–69
  motivational outcomes of, 70
  motivational regulation and, 68–70
  research on, 66–67
  self-regulated learning and, 66–71
  surface processing related to, 68
Personal agency beliefs (PABs)
  emotion working with, 135
  in MST, 131, 133–134
  in social situations, 133
  social vulnerability and, 134
Personality, 291–292
  affect and, 267–268
  as determinant of happiness/sadness, 266–267
  effectance/intrinsic motivation focus in research on, 305–306
  in homeostasis model, 255–256
  homeostatic system influence on, 265, 267
  motivation's genetic link to, 271
  needs influenced by, 284–285
  needs/motivation and, 271–273
  negative/positive affectivity and, 267–268
  neuroticism/extraversion dimensions of, 267
  perceived control for, 275
  relationship strength of SWB with, 269–271
  self-esteem's component of, 279–280

SWB and, 265, 266–273, 287
SWB maintained at level of, 255–256
SWB's direct/indirect links with, 265, 268–269
traits, 306
Policy
  balance for educational, 108
  implications for educational, 107–112
  isolation/barriers to inclusion in, 109–110
  living systems framework for educational, 108–109
  special education and, 108

Q

Quality-of-life
  core domains as motivational states of, 303
  current understanding of concept, 304–305
  domains of, 304–305, 305
  generalized hierarchy of, 310–312, 310–311
  individual implications of motivational perspective of, 309–312, 310–311
  meaning of, 304
  motivational aspects of core domains of, 306–308, 307
  as motivational construct, 316–317
  motivational perspective of, 309–316, 310–311, 313
  motivational strategies and, 308–309
  personalized hierarchy of, 312–313, 313
  policy implications of, 316
  self-determination correlation to, 314–315

R

Reading
  acquisition of skills of, 166
  applications of skills of, 163–164
  cognitive/motivational factors in development of subnormal achievement in, 162–177, 167, 168, 169, 171–172, 176, 177
  in Finnish culture, 174
  formation of cognitive prerequisites/subskills of, 162

  longitudinal studies on competencies formation in, 164–177, 167, 168, 169, 171–172, 176, 177
  motivation developmental interaction with, 165–170, 167, 168, 169
  motivational vulnerability development/difficulties with, 170–173, 171–172
  motivational-emotional vulnerability and, 171–172
  problems, 162–163
  progression/regression in, 165
  requirements of skilled, 163
  scaffolding/skill acquisition of, 162
  subskills of, 162–163
  task orientation and, 175, 177
  voluntary, 164
Regulation. *See* External regulation; Identified regulation; Integrated regulation
Relationships
  caring as central to, 99
  exceptional students' social, 206–207
  in learning environment, 103
  MR and, 127
  peer, 207
  positive significant/non-significant, 276
  social, 105
  student/teacher, 108, 111–112
  support perceptions and, 206
Respect
  encouragement of mutual, 214–215
  teacher promoted, 215
Responsibility
  choices and, 96
  developing personal/social, 96–97

S

Scaffolding
  controlling strategies in, 150–151
  dosing/fading in, 149–150
  early parenting and, 180
  interactional imbalance/dysfunctionality conceived in, 150–153
  interactions in, 157
  parent/teachers responses in, 152–153
  parent/teachers support in, 152
  process of, 149–150, 149
  as reciprocal, 153

Scaffolding (*cont.*)
  social balancing mechanisms and, 161
  socially mediated development of
    cognition/motivation and,
    148–161, 149, 155
SDT. *See* Self-determination theory
Self-advocacy, 22
Self-affirmations, 47
Self-Consistency Theory, 278–279
Self-determination, 1, 306
  characteristics of actions of, 314
  components of, 315
  definitions of, 22
  interventions for individuals with
    MR, 21–24
  interventions to facilitate, 22
  intrinsically motivated behaviors
    representing prototype of, 4
  for learning, 16–17
  motivation relationship with, 316
  personal control and, 23–24
  promotion of, 2
  quality-of-life correlation to, 314–315
Self-determination theory (SDT), 25, 313
  acquisition/integration/use of information
    in, 14–15
  competence/autonomy/relatedness as needs
    in, 9–10
  developmental perspective of, 21
  extrinsic motivation in, 5–6
  integration in, 13–14
  intention in, 2–3
  internalization in, 6, 13–14
  motivation in, 2–3
  personal control and, 23–24
  possible implications for MR field
    of, 19–24
  as process model, 22
  self-determined/controlled behaviors
    in, 3–4
  types of extrinsic regulation in, 6–9
  use of, 1
  volition/self-initiation supported by, 24
Self-determined behavior, controlled
    behavior *vs.*, 3–4
Self-Enhancement Theory, 278–279
Self-esteem
  as cognition, 276–277
  high/low, 278–279
  as homeostatic device, 277–278
  intellectual disabilities and, 277
  motivation and, 278–280
  personality component of, 279–280
  research on, 276
  as SWB determinant, 277
Self-experimentation, 52
Self-observation, 52
Self-regulated learning, 31
  approaching/avoiding goals
    influence on, 59
  assumptions of, 32–33
  behavioral reflection for, 53
  cognition area of, 34, 35–43
  cognitive control/regulation in, 39–40
  context regulation for, 34, 53–57
  defining, 33
  general framework for, 32–33, 34, 35–37
  goal orientation and, 57–71, 57–72, 59
  for individuals with LD, 41–43
  mastery goals and, 62–66
  models of, 32–33, 35, 39–40, 45
  performance goals and, 66–71
  personal interest and, 45
  phases/areas for, 33, 34, 35–36
  prior knowledge and, 37
  promoting, 181
  strategies for, 40, 55
  task negotiation in, 55
  time management and, 51–52
  value beliefs in, 45
Self-regulation, 306
  of behavior, 50–53
  development of, 148
  emotions and, 48, 135
  extrinsic motivation and, 50
  intrinsic motivation and, 50
  learning and integrated, 14–15
  self-evaluation for, 40–41
  social cognitive models of, 59
  strategies for, 55
  task oriented students' strategies of, 156
  task-focused activities and, 148
  training in, 43
  through utilizing ZPD, 148–149
Self-talk, 52
Self-worth, 48
  as protection mechanism, 67
Social competence. *See also* Social
    incompetence
  contribution to academic goals, 121

INDEX 331

defining, 226
emotion regulation contribution to, 135
examples of, 124–125
motivation and, 140–141
MR and, 225
self-reports of loneliness and, 231–232
Social contexts
 internalization and, 13–14
 intrinsic motivation and, 10–13
 intrinsic motivation/autonomous
  self-regulation facilitated by, 14–15
 intrinsic/extrinsic motivation and, 1, 9
Social dependence orientation
 approach directed activity of children
  with, 160
 coping categories representing, 161
 coping strategies of, 160–161
 instructor as focus in, 155, 159
 learning tasks' superficial processing in, 160
 reading skills and, 166–167, 167
 student/teacher relations of students
  with, 160
Social difficulties
 of children with development
  disabilities, 234
 in development disabilities, 230–231
 sources of, 234–235
Social incompetence. *See also* Social
  competence
 action model used to explain, 125–139, 126
 emotion regulation contribution to, 135
 everyday intelligence contribution
  to, 128–130
 examples of, 123–124, 124
 as failure to navigate specific difficult
  social situations, 126–127
 motivation's contribution to, 126, 131–137
 as MR's defining characteristic, 121
 neurological basis of, 141
 outcome standpoint of, 125–126
 of people with MR, 140
 physical incompetence and, 138–139
 Pinocchio as case study of, 122–139, 124
 remediation of, 139–142
 situational factors contributing to, 127–128
Social intelligence. *See* Social competence
Social interaction, motivation/cognition
 development dependence on, 148
Social isolation, of people with development
 disabilities, 225

Social mediation, higher mental functions
 development through, 148–149
Social motivation
 approaches to, 203
 of exceptional students, 206–207
 social efficacy and, 204–205
Social proof, for acceptable behavior, 128
Social status, 240–241
Social transactions, 130
 mutuality/reciprocity of, 153
Social vulnerability, 134
Special education. *See also* Education;
 Learning disabilities; Mental
 retardation
 backgrounds of students in, 85–86
 barriers to integration of motivation
  research and, 193–196
 classroom environment in, 213–215
 early adolescents' motivation in classes of,
  208–215, 210–211
 extrinsic rewards use in, 199
 goal orientation and, 209, 210
 goal theory in, 200–201
 individual attention for, 99
 integrating motivation research
  with, 196–197
 motivation research integrated in field
  of, 192
 motivation/achievements of students
  in, 98–99
 motivation/teacher relationships/
  engagement correlations in classes
  of, 210, 211
 policies of, 108
 rights of children receiving, 108
 specialization in, 193
 successful programs of, 86
 terminology in field of, 194–195
SQOL. *See* Subjective Quality of Life
Students. *See* Exceptional students; Learners;
 Non-exceptional students
Subjective Quality of Life (SQOL), 257
 ComQol measurement of, 260
 normative values of, 259–261, 259
 past/present estimations of, 286
Subjective well-being (SWB)
 adaptation in homeostatic model
  of, 285–288
 cognitive buffering system of, 273–281
 cognitive component of, 257

Subjective well-being (SWB) (*cont.*)
  defining, 256
  depression level of, 290–291
  extraversion/neuroticism for, 268, 273
  extrinsic indicators correlation to, 262–264
  extrinsic influence on, 262–263, 263
  generic *vs.* specific instrumentation for measuring, 258–259
  homeostasis model for, 261–266, 263, 265
  homeostatic maintenance/failure of, 288–291
  homeostatic system correlation to, 264
  individuals' homeostasis of, 261–262
  as intellectual disabled peoples' outcome measure, 264
  joy level of, 289–290
  levels predictability of, 261
  as maintained by brain, 265
  maintenance mechanisms for, 256
  maintenance of, 273
  met needs as buffers of, 265, 284–285
  met/unmet needs link to, 281–283
  motivation from challenges to, 255
  nomenclature/measurement issues with, 256–258
  normal levels of, 291–292
  optimism as maintaining, 280–281, 286
  perceived control in, 274–275
  perceived health as component of, 264
  personal wealth and, 284
  personality and, 266–273, 287
  personality as level maintaining, 255–256
  personality influence on, 265, 266–267
  personality's direct/indirect links with, 265, 268–269
  relationship strength of personality with, 269–271
  reward sensitivity linked to, 273
  self-esteem as determinant of, 277
  self-report measuring of, 258
  shift in control of, 270–271
  specific prediction of, 263–264
  stability of, 282
  temporal stability of, 262
  velocity goal of, 289
Subnormal cognitive performance. *See also* Learning disabilities; Mental retardation
  comprehensive systemic view of, 145
  defining, 146–147
  symptoms associated with, 146
  trait-type conceptualization as distinctive factor among, 147
Support, perceptions of, 205–206
SWB. *See* Subjective well-being

T

Task orientation
  adaptive focus of children with, 154, 156
  approach directed activity of, 154
  cognitive/self-regulatory strategies of students with, 156
  reading skills and, 166–167, 167, 175, 177
Teachers
  failure caused anger of, 173
  learner-centered, 95
  loneliness helped by, 244
  motivator role of, 105–106
  personal domain/spiritual condition of, 112
  relationships to students with LD, 207
  respect promoted by, 215
  response to poor readers, 172–173
  as social dependence orientation focus, 155, 159
  student interaction, 180
  student learning responsibility of, 107
  student relationship with, 108, 111–112
  support perceptions from, 205

W

Writing, motivational vulnerability development difficulties with, 170–173

Z

Zone of proximal development (ZPD). *See also* Development
  adult guidance adjusted to, 150
  independent functioning in, 178
  self-regulation through utilizing, 148–149

Contents of Previous Volumes

Volume 1

A Functional Analysis of Retarded Development
SIDNEY W. BIJOU

Classical Conditioning and Discrimination Learning Research with the Mentally Retarded
LEONARD E. ROSS

The Structure of Intellect in the Mental Retardate
HARVEY F. DINGMAN AND C. EDWARD MEYERS

Research on Personality Structure in the Retardate
EDWARD ZIGLER

Experience and the Development of Adaptive Behavior
H. CARL HAYWOOD AND JACK T. TAPP

A Research Program on the Psychological Effects of Brain Lesions in Human Beings
RALPH M. REITAN

Long-Term Memory in Mental Retardation
JOHN M. BELMONT

The Behavior of Moderately and Severely Retarded Persons
JOSEPH E. SPRADLIN AND FREDERIC L. GIRARDEAU

Author Index-Subject Index

Volume 2

A Theoretical Analysis and Its Application to Training the Mentally Retarded
M. RAY DENNY

The Role of Input Organization in the Learning and Memory of Mental Retardates
HERMAN H. SPITZ

Autonomic Nervous System Functions and Behavior: A Review of Experimental Studies with Mental Defectives
RATHE KARPER

Learning and Transfer of Mediating Responses in Discriminating Learning
BRYAN E. SHEPP AND FRANK D. TURRISI

A Review of Research on Learning Sets and Transfer or Training in Mental Defectives
MELVIN E. KAUFMAN AND HERBERT J. PREHM

Programming Perception and Learning for Retarded Children
MURRAY SIDMAN AND LAWRENCE T. STODDARD

Programming Instruction Techniques for the Mentally Retarded
FRANCES M. GREENE

Some Aspects of the Research on Mental Retardation in Norway
IVAR ARNIJOT BJORGEN

Research on Mental Deficiency During the Last Decade in France
R. LAFON AND J. CHABANIER

Psychotherapeutic Procedures with the Retarded
MANNY STERNLIGHT

Author Index-Subject Index

Volume 3

Incentive Motivation in the Mental Retardate
PAUL S. SIEGEL

Development of Lateral and Choice-Sequence Preferences
IRMA R. GERJUOY AND JOHN J. WINTERS, JR.

Studies in the Experimental Development of Left-Right Concepts in Retarded Children Using Fading Techniques
SIDNEY W. BIJOU

Verbal Learning and Memory Research with Retardates: An Attempt to Assess Developmental Trends
L. R. GOULET

Research and Theory in Short-Term Memory
KEITH G. SCOTT AND MARCIA STRONG SCOTT

Reaction Time and Mental Retardation
ALFRED A. BAUMEISTER AND GEORGE KELLAS

Mental Retardation in India: A Review of Care, Training, Research, and Rehabilitation Programs
J. P. DAS

Educational Research in Mental Retardation
SAMUEL L. GUSKIN AND HOWARD H. SPICKER

Author Index-Subject Index

Volume 4

Memory Processes in Retardates and Normals
NORMAN R. ELLIS

A Theory of Primary and Secondary Familial Mental Retardation
ARTHUR R. JENSEN

Inhibition Deficits in Retardate Learning and Attention
LAIRD W. HEAL AND JOHN T. JOHNSON, JR.

Growth and Decline of Retardate Intelligence
MARY ANN FISHER AND DAVID ZEAMAN

The Measurements of Intelligence
A. B. SILVERSTEIN

Social Psychology and Mental Retardation
WARNER WILSON

Mental Retardation in Animals
GILBERT W. MEIER

Audiologic Aspects of Mental Retardation
LYLE L. LLOYD

Author Index-Subject Index

Volume 5

Medical-Behavioral Research in Retardation
JOHN M. BELMONT

Recognition Memory: A Research Strategy and a Summary of Initial Findings
KEITH G. SCOTT

Operant Procedures with the Retardate: An Overview of Laboratory Research
PAUL WEISBERG

Methodology of Psychopharmacological Studies with the Retarded
ROBERT L. SPRAGUE AND JOHN S. WERRY

Process Variables in the Paired-Associate Learning of Retardates
ALFRED A. BAUMEISTER AND GEORGE KELLAS

Sequential Dot Presentation Measures of Stimulus Trace in Retardates and Normals
EDWARD A. HOLDEN, JR.

Cultural-Familial Retardation
FREDERIC L. GIRARDEAU

German Theory and Research on Mental
 Retardation: Emphasis on Structure
LOTHAR R. SCHMIDT AND
 PAUL B. BALTES

Author Index-Subject Index

Volume 6

Cultural Deprivation and Cognitive
 Competence
J. P. DAS

Stereotyped Acts
ALFRED A. BAUMEISTER AND
 REX FOREHAND

Research on the Vocational Habilitation of the
 Retarded: The Present, the Future
MARC W. GOLD

Consolidating Facts into the Schematized
 Learning and Memory System of Educable
 Retardates
HERMAN H. SPITZ

An Attentional-Retention Theory of Retardate
 Discrimination Learning
MARY ANN FISHER AND DAVID
 ZEAMAN

Studying the Relationship of Task Performance
 to the Variables of Chronological Age, Mental
 Age, and IQ
WILLIAM E. KAPPAUF

Author Index-Subject Index

Volume 7

Mediational Processes in the Retarded
JOHN G. BORKOWSKI AND
 PATRICIA B. WANSCHURA

The Role of Strategic Behavior in Retardate
 Memory
ANN L. BROWN

Conservation Research with the Mentally
 Retarded
KERI M. WILTON AND
 FREDERIC J. BOERSMA

Placement of the Retarded in the Community:
 Prognosis and Outcome
RONALD B. MCCARVER AND
 ELLIS M. CRAIG

Physical and Motor Development of Retarded
 Persons
ROBERT H. BRUININKS

Subject Index

Volume 8

Self-Injurious Behavior
ALFRED A. BAUMEISTER AND
 JOHN PAUL ROLLINGS

Toward a Relative Psychology of Mental
 Retardation with Special Emphasis on
 Evolution
HERMAN H. SPITZ

The Role of the Social Agent in Language
 Acquisition: Implications for Language
 Intervention
GERALD J. MAHONEY AND
 PAMELA B. SEELY

Cognitive Theory and Mental
 Development
EARL C. BUTTERFIELD AND
 DONALD J. DICKERSON

A Decade of Experimental Research in Mental
 Retardation in India
ARUN K. SEN

The Conditioning of Skeletal and Autonomic
 Responses: Normal-Retardate Stimulus Trace
 Differences
SUSAN M. ROSS AND LEONARD E. ROSS

Malnutrition and Cognitive Functioning
J. P. DAS AND EMMA PIVATO

Research on Efficacy of Special Education for the
 Mentally Retarded
MELVINE E. KAUFMAN AND
 PAUL A. ALBERTO

Subject Index

Volume 9

The Processing of Information from Short-Term Visual Store: Developmental and Intellectual Differences
LEONARD E. ROSS AND
THOMAS B. WARD

Information Processing in Mentally Retarded Individuals
KEITH E. STANOVICH

Mediational Process in the Retarded: Implications for Teaching Reading
CLESSEN J. MARTIN

Psychophysiology in Mental Retardation
J. CLAUSEN

Theoretical and Empirical Strategies for the Study of the Labeling of Mentally Retarded Persons
SAMUEL L. GUSKIN

The Biological Basis of an Ethic in Mental Retardation
ROBERT L. ISAACSON AND
CAROL VAN HARTESVELDT

Public Residential Services for the Mentally Retarded
R. C. SCHEERENBERGER

Research on Community Residential Alternatives for the Mentally Retarded
LAIRD W. HEAL, CAROL K. SIGELMAN, AND HARVEY N. SWITZKY

Mainstreaming Mentally Retarded Children: Review of Research
LOUIS CORMAN AND
JAY GOTTLIEB

Savants: Mentally Retarded Individuals with Special Skills
A. LEWIS HILL

Subject Index

Volume 10

The Visual Scanning and Fixation Behavior of the Retarded
LEONARD E. ROSS AND
SUSAM M. ROSS

Visual Pattern Detection and Recognition Memory in Children with Profound Mental Retardation
PATRICIA ANN SHEPHERD AND
JOSEPH F. FAGAN III

Studies of Mild Mental Retardation and Timed Performance
T. NETTELBECK AND N. BREWER

Motor Function in Down's Syndrome
FERIHA ANWAR

Rumination
NIRBHAY N. SINGH

Subject Index

Volume 11

Cognitive Development of the Learning-Disabled Child
JOHN W. HAGEN, CRAIG R. BARCLAY, AND BETTINA SCHWETHELM

Individual Differences in Short-Term Memory
RONALD L. COHEN

Inhibition and Individual Differences in Inhibitory Processes in Retarded Children
PETER L. C. EVANS

Stereotyped Mannerisms in Mentally Retarded Persons: Animal Models and Theoretical Analyses
MARK H. LEWIS AND
ALFRED A. BAUMEISTER

An Investigation of Automated Methods for Teaching Severely Retarded Individuals
LAWRENCE T. STODDARD

Social Reinforcement of the Work Behavior of Retarded and Nonretarded Persons
LEONIA K. WATERS

Social Competence and Interpersonal Relations between Retarded and Nonretarded Children
ANGELA R. TAYLOR

The Functional Analysis of Imitation
WILLIAM R. MCCULLER AND
    CHARLES L. SALZBERG

Index

Volume 12

An Overview of the Social Policy of
    Deinstitutionalization
BARRY WILLER AND
    JAMES INTAGLIATA

Community Attitudes toward Community
    Placement of Mentally Retarded
    Persons
CYNTHIA OKOLO AND SAMUEL GUSKIN

Family Attitudes toward Deinstitutionalization
AYSHA LATIB, JAMES CONROY, AND
    CARLA M. HESS

Community Placement and Adjustment of
    Deinstitutionalized Clients: Issues and
    Findings
ELLIS M. CRAIG AND
    RONALD B. MCCARVER

Issues in Adjustment of Mentally Retarded
    Individuals to Residential Relocation
TAMAR HELLER

Salient Dimensions of Home Environment
    Relevant to Child Development
KAZUO NIHIRA, IRIS TAN MINK, AND
    C. EDWARD MEYERS

Current Trends and Changes in Institutions for
    the Mentally Retarded
R. K. EYMAN, S. A. BORTHWICK, AND
    G. TARJAN

Methodological Considerations in Research on
    Residential Alternatives for Developmentally
    Disabled Persons
LAIRD W. HEAL AND
    GLENN T. FUJIURRA

A Systems Theory Approach to
    Deinstitutionalization Policies
    and Research
ANGELA A. NOVAK AND
    TERRY R. BERKELEY

Autonomy and Adaptability in Work Behavior of
    Retarded Clients
JOHN L. GIFFORD, FRANK R. RUSCH,
    JAMES E. MARTIN, AND
    DAVID J. WHITE

Index

Volume 13

Sustained Attention in the Mentally Retarded:
    The Vigilance Paradigm
JOEL B. WARM AND
    DANIEL B. BERCH

Communication and Cues in the Functional
    Cognition of the Mentally Retarded
JAMES E. TURNURE

Metamemory: An Aspect of Metacognition in the
    Mentally Retarded
ELAINE M. JUSTICE

Inspection Time and Mild Mental
    Retardation
T. NETTELBECK

Mild Mental Retardation and Memory
    Scanning
C. J. PHILLIPS AND T. NETTELBECK

Cognitive Determinants of Reading in Mentally
    Retarded Individuals
KEITH E. STANOVICH

Comprehension and Mental Retardation
LINDA HICKSON BILSKY

Semantic Processing, Semantic Memory, and
    Recall
LARAINE MASTERS GLIDDEN

Proactive Inhibition in Retarded Persons:
    Some Clues to Short-Term Memory
    Processing
JOHN J. WINTERS, JR.

A Triarchic Theory of Mental Retardation
ROBERT J. STERNBERG AND
    LOUIS C. SPEAR

Index

Volume 14

Intrinsic Motivation and Behavior Effectiveness in Retarded Persons
H. CARL HAYWOOD AND HARVEY N. SWITZKY

The Rehearsal Deficit Hypothesis
NORMAN W. BRAY AND LISA A. TURNER

Molar Variability and the Mentally Retarded
STUART A. SMITH AND PAUL S. SIEGEL

Computer-Assisted Instruction for the Mentally Retarded
FRANCES A CONNERS, DAVID R. CARUSO, AND DOUGLAS K. DETTERMAN

Procedures and Parameters of Errorless Discrimination Training with Developmentally Impaired Individuals
GIULO E. LANCIONI AND PAUL M. SMEETS

Reading Acquisition and Remediation in the Mentally Retarded
NIRBHAY N. SINGH AND JUDY SINGH

Families with a Mentally Retarded Child
BERNARD FARBER AND LOUIS ROWITZ

Social Competence and Employment of Retarded Persons
CHARLES L. SALZBERG, MARILYN LIKINS, E. KATHRYN MCCONAUGHY, AND BENJAMIN LINGUGARIS/KRAFT

Toward a Taxonomy of Home Environments
SHARON LANDESMAN

Behavioral Treatment of the Sexually Deviant Behavior of Mentally Retarded Individuals
R. M. FOXX, R. G. BITTLE, D. R. BECHTEL, AND J. R. LIVESAY

Behavior Approaches to Toilet Training for Retarded Persons
S. BETTISON

Index

Volume 15

Mental Retardation as Thinking Disorder: The Rationalist Alternative to Empiricism
HERMAN H. SPITZ

Developmental Impact of Nutrition on Pregnancy, Infancy, and Childhood: Public Health Issues in the United States
ERNESTO POLLITT

The Cognitive Approach to Motivation in Retarded Individuals
SHYLAMITH KREITLER AND HANS KREITLER

Mental Retardation, Analogical Reasoning, and the Componential Method
J. MCCONAGHY

Application of Self-Control Strategies to Facilitate Independence in Vocational and Instructional Settings
JAMES E. MARTIN, DONALD L. BURGER, SUSAN ELIAS-BURGER, AND DENNIS E. MITHAUG

Family Stress Associated with a Developmentally Handicapped Child
PATRICIA M. MINNES

Physical Fitness of Mentally Retarded Individuals
E. KATHRYN MCCONAUGHY AND CHARLES L. SALZBERG

Index

Volume 16

Methodological Issues in Specifying Neurotoxic Risk Factors for Developmental Delay: Lead and Cadmium as Prototypes
STEPHEN R. SCHROEDER

The Role of Methylmercury Toxicity in Mental Retardation
GARY J. MYERS AND DAVID O. MARSH

Attentional Resource Allocation and Mental Retardation
EDWARD C. MERRILL

Individual Differences in Cognitive and Social Problem-Solving Skills as a Function of Intelligence
ELIZABETH J. SHORT AND STEVEN W. EVANS

Social Intelligence, Social Competence, and Interpersonal Competence
JANE L. MATHIAS

Conceptual Relationships between Family Research and Mental Retardation
ZOLINDA STONEMAN

Index

Volume 17

The Structure and Development of Adaptive Behaviors
KEITH F. WIDAMAN, SHARON A. BORTHWICK-DUFFY, AND TODD D. LITTLE

Perspectives on Early Language from Typical Development and Down Syndrome
MICHAEL P. LYNCH AND REBECCA E. EILERS

The Development of Verbal Communication in Persons with Moderate to Mild Mental Retardation
LEONARD ABBEDUTO

Assessment and Evaluation of Exceptional Children in the Soviet Union
MICHAEL M. GERBER, VALERY PERELMAN, AND NORMA LOPEZ-REYNA

Constraints on the Problem Solving of Persons with Mental Retardation
RALPH P. FERRETTI AND AL R. CAVALIER

Long-Term Memory and Mental Retardation
JAMES E. TURNURE

Index

Volume 18

Perceptual Deficits in Mildly Mentally Retarded Adults
ROBERT FOX AND STEPHEN OROSSIII

Stimulus Organization and Relational Learning
SAL A. SORACI, JR. AND MICHAEL T. CARLIN

Stimulus Control Analysis and Nonverbal Instructional Methods for People with Intellectual Disabilities
WILLIAM J. MCILVANE

Sustained Attention in Mentally Retarded Individuals
PHILLIP D. TOMPOROWSKI AND LISA D. HAGER

How Modifiable Is the Human Life Path?
ANN M. CLARKE AND ALAN D. B. CLARKE

Unraveling the "New Morbidity": Adolescent Parenting and Developmental Delays
JOHN G. BORKOWSKI, THOMAS L. WHITMAN, ANNE WURTZ PASSINO, ELIZABETH A. RELLINGER, KRISTEN SOMMER, DEBORAH KEOUGH, AND KERI WEED

Longitudinal Research in Down Syndrome
JANET CARR

Staff Training and Management for Intellectual Disability Services
CHRIS CULLEN

Quality of Life of People with Developmental Disabilities
TREAVOR R. PARMENTER

Index

Volume 19

Mental Retardation in African Countries: Conceptualization, Services, and Research
ROBERT SERPELL, LILIAN MARIGA, AND KARYN HARVEY

Aging and Alzheimer Disease in People with Mental Retardation
WARREN B. ZIGMAN, NICOLE SCHUPF, APRIL ZIGMAN, AND WAYNE SILERMAN

Characteristics of Older People with Intellectual Disabilities in England
JAMES HOGG AND STEVE MOSS

Epidemiological Thinking in Mental Retardation: Issues in Taxonomy and Population Frequency
TOM FRYERS

Use of Data Base Linkage Methodology in Epidemiological Studies of Mental Retardation
CAROL A. BOUSSY AND KEITH G. SCOTT

Ways of Analyzing the Spontaneous Speech of Children with Mental Retardation: The Value of Cross-Domain Analyses
CATHERINE E. SNOW AND BARBARA ALEXANDER PAN

Behavioral Experimentation in Field Settings: Threats to Validity and Interpretation Problems
WILLY-TORE MRCH

Index

Volume 20

Parenting Children with Mental Retardation
BRUCE L. BAKER, JAN BLACHER, CLAIRE B. KOPP, AND BONNIE KRAEMER

Family Interactions and Family Adaptation
FRANK J. FLOYD AND CATHERINE L. COSTIGAN

Studying Culturally Diverse Families of Children with Mental Retardation
IRIS TAN MINK

Older Adults with Mental Retardation and Their Families
TAMAR HELLER

A Review of Psychiatric and Family Research in Mental Retardation
ANN GATH

A Cognitive Portrait of Grade School Students with Mild Mental Retardation
MARCIA STRONG SCOTT, RUTH PEROU, ANGELIKA HARTL CLAUSSEN, AND LOIS-LYNN STOYKO DEUEL

Employment and Mental Retardation
NEIL KIRBY

Index

Volume 21

An Outsider Looks at Mental Retardation: A Moral, a Model, and a Metaprincipal
RICHARD P. HONECK

Understanding Aggression in People with Intellectual Disabilities: Lessons from Other Populations
GLYNIS MURPHY

A Review of Self-Injurious Behavior and Pain in Persons with Developmental Disabilities
FRANK J. SYMONS AND TRAVIS THOMPSON

Recent Studies in Psychopharmacology in Mental Retardation
MICHAEL G. AMAN

Methodological Issues in the Study of Drug Effects on Cognitive Skills in Mental Retardation
DEAN C. WILLIAMS AND KATHRYN J. SAUNDERS

The Behavior and Neurochemistry of the Methylazoxymethanol-Induced Microencephalic Rat
PIPPA S. LOUPE, STEPHEN R. SCHROEDER, AND RICHARD E. TESSEL

Longitudinal Assessment of Cognitive-Behavioral Deficits Produced by the Fragile-X Syndrome
GENE S. FISCH

Index

Volume 22

Direct Effects of Genetic Mental Retardation Syndromes: Maladaptive Behavior and Psychopathology
ELIZABETH M. DYKENS

Indirect Effects of Genetic Mental Retardation Disorders: Theoretical and Methodological Issues
ROBERT M. HODAPP

The Development of Basic Counting, Number, and Arithmetic Knowledge among Children Classified as Mentally Handicapped
ARTHUR J. BAROODY

The Nature and Long-Term Implications of Early Developmental Delays: A Summary of Evidence from Two Longitudinal Studies
RONALD GALLIMORE, BARBARA K. KEOGH, AND LUCINDA P. BERNHEIMER

Savant Syndrome
TED NETTLEBECK AND ROBYN YOUNG

The Cost-Efficiency of Supported Employment Programs: A Review of the Literature
ROBERT E. CIMERA AND FRANK R. RUSCH

"The Child That Was Meant?" or "Punishment for Sin?": Religion, Ethnicity, and Families with Children with Disabilities
LARAINE MASTERS GLIDDEN, JEANNETTE ROGERS-DULAN, AND AMY E. HILL

Index

Volume 23

Diagnosis of Autism before the Age of 3
SALLY J. ROGERS

The Role of Secretin in Autistic Spectrum Disorders
KAROLY HORVATH AND J. TYSON TILDON

The Role of Candidate Genes in Unraveling the Genetics of Autism
CHRISTOPHER J. STODGELL, JENNIFER L. INGRAM, AND SUSAN L. HYMAN

Asperger's Disorder and Higher Functioning Autism: Same or Different?
FRED R. VOLKMAR AND AMI KLIN

The Cognitive and Neural Basis of Autism: A Disorder of Complex Information Processing and Dysfunction of Neocortical Systems
NANCY J. MINSHEW, CYNTHIA JOHNSON, AND BEATRIZ LUNA

Neural Plasticity, Joint Attention. and a Transactional Social-Orienting Model of Autism
PETER MUNDY AND A. REBECCA NEAL

Theory of Mind and Autism: A Review
SIMON BARON-COHEN

Understanding the Language and Communicative Impairments in Autism
HELEN TAGER-FLUSBERG

Early Intervention in Autism: Joint Attention and Symbolic Play
CONNIE KASARI, STEPHANNY F. N. FREEMAN, AND TANYA PAPARELLA

Attachment and Emotional Responsiveness in Children with Autism
CHERYL DISSANAYAKE AND MARIAN SIGMAN

Families of Adolescents and Adults with Autism: Uncharted Territory
MARSHA MAILICK SELTZER, MARTY WYNGAARDEN KRAUSS, GAEL I. ORSMOND, AND CARRIE VESTAL

Index

Volume 24

Self-Determination and Mental Retardation
MICHAEL L. WEHMEYER

International Quality of Life: Current
  Conceptual, Measurement, and
  Implementation Issues
KENNETH D. KEITH

Measuring Quality of Life and Quality of
  Services through Personal Outcome
  Measures: Implications for Public Policy
JAMES GARDNER,
  DEBORAH T. CARRAN, AND
  SYLVIA NUDLER

Credulity and Gullibility in People with
  Developmental Disorders: A Framework for
  Future Research
STEPHEN GREENSPAN, GAIL LOUGHLIN,
  AND RHONDA S. BLACK

Criminal Victimization of Persons with Mental
  Retardation: The Influence of Interpersonal
  Competence on Risk
T. NETTELBECK AND C. WILSON

The Parent with Mental Retardation
STEVE HOLBURN, TIFFANY PERKINS,
  AND PETER VIETZE

Psychiatric Disorders in Adults with Mental
  Retardation
STEVE MOSS

Development and Evaluation on Innovative
  Residential Services for People with Severe
  Intellectual Disability and Serious
  Challenging Behavior
JIM MANSELL, PETER MCGILL, AND
  ERIC EMERSON

The Mysterious Myth of Attention Deficits and
  Other Defect Stories: Contemporary Issues in
  the Developmental Approach to Mental
  Retardation
JACOB A. BURACK, DAVID W. EVANS,
  CHERYL KLAIMAN, AND
  GRACE IAROCCI

Guiding Visual Attention in Individuals with
  Mental Retardation
RICHARD W. SERNA AND
  MICHAEL T. CARLIN

Index

Volume 25

Characterizations of the Competence of Parents
  of Young Children with Disabilities
CARL J. DUNST, TRACY HUMPHRIES,
  AND CAROL M. TRIVETTE

Parent–Child Interactions When Young Children
  Have Disabilities
DONNA SPIKER, GLENNA C. BOYCE,
  AND LISA K. BOYCE

The Early Child Care Study of Children with
  Special Needs
JEAN F. KELLY AND
  CATHRYN L. BOOTH

Diagnosis of Autistic Disorder: Problems and
  New Directions
ROBYN YOUNG AND NEIL BREWER

Social Cognition: A Key to
  Understanding Adaptive Behavior
  in Individuals with Mild Mental
  Retardation
JAMES S. LEFFERT AND
  GARY N. SIPERSTEIN

Proxy Responding for Subjective Well-Being: A
  Review
ROBERT A. CUMMINS

People with Intellectual Disabilities from Ethnic
  Minority Communities in the United States
  and the United Kingdom
CHRIS HATTON

Perception and Action in Mental Retardation
W. A. SPARROW AND ROSS H. DAY

Volume 26

A History of Psychological Theory and
  Research in Mental Retardation since World
  War II
DONALD K. ROUTH AND STEPHEN R.
  SCHROEDER

Psychopathology and Intellectual Disability:
  The Australian Child to Adult
  Longitudinal Study
BRUCE J. TONGE AND STEWART L.
  EINFELD

Resilience, Family Care, and People with Intellectual Disabilities
GORDON GRANT, PAUL RAMCHARAN, AND PETER GOWARD

Prevalence and Correlates of Psychotropic Medication Use among Adults with Developmental Disabilities: 1970–2000
MARIA G. VALDOVINOS AND STEPHEN R. SCHROEDER

Integration as Acculturation: Developmental Disability, Deinstitutionalization, and Service Delivery Implications
M. KATHERINE BUELL

Cognitive Aging and Down Syndrome: An Interpretation
J. P. DAS

Index

Volume 27

Language and Communication in Individuals with Down Syndrome
ROBERT S. CHAPMAN

Language Abilities of Individuals with Williams Syndrome
CAROLYN B. MERVIS, BYRON F. ROBINSON, MELISSA L. ROWE, ANGELA M. BECERRA, AND BONITA P. KLEIN-TASMAN

Language and Communication in Fragile X Syndrome
MELISSA M. MURPHY AND LEONARD ABBEDUTO

On Becoming Competent Communicators: The Challenge for Children with Fetal Alcohol Exposure
TRUMAN E. COGGINS, LESLEY B. OLSWANG, HEATHER CARMICHAEL OLSON, AND GERALYN R. TIMLER

Memory, Language Comprehension, and Mental Retardation
EDWARD C. MERRILL, REGAN LOOKADOO, AND STACY RILEA

Reading Skills and Cognitive Abilities of Individuals with Mental Retardation
FRANCES A. CONNERS

Language Interventions for Children with Mental Retardation
NANCY C. BRADY AND STEVEN F. WARREN

Augmentative and Alternative Communication for Persons with Mental Retardation
MARYANN ROMSKI, ROSE A. SEVCIK, AND AMY HYATT FONSECA

Atypical Language Development in Individuals with Mental Retardation: Theoretical Implications
JEAN A. RONDAL

Index

RC
570
.15

SOUTH UNIVERSITY
709 MALL BLVD.
SAVANNAH, GA 31406